IT COULD BE

ALLERGY

AND IT CAN BE

CURED

Dedication

This book is dedicated to all those who seek the knowledge needed to maintain optimum health, and to all those who suffer ill health but have not given up the search for answers.

IT COULD BE
ALLERGY
AND IT CAN BE
CURED

PHILLIP ALEXANDER ND

ETHICARE PTY LTD

Acknowledgements

This work would not have been possible without the help of some very fine and talented people: James Young, who edited, designed and typeset the book; Stan Lamond, who designed the cover; Di Harriman, who compiled the index; Paula Jackson, who told her own story; and Ted Kaye, who took the photo-graphs.

A special thanks to my three colleagues: Ludmilla Mallory for the recipes; Kerry Dawe for compiling the list of questions in Chapter 15 and for her advice on cover design; and to Michelle Dytor for taking care of my patients while I wrote, for being the photographic model and for her editorial input. Through their constructive criticism and recommendations, Ludmilla, Kerry and Michelle have brought a female perspective to this work, giving it a balance it would not have had otherwise.

Very special thanks go to all those who have taught me so much about this subject: my lecturers in college, the distinguished overseas physicians and scientists whose lectures I've attended and, most important of all, my patients, for they have taught me more than anybody. Thanks also go to those patients who have allowed the use of their case histories.

My thanks go to Mr Hans Selye for allowing the reproduction (on page 156) of a quote from his book, *The Stress of Life*, McGraw-Hill, New York, 1978.

This revised fourth edition published by Ethicare Pty Ltd, 29/22 Fisher Rd, Dee Why NSW 2099, Australia. Telephone (02) 9981 2225 or (02) 9982 7135
First published in 1988 by Davont Pty Ltd as *Your Allergies Can Be Cured*
Second edition 1990
Third edition 1994
Reprinted 1995
Reprinted 2002
Copyright © Ethicare Pty Ltd 1988, 1990, 1994, 1995, 1997, 1999, 2000, 2002
Edited, designed and typeset by James Young
Index by Di Harriman
Cover design by Stan Lamond
Photographs by Photo Associates
Photographic model: Michelle Dytor
Printed in Australia by McPherson's Printing Group

National Library of Australia
Cataloguing-in-Publication data

Alexander, Phil.
  It could be allergy and it can be cured.

  Bibliography.
  Includes index.
  ISBN 0 646 18119 X.

  1. Food allergy—Diet therapy. I. Title.

641.563

Contents

Important notice

This book is a self-help treatment book. However, the treatment programs outlined in it are to be, at all times, supervised by a doctor or other health professional. The author does not recommend that you treat yourself, by yourself.

Should you choose to supervise your own treatment, which is your right, you must take full responsibility for the outcome.

Introduction

The big medical discovery of the 70s was that allergies can cause more than just sneezes, skin rashes and asthma, and that many people suffer from them without knowing it. Through the 80s more and more symptoms of disease were found to have an allergy component as part of their cause. Such seemingly unrelated conditions as high blood pressure, heart attacks, depression, hyperactivity, poor memory, lack of energy, bedwetting in adults, irritable bowel, hearing loss and many more were found to be caused by allergy when no other cause could be found.

Concurrent with this diagnostic breakthrough was the discovery that a change of diet could balance the metabolism of the body and cure allergies. The allergy sufferer no longer has to spend a lifetime on cortisone drugs, antihistamines, fluid tablets, puffers and nasal sprays to ameliorate the symptoms of allergies.

This book is the sum total of everything I've learnt as a result of curing my own allergies and spending twenty-two years in private practice taking care of allergy sufferers, most of whom didn't realise thay were suffering from allergy. It contains a simple, yet effective, dietary regime that addresses the cause rather than the symptoms of allergy. The program breaks new ground in the treatment of allergy and in its own way helps to roll back the frontiers of science. It is a boon to both diagnosed allergy sufferers and those who've been consigned to the 'too-hard basket' by doctors.

It has been rewarding for me to work with people so afflicted by allergy they couldn't think clearly and so in pain from their allergies they couldn't move freely. To witness their determination to win and their strict adherence to the treatment program has been a great inspiration. Through sheer persistence and despite all odds these people have managed to get well.

Observing human triumph over adversity is an edifying experience. It makes one realise that nothing is impossible.

The tried and tested treatment regime in this book has worked for many people and I have no doubt that their triumph can be your triumph too.

Phillip Alexander
Sydney, 1995

Paula's story

'Even your body knows its heritage and its rightful needs and will not be deceived.
And your body is the harp of your soul,
And it is yours to bring forth sweet music from it or confused sounds.'

Kahlil Gibran, *The Prophet*

As a 23-year-old woman living in the 80s, I have, like many other people, tried to eat well and get some exercise. The media had made me very body conscious, and if I didn't keep my weight down, I became depressed, felt unattractive and my self-esteem plummeted. In order to keep it down, I had to eat very small amounts. I became convinced that I had a fat-storing metabolism and to keep my weight down I had to eat very little.

Like many women, I have agonised over my body, spending literally hundreds of dollars on cellulite treatments, and there have been many years of not a morsel passing my lips without a calorie count. Looking back on it, it was an awfully stressful, anti-social way to be treating food. You could say I was at war with my body.

At 60 kg (9 st 7 lb) in July 1987, I decided to go on one of my severe diets, which consisted of cereal and skim milk for breakfast, Ryvita, salmon and salad for lunch and steamed vegetables for dinner. By November I had lost 6.5 kg (1 st). I experienced weakness and hunger pains, but the psychological high I was on overrode feelings of drowsiness and lethargy.

At this time, I was studying part-time and had taken over the job of Section Head in a nursery caring for children under three years of age. Wanting to achieve recognition from my colleagues, I set myself the task of getting the nursery into good working order. Basically, I put my needs last and burnt the candle at both ends. I began a downhill run and by March 1988 I had deteriorated physically and mentally and needed a week off work for what the doctor diagnosed as stress. The week off work helped alleviate the severe headaches and back pain, but on returning to work I still did not feel 100 per cent better.

I spent the Easter weekend at my parents' property on the

outskirts of Bathurst, and all Mum's lovely cooking went down very well. So well, in fact, that within three weeks I had gained the 6.5 kg (1 st) I had lost and kept off over a nine month period. I was unable to start dieting again; I was tired of it all. Depression set in severely.

I was also extremely sensitive and emotional. I would snap at people without meaning to. Regarding the poor concentration and loss of memory, I can tell you, when you're twenty-three and find it impossible to recall one bit of conversation you had ten minutes earlier, it's very scary.

At the time I consulted Phil Alexander in May 1988, I was beginning to doubt my professional capabilities. Talking to Phil was very encouraging. Yes, he told me, I would recover, my symptoms would be alleviated; but I must rest, as I was suffering from stress as well. He told me that my sinusitis and resultant bad breath was of physiological, not psychological, origin and gave me a referral to an allergy clinic for tests.

Although I wasn't allergic to any foods, I was allergic to moulds, house dust mites, grasses and pollens. Phil placed me on the Anti-Candida Program, with the prescribed drug Nystatin to kill off the candida yeast over-growth in my body, and a vitamin supplement to help balance my out-of-kilter metabolism, unbalanced by my many years of crash/semi-starvation diets. To think that for years I thought I was doing the right thing by my body. How wrong I was!

The meals set out for me were incredibly substantial and I thought I would put on weight. Not so at all. Although the first week of my Anti-Candida Program was unpleasant, with headaches, sinusitis and stomach pain (all candida yeast withdrawal symptoms), I lost 2.25 kg (5 lb) of fluid in five days, as I had more of a fluid problem than a fat problem. After a fortnight I felt 100 per cent better and had lost another 1.5 kg (3 lb). I was sitting down to beautiful meals each night and I was very hungry in between meals. There was no bloating associated with eating and my metabolism was speeding up considerably. As well as sticking to the program religiously, I kept my house free of mould and dust and made sure I got plenty of rest.

By the time I went back to see Phil, after four weeks on my program, I was so excited I literally bounded into his office so eager to tell him how wonderful I was feeling, how much energy I had. I had lost 4.5 kg (10 lb) altogether, and the high I was experiencing was indescribable, very different from the highs I had experienced when I had lost weight before.

Phil was pleased for me and instructed me to carry on as I was. During the second month my appetite decreased a little and I no longer needed rice wafers in between meals. It was at this time that I came down with inflamed back muscles, due to heavy lifting. As rotten as I was feeling physically, I still felt mentally well and made

10

sure I didn't spend my days off work feeling sorry for myself. I kept busy with sewing and recovered rapidly without the aid of prescribed drugs from my doctor. I wondered if I would have recovered as well two months earlier, before my program.

To sum it all up, after being at war with my body for four years, I am discovering what it is like to have energy, not feel over-stressed, feel restored after a good night's sleep and be happy. When people ask me if the program is working for me, I tell them that I am an entirely different person from what I was two and a half months ago. That is the absolute truth too! I feel attractive, confident; my self-esteem is riding high and I am learning not to compare myself to other women, to love me and my body for what it is.

I am discovering new, tasty nutritious meals and there are no guilt feelings attached to sitting down and eating a beautiful veal and vegie casserole. Farewell to calorie counting forever!

What is so exciting for me is that I am still in the healing process. I have some way to go, but I am already reaping the benefits. People are commenting on how well I look—my skin, my hair, my eyes. My parents are thrilled and relieved to see that, at last, the answer to my problem has been found. My boyfriend tells me how attractive I have been looking lately and I know my state of physical, and mental/emotional health will improve more. Like my newly found love of cooking and eating, I am exercising more because I have the energy and really want to. I don't feel I have to—there is now a challenge to be the healthiest person I can. My current exercise is martial arts and I love it more now that I am on my anti-allergy program. I feel better than I did when I lost weight on a diet at the ladies' gym and was doing four aerobic classes a week, as well as weights.

I shudder to think what would have happened to my health if I had not investigated further the real cause of my complaints. I'm sure I would have crash dieted more, and in doing so deteriorated more, perhaps irreparably. I stick with this program and take it seriously, and so I should. This is my life and my body, the only one I have been given. I will not break this program.

Realising how biochemically different I am I would never again pick a diet that doesn't have the research and experience of a practising physician backing it. Never again would I skip a meal. When I see young women skipping meals and eating minuscule amounts, I now try to explain what they are doing to themselves. They don't listen, because they think they know it all, and know their body's needs just like I thought I did.

Thanks to the expertise and knowledge of the author of this book, I am learning to love me, and love my body for what it is. I am healthy, alive, vital, energetic and attractive. I am indebted to Phil Alexander for all his help in making what really is the 'new me'.

I hope readers will see me as a success story and an inspiration to overcome their complaints.

As I re-read my words, the excitement and challenge builds up in me more. I really believe in what I am doing. It all may be hard for you to comprehend, it is even hard for me sometimes, but if you have success in overcoming your allergies, you will understand the message I am conveying.

Paula Jackson, 1988

POSTSCRIPT—1990

Paula is still fit and well though she's been through a rough patch that saw her health decline for a while. Like so many people who've regained their vitality, Paula began to embrace life with great enthusiasm. Too much enthusiasm in fact. She burnt herself out. Tiredness, aches and pains, fluid retention and confusion began to return. Not because of allergy and candida infection this time, but because of fatigue. Paula, like so many others, believed her new found energy was boundless and in an effort to make up for lost time began doing all those things she was too tired to do before. Admittedly pre-wedding nerves and adjusting to married life played it's part but the major cause of her symptoms was overdoing it.

We human beings have a very short memory of matters pertaining to our former ill health. We easily forget what it was like to be down and Paula fell into this trap. She now realises that although the spirit may be willing the flesh has limitations. She has now learned to pace herself by recognising her particular early warning symptoms of stress and slowing down before these symptoms become full blown.

UPDATE—1995

Paula is now 30 and feeling better than she did at age 19. She's married, pregnant, works part time and has a healthy two-year-old boy who shows all the signs of being an advanced, even gifted, child. All this she attributes to her continued adherence to the Metabolism-Balancing Program and supplements. She maintains high energy levels, trouble-free pregnancies (no toxaemia) and optimal weight levels during and between pregnancies. The learning experience of overcoming her previous illness has put her in tune with her body and there has been no return of her candida and allergy symptoms.

Justin's story

Justin (10) suffering from severe conjunctivitis leading to blindness. Allergic to barley, lamb, airborne moulds, house dust, dust mites and grasses.

J ustin's story has been included at the request of his mother who is determined that no other mother should experience the heartache and anguish of the possibility of losing a child to blindness. Because Justin's story was still unfolding it was not written until the day before the 1988 edition of this book went to print.

It was after one of my many public seminars on how to cure allergies that I first met Justin. After question time, while I was packing up to leave, a woman (Robyn) approached me with a little boy who was wearing dark glasses. At first glance I thought she was going to ask me about her swollen red eyes that looked allergic. As she got closer I could see she had been crying and when she spoke there was great anguish in her voice.

'They say my little boy will be blind in twelve months and I can't accept that,' she said. 'After listening to your talk tonight I can see that I was right all along. You don't have to learn to live with allergies and surrender to dangerous drugs.'

Robyn took Justin's sunglasses off to reveal the worst case of conjunctivitis I'd ever seen. He looked as though he'd been beaten up. His eyes were black and blue with streaks of red where he had been scratching. They were so swollen they were almost closed. Only the narrowest of slits still remained and they were partly covered with the goo that was oozing out of his inflamed eyes.

Robyn went on to tell me that the eyes had become suddenly inflamed three years ago and that the doctor had diagnosed Justin as being severely allergic. Many drugs had been tried in a vain effort to reduce the allergic inflammation of Justin's eyes. As a last resort the doctor prescribed the cortisone drugs Maxidex and Predsol claiming they were to be administered as drops into Justin's eyes each day. The doctor was quite concerned about the side effects of the drugs (prolonged use of them causes cataracts and eventually blindness). Despite this he insisted that cortisone was the only treatment medical science had that would reduce the inflammation enough for Justin to be able to open his eyes and

13

that he and Robyn had no choice but to accept the inevitability of Justin's eventual blindness. So concerned was the doctor over Justin's prospects that he referred him to a professor in Sydney in the hope that more could be done for him.

The professor was taken aback by the severity of Justin's condition and would always have colleagues and students there to observe Justin at each visit. To use Robyn's expression, 'the professor would beat around the bush and not give me any straight answers.' He told her to continue with the cortisone drugs and was very vague when questioned about their side effects. He just didn't want to talk about them.

Justin began making regular trips down to Sydney to see the professor and each time he would chastise Robyn for taking Justin to homeopaths, herbalists and nutritionists. Robyn, for her part, refused to give in and wasted no time telling the professor she was going to try everything before she accepted the fate of Justin's blindness. Deep down she knew there was an answer.

Not long after, while sweeping out her laundry, she noticed, by chance, an advertisement for one of my free public seminars on 'Your allergies can be cured'. She saw it on the sheet of newspaper she was using to wrap up the sweepings from the laundry floor.

Grasping at straws but determined not to accept defeat she made it to the seminar to hear what she described as 'common-sense on this subject for the first time'. She told me later that on hearing of the effects dietary change could have on curing allergies she realised Justin was going to be OK and that the sense of relief was so overwhelming she had trouble containing her emotions.

Robyn brought Justin to see me within a day or two of the talk. He was tested and showed up to be allergic to barley, lamb, malt and airborne moulds, which meant he had to go off all mould- and yeast-containing foods (see 'Food tables' at the back of the book). He was also allergic to house dust, dust mites, and grasses, particularly rye grass, which meant he couldn't eat rye bread or Ryvita. Because Robyn had a history of vaginal thrush while carrying Justin and because he had oral thrush as a baby he was treated for *Candida albicans* yeast infection as well.

On the combined Anti-Candida/Anti-Allergy Program and Nystatin, *Lactobacillus acidophilus* capsules and a complete multi-vitamin and mineral formula supplement containing the six essential minerals—calcium, magnesium, potassium, iron, zinc and manganese—to build up his damaged eye tissue he made a remarkable recovery. Within a week of being on the program he was off the cortisone as his eyes were 50 per cent better. He is now 70–80 per cent better depending on how tired he is and whether or not there is a strong, dry westerly wind blowing the rye grass in from the grazing lands. He has not used the cortisone since being on the program and hardly ever needs to rub his eyes. Justin is a good example of how changes in diet can reduce one's sensitivity to airborne and inhalant allergies as he's able to play on newly mown grass and in the bush without any flare-ups of his condition.

Justin is still waiting on delivery of the dust mite cover for his pillow and mattress. This will improve his condition further as at present the dust mites that live in his pillow by day and come out to feed on his skin at night are gaining entry to his eyes and perpetuating the inflammation there.

The damage the cortisone has done to Justin's eyes is also contributing to the present plateau in his rate of improvement. It will take some time to replace the collagen, elastin and delicate eye tissues destroyed by the cortisone. Fortunately, the vitamin and mineral formula will speed up this process of tissue regrowth.

On last contact with Robyn she remarked how much stronger and healthier his eyes are becoming with each passing month. Whether Justin becomes 100 per cent symptom free is hard to say as it's difficult to accurately assess how much damage the cortisone has done to the delicate eye tissue. Even if he never progresses beyond 80 per cent improvement, he's as good as cured as his eyes no longer hold him back and he's now functioning on all levels without the use of drugs. He is now able to plan a future without the limitations of blindness and has the opportunity and freedom to be whatever he wants to be.

The thing that impresses me most about Justin is that he's as dedicated to the program as Robyn. He exhibits great self-discipline for one so young and will not break the program for anything. He refuses all junk food, stays away from the school canteen, doesn't swap lunches with the other kids and takes his own special food to birthday parties. He doesn't succumb to the pressure of well-meaning adults who offer him foods that are contrary to his program. The words, 'Oh, come on. Surely a little bit won't hurt you,' leave him unmoved. He and Robyn cope brilliantly with the whingers and knockers who 'pooh-pooh' the program despite the dramatic improvement they see in Justin's condition. It seems to me that Justin's potential tragedy is building great strength of character that will stand him in good stead in adulthood.

Although Justin is not completely out of the woods yet he is well on the way. He still gets the odd headache, stuffy nose and itchy eyes, usually when he's hungry and fighting with his sister. Such emotional upheaval causes neurokinin to be released into the skin and mucous membranes of his eyes, head and nose and this inflames the delicate tissues there (see section on acne in Chapter 6 for more information on neurokinin).

Only time will tell how Justin's saga ends, though for my part I'm confident the ending will be a happy one.

POSTSCRIPT—1990

Justin made a 100 per cent recovery. The cortisone-damaged tissues completely repaired themselves and he was free of all his symptoms. He stayed on all his supplements during the food reintroduction process. Happily he had lost his sensitivity to all the foods he was previously allergic to. Now that he was back on the Metabolism-Balancing Program (with no more than 5 per cent junk food) I asked him to stay on the supplements. I explained to him that I was worried his resistance may drop if he went off them and he agreed to co-operate.

For fifteen months everything was fine. Justin was eating what he liked and there was no sign of his symptoms returning. It was about this time that he rebelled against taking the supplements. Without warning he put his foot down and refused to take any more. Slowly but surely his symptoms began to return though not to their previous degree of intensity. As distressed as she is Robyn can't get through to him and this is the way it'll be for a little while. Justin has reached that pre-pubescent stage that many boys go through when the male sex hormone testosterone hits the blood-stream for the first time. They lose their niceness and if they don't have an adult male around to keep them in line can become stroppy and rebellious.

All that can be done now is to wait for him to settle down. I've learned that pushing kids who are in this life phase is the wrong way to go. They've got to come around in their own time. Justin knows what has to be done to regain his health and when he's sick of being sick he'll do it. Only this time it will be his idea and his decision. Right now he's preoccupied with the important task of developing and advertising his individuality. When the novelty wears off he'll go back onto the Metabolism-Balancing Program and supplements. I've seen this happen many times and have no doubt it will happen in Justin's case too.

UPDATE—1995

Justin's eyes, for the main part, are good. Since 1990, he put himself back on the supplements for a while and his eyes cleared up completely. Now that he's left school, his old routine has been broken by his new work environment, friends and freedoms. As a result, he's forgetting to take his supplements. For the main part he's OK, but if he binges on junk food, his eyes flare up, though not as badly as before.

16

1.
Portrait of an allergy sufferer

'The most beautiful experience we can have is the mysterious.'

Albert Einstein, *The Living Philosophies*

My own allergy story, like most others, began in childhood. I was dogged by skin rashes and a perennially stuffy nose that deteriorated into three to four severe month long head colds every year. I can still vividly remember going to school with various coloured creams on my face and being teased by the other kids.

I also suffered from a nervous squint which turned to rapid blinking when I was under stress, such as facing a fast ball at cricket or facing the teacher over some misdemeanour. I suffered from periodic attacks of anxiety that left me depressed. Because I considered this to be normal I never mentioned it to anyone.

By the time I reached high school I'd added severe acne to the rashes that came and went from my face, chest, back and arms. Antibiotics and various creams were prescribed for the acne. The antibiotics always made me feel off colour and after some time on them I began to suffer from an anal itch, that I was more nervous than before and that I had trouble concentrating in class and remembering what I had studied. My stuffy nose was still a problem and my acne wasn't that much better.

By the age of eighteen I was fed up. My skin and nose were no better and I seemed to spend all my time studying to achieve the same marks my mates were getting with half the effort. My acne had given me an inferiority complex and I couldn't talk to girls without the nervous blinking. My doctor told me I had a periodic allergy and prescribed antihistamines to be taken whenever my skin flared up or my nose became unbearably stuffy. I was told that my allergies were something that I just had to live with.

SELF-HELP

I decided that this wasn't good enough and if my doctor couldn't help me then I'd help myself. On passing my entrance exam I enrolled in medicine at the university with the intention of becoming the sort of doctor who could do something about acne and allergies. Filled with crusading zeal and convinced I'd find all the answers I read every book I could find on those subjects.

My quest for knowledge took me from the medical school library to the public library where I read *Let's Get Well* by Adelle Davis. Her book described in detail how allergic people needed greater quantities of vitamins and minerals than non-allergic people to keep their metabolisms balanced and to strengthen the walls of their cells against the entry of allergenic substances. Impressed by the research evidence she submitted and the successful treatment she quoted I decided to give it a go.

I immediately changed my diet from the typical student fare of beer, salted peanuts and take-away foods to fresh fruit and vegetables and properly prepared, balanced meals. I added to my program supplements of full spectrum vitamins and minerals.

Within six weeks there was a noticeable improvement in my acne and nervousness. As the months rolled by my skin became steadily better as did my concentration, memory, self-confidence and energy levels. Although I was still getting my periodic skin rashes, especially when I drank beer, they weren't as itchy and for the first winter on record my stuffy nose didn't develop into a cold or 'flu.

Enthused by my new level of well-being, I began quoting Adelle Davis to anyone who would listen. Disappointingly, my peers and lecturers weren't the least bit interested in what I had to say. Undaunted, I continued to preach the virtues of diet for the treatment of acne, allergies and flagging mental and physical vitality. Before long I was labelled a fanatic and when I remonstrated that nutrition should be taught at medical school, I was labelled a rabble-rouser and put on notice to behave.

This antipathy on the part of the establishment was beginning to take its toll and I was having trouble getting my enthusiasm up to study. I began sleeping in and missing lectures. I couldn't bring myself to open a pharmacology textbook, let alone read one. I was disillusioned and depressed. I was losing faith in modern science and what I was being taught and for the first time doubted I'd find the answers I was looking for.

The final straw was the conversation I had with a sixth year medical student at a party one night. This character boasted about how much money he was going to earn when he went into private practice. He was going to specialise in allergies, especially allergic skin conditions. 'Why?' I asked. 'Because your patients never die and they never get better. They just keep on coming back year after year spending money with you,' he replied.

His words both flabbergasted and depressed me. What did I have to look forward to? I hadn't even sat my intermediate exams. Clearly five years of more study wasn't going to teach me what I wanted to know.

I left university and after a couple of years working on building sites, digging graves in a cemetery and working on garbage trucks, I had enough money to put myself through naturopath college.

FINDING THE CURE

Naturopathy taught me how to treat the cause rather than the symptoms of a disease and that to treat allergies you must first have allergy tests, find out what you are allergic to and remove it from your food and environment. No one had ever said that to me before. I threw away my antihistamines and antibiotics, took the allergy tests and removed all allergenic foods from my diet. So effective was the program that my remaining acne, itchy skin, stuffy nose, nervousness, anxiety and depression disappeared completely within three months and I didn't need to take the oral desensitising vaccine for my inhalant allergies. There was no doubt in my mind that the metabolism-balancing effect of Adelle Davis' vitamin and mineral regime, which had reduced the intensity of all my symptoms, enabled my body to respond as successfully as it did.

Reintroduction of my former allergy foods saw a return of all my symptoms only if I was under stress from over-work, late nights, too much sport, skipping meals or not taking my vitamins. Under stress, a glass of wine or a slice of bread would give me a few pimples, a slightly itchy skin and a reasonably stuffy nose. The only time my nervousness, anxiety or depression returned was when I was off my vitamins and minerals for a fortnight or more.

This was the pattern of my life for a number of years until I discovered I had a *Candida albicans* yeast infection in my intestines. By going on the Anti-Candida Program I eradicated the yeast and found that the anal itch I'd suffered since first taking antibiotics and the distended abdomen I'd never been able to diet or exercise away disappeared. All my symptoms disappeared and I'm happy to say they have never returned.

Since beating the candida infection I find that smoke-filled restaurants don't stuff up my nose any more and I can eat and

19

drink what I like, without any hint of my symptoms returning, even if I am stressed or it's late and I'm tired. Because I must religiously take my vitamins and minerals to achieve this, some would argue that I'm technically not cured of my allergies. Because taking extra food in pill form is no hassle to me (I've accepted that the metabolism of an allergic person requires more vitamins and minerals than the non-allergic person) and because I'm free to go where I like, eat and drink what I like, and have been for years, I feel as though I'm very much cured. To me, a cure is total freedom from debilitating symptoms and skin that is smooth, supple and free of acne scars.

Unravelling the mystery of my allergies has been a great adventure. I have learnt much and have matured in many ways because of it. I'm sure this book will help make the unravelling of your allergy mystery an adventure too!

2.
Allergies

'Not only will men of science have to grapple with the sciences that deal with man, but—and this is a far more difficult matter— they will have to persuade the world to listen to what they have discovered. If they cannot succeed in this difficult enterprise, man will destroy himself by his halfway cleverness.'

Bertrand Russell, 1872–1970

WHAT IS AN ALLERGY?

An allergy is an *over-reaction* of the body's immune system in its efforts to protect the body against what it (the immune system) perceives to be a threat. When resistance is down, sensitivities are up and allergies easily develop.

ALLERGIES AND THE IMMUNE SYSTEM

The immune system is the body's main line of defence against invading foreign substances that can damage it. It is made up of the white blood cells, known as lymphocytes. These are clumped together in lymphoid tissue, which is found in the spleen, the lining of the small and large intestines and the lymph nodes of the neck, armpits and groin. The lymph nodes are well evident during periods of infection when they swell up and are frequently referred to as 'swollen glands'.

When a foreign substance enters the body, the lymphocytes become sensitised by its presence and produce special proteins, called antibodies, which circulate in the blood until they make contact with and destroy the foreign substance.

Collectively, these foreign substances are known as antigens and may come in many different shapes and forms—viruses, bacteria, fungi, toxic chemicals from polluted water and air, and the preservatives and colourings in artificial foods. Evidence suggests that the major toxin (acetaldehyde) released into the blood by the yeast *Candida albicans* is a potent antigen.

21

In rendering the antigen harmless to the body, the antibodies have given us an immunity to that antigen. Once sensitised by an antigen, the lymphocytes remember that antigen and, in some cases, are able to successfully produce antibodies against it for the rest of our lives. In this way we enjoy lifelong immune protection from that substance. The diseases measles and chicken pox are good examples. Once contracted in childhood, our resistance to them usually becomes so great that they seldom bother us again through life.

Unfortunately, not all immune systems function perfectly all of the time. Sometimes there are imbalances in the immune system (resulting from imbalances in the body's metabolism) that give rise to excesses in the immune reaction. These excesses cause side effects and these side effects are known as allergic reactions.

Allergic reactions occur when there is an excess of histamine released into the blood and tissues.

HISTAMINE

Histamine is a chemical that is released by the white blood cells (basophils), the blood platelets and the mast cells in that area of the body that a foreign substance is residing. Histamine's job is to (1) dilate the blood vessels so that extra lymphocytes can arrive quickly on the scene, and (2) speed up the metabolic rate of all the cells in the area, that they may have the energy to protect themselves from and, in the case of lymphocytes, defeat the foreign body (virus, bacteria, fungus, etc.). In this way histamine acts as a normal part of the immune reaction and is vital if we are to survive invasion by infectious agents. Normal amounts of histamine dilate the blood vessels only as much as is needed to supply the required number of lymphocytes to do the job. The arrival of the extra lymphocytes, the dilation of the blood vessels and the increased metabolic rate of the cells in the area, produces only a mild inflammation which, for the main part, goes unnoticed.

If too much histamine is released there is an excessive inflammatory reaction that leads to tissue damage. In these circumstances the immune mechanisms are protecting us at the cost of tissue damage and excessive inflammation (swelling, redness, pain).

Allergic reactions take place in those people whose immune systems habitually over-react to certain antigens. Any antigen that causes such an over-reaction of the immune system is known as an allergen. However individual and different allergic people may be, they all have one thing in common: an immune system that over-reacts to antigens/allergens, such as foods, grasses, pollens, moulds, dust mites, dust, etc., that are normally not life threatening.

THE ALLERGIC REACTION: HOW IT HAPPENS

It's no coincidence that most allergies, especially adult onset allergies, start after a bout of glandular fever, 'flu, hepatitis, surgical operation or crash diet. All of these factors are stressors that leave the body tired and the immune system depressed. The exact mechanisms by which allergic reactions take place are enormously complex and, for the main part, poorly understood. What is clearly recognised and agreed upon though, is that an excess of histamine released from the basophils, blood platelets and mast cells causes an inflammation at the point of release, and that this inflammation gives rise to the definitive symptoms of an allergy.

The allergy takes its name from the tissue the inflammation takes place in. If the inflammation takes place in the windpipe, it's called asthma; in the nose, rhinitis, sinusitis or hayfever. Histamine inflammation in the joints gives rise to arthritis and in the eyes to conjunctivitis. Because histamine can be released into any tissue of the body, the symptoms of allergy are many and varied. Many people experience allergic reactions in more than one tissue at a time.

Because we're all so biochemically unique, we can manifest our allergies in slightly different ways. For instance, histamine inflammation in the brain can give rise to depression in some people, poor concentration in others and dizzy spells, drowsiness and fatigue in others. Histamine inflammation in the skin can manifest as eczema in some, psoriasis in others, hives in others and adult acne in many others.

The difference between a normally reacting immune system and an over-reacting immune system is that an over-reacting immune system wants to protect us against foreign bodies that are not normally life threatening. Pollens, grasses, dusts, dust mites, moulds and foods do not pose the threat to us that viruses, bacteria and internally growing fungi do.

What causes an immune system to become over-reactive? Stress of any sort will do it (see Chapter 11, 'Stress'). The stresses of cold, trauma, over-work, over-exercise, over-socialising, over-commitment, significant loss and infection (bacterial, viral or fungal) can all do it. Especially if you've experienced two or more of them over a prolonged period of time. Prolonged stress makes us tired. When the body is tired, every one of its 60 trillion cells, including those of the immune system, is tired. When we're tired, we tend to be more sensitive than usual and over-react to things that wouldn't normally bother us. We become short tempered and intolerant. We perceive things negatively and flare up at imagined insults and react aggressively to imagined challenges. So it is with the cells of the immune system. When the body is stressed and tired, the immune system flares up at things that don't normally pose a threat to us and an excess of histamine is released. Not all tired immune systems react this way—there has to be a genetic predisposition to over-reaction before the allergic mechanism can be triggered.

Singularly, the greatest stress the cells of the immune system (and indeed the rest of the body) can experience, is the withholding from them of essential nutrients (oxygen, water, vitamins, minerals, protein, essential fatty acids, carbohydrate). In addition to making a cell tired, nutrient deficiencies create imbalances in its metabolism. An unbalanced metabolism gives rise to unbalanced behaviour by the cell. This erratic behaviour of the immune system cells that gives rise to allergic reactions is a good example of metabolic imbalances created by nutrient deficiency. (See Chapter 16, 'Scientific explanations—The metabolism'.)

ALLERGY SUFFERERS

Allergy sufferers are said to be strongly immunised against an antigen and have far more antibodies in their blood than non-allergic people. Although allergic diseases themselves are not inherited, the tendency for the immune system to over-react to an antigen can be passed on from parent to child.

If one parent is allergic there is a 50 per cent chance any offspring will be. If both parents are allergic there is a 75 per cent chance offspring will be. Allergy sufferers differ from non-allergic people in that they have antibodies permanently attached to the basophils and mast cells in their bodies. Because it is the *tendency* to allergic reaction that is passed on, all allergies can be successfully treated. This is because the allergy itself is carried in the blood and once the allergens have been identified and removed from the diet and environment it's only a matter of time before those remaining in the blood are eliminated through the kidneys. When this happens the allergy, be it arthritis, psoriasis, asthma, eczema, sinusitis, hayfever, fluid retention or depression, will disappear.

So just because your grandmother and mother suffered from any one of the allergy symptoms listed in this book, it doesn't mean you have to.

Because allergies are carried in the blood, an allergic pregnant mother can prevent allergies developing in her child by removing from her diet and environment those things she's allergic to. Although the mother may well pass on the genetic predisposition to allergy, the actual allergy won't be passed on. Perhaps the greatest advantage to the child of the mother who has her allergies treated in pregnancy or before, is the removal of the possibility of experiencing more severe allergies than the parents. Dr Pottenger noted (see Dr Pottenger's experiments on cats later in this chapter) that each new generation of cats had more severe allergies than their parents. Many of his third generation cats died from complications of their condition. So poor was their health that only three of the one hundred third generation asthmatic cats lived to begin breeding the subsequent healthy generation.

Many a parent of allergic children I have treated has remarked that they were never as allergic as their children when they were young. However, many mothers experienced a worsening of their allergies after the stress of childbirth or the stress of pregnancy termination. Childbirth sees a massive loss to the body of fluid, oxygen, vitamins and minerals in the placenta and amniotic fluid. Breastfeeding sees a further loss of these nutrients. Pregnancy termination sees the same loss in the blood and dead foetus. In my experience these mothers do not overcome their allergies unless their diets are supplemented with a complete multi-vitamin and mineral formula, particularly if they're breastfeeding.

THE ROLE OF NUTRITION

Inadequate nutrition is perhaps the greatest single factor in determining whether you will develop allergies or not. So strong is the influence of nutrition that it can prevent the onset of allergies in those who are genetically predisposed to them.

My experience with treating allergy sufferers confirms the link between allergy and nutrition. Patients of mine who have gone on the Metabolism-Balancing Program and supplementary vitamins and minerals for six to eight weeks have experienced a marked reduction in the number of substances they were allergic to. Before- and after-program allergy tests have confirmed this. Most of these patients have remarked that their allergies originally started with or returned when they went on a weight loss diet (usually a crash diet). The men remark that drinking beer can sometimes cause their allergies (stuffy nose, asthma, skin complaints) to flare up but only when they've been skipping meals and are tired and run down.

Many notable scientists have accumulated significant evidence supporting the link between allergies and our highly processed modern diet. The late Weston Price, in his excellent study, *Nutrition and Physical Degeneration,* notes that allergies are almost never found in primitive peoples living a simple lifestyle and eating a natural diet. Dr Price points out that the typical modern diet, high in sugar, white bread, canned vegetables and processed meats, does not provide sufficient nutrition and therefore lowers resistance to allergies. Dr Carl Pfeiffer, Director and Chief Neuropharmacologist at the Brain Bio Centre in Princeton, New Jersey, has discovered that susceptibility to allergies in babies can be due to a lack of an adequate supply of vitamin B6 and zinc in the mother's diet during pregnancy. White flour and sugared foods are practically devoid of vitamin B6 and zinc. Over sixty different enzymes found in the cells of the liver, small intestine and brain are made, in part, from vitamin

B6 and zinc. A deficiency in enzymes means imbalances in the body's metabolism and subsequent imbalances in the immune system.

Enzymes are made from proteins, vitamins and minerals. If these are scarce, the enzymes wear out and are not replaced. Imbalances in the metabolism and allergies thus ensue. In vitamin A and D deficient people, allergies tend to manifest themselves in the upper respiratory tract, nose, throat, bronchial tubes and the skin (acne, eczema, psoriasis, hives, rosacea). In vitamin B6, vitamin C, zinc and manganese deficiencies the allergies appear in the brain, giving rise to anything from mild depression to manic depressive psychosis and schizophrenia. Calcium, magnesium and potassium deficiencies frequently manifest as asthma.

In many cases, sound nutrition will significantly reduce the intensity of the allergy and in some cases will completely cure it. Dr Francis Pottenger (University of Southern California and The Price–Pottenger Institute of Research) produced allergies in cats by feeding them a poor diet. Allergies began to appear in the first generation of cats and by the second generation, 60 per cent of the cats were allergic—by the third generation 100 per cent of the cats were allergic. He was credited with having the only asthmatic cats on record. He began feeding his third generation cats on a well-balanced diet and by the fourth generation the allergies had completely disappeared.

Another interesting experiment first conducted by Dr Roger Williams (University of Texas) and later duplicated by Dr U. D. Register (Loma Linda University, California) determined the effects of diet on the metabolism of rats. One group of rats (Group A) was fed the typical American teenage diet of glazed doughnuts, crackers and cola drinks (junk). A second group (Group B) were fed a wholegrain diet of oats, wheat, rice, fresh fruit and vegetables as well as nuts, seeds and cottonseed oil. Neither group of rats was over-exercised or psychologically stressed. In each case the rats were given one pail containing only water and one pail of 90 per cent water and 10 per cent alcohol. Group A rats became aggressive and antisocial. They hardly touched the water only pail and drank liberally from the pail containing the alcohol. Group B rats remained friendly and social. They hardy touched the alcohol-containing pail and drank liberally from the water pail.

Over a period of months Group A rats were consuming the equivalent of what would be a quart of 100 proof whisky a day for an adult man. Adding a multi-vitamin and mineral supplement greatly reduced alcohol intake in Group A rats within a week. Adding the unrefined diet of Group B rats to the supplement reduced alcohol intake to that of the Group B level. The initial aggressive behaviour displayed by Group A rats is typical of someone with allergies manifesting in the brain. Were the Group A rats attempting to anaesthetise themselves against the distressing emotions derived from newly developed brain allergies to refined foods? The work of Theron Randolph MD on alcoholism in humans (*The Role of Specific Alcoholic Beverages*, pages 321–33) suggests they could be. Certainly all three scientists agree that significant imbalances had been created in the metabolisms of the rats which developed the biological thirst for alcohol.

Dr Pottenger's other experiments revealed that people with a milk allergy wear down their intestinal villi, the tiny finger-like projections that stick out from the lining of the intestine through which food is absorbed, each time they drink milk. These villi can take months to regrow. Worn down villi mean you absorb less vitamins and minerals no matter how nutritious your diet is.

In its study on the nutritional status of Australians handed down in 1988, the Federal Department of Health concluded that Australian women (due to childbirth, terminations and menstruation) tend to be deficient in iron, zinc and calcium. These are three of the principal nutrients needed by the immune system cells to maintain the balance of their metabolisms and keep their energy levels up. Clearly the Aussie diet is not invigorating us as well as it used to. In its 1944 report, the Federal Department of Health found no deficiencies in Australians. There were less refined, convenience foods in 1944 and less allergies too.

OVER-EXPOSURE: THE OVER-BIG STRESS

Over-exposure to a given food/food chemical in our diet, or substance in our environment (mainly chemicals) can so irritate tired, poorly nourished immune system cells as to incite their over-reaction to that food or substance.

CYCLIC ALLERGIES

Cyclic allergies are those that develop as a result of over-exposure to a food, chemical, pollutant, fume, gas, pollen or grass. Cyclic allergies account for 95 per cent of all allergies (the remaining 5 per cent are fixed) and can usually be overcome if you haven't been exposed to the allergen for too long. The majority of cyclic allergies begin as a result of over-exposure to a chemical or food. Many children are born with a cyclic allergy as their mothers were suffering from a cyclic allergy during pregnancy. As time goes by the sensitivity can spread to other foods and chemicals and on to grasses, pollens, dusts, yeasts, fungi and dust mites. Ninety days' avoidance of the allergenic substance is usually enough to desensitise the body to that substance.

STRESS AND OVER-EXPOSURE

People are more prone to develop over-exposure allergies if they are tired, under stress or suffering from a cold, 'flu or other infection.

For instance, anyone over-indulging in alcohol while suffering from the 'flu, the effect of over-work or the stress of a broken relationship can develop a sensitivity to the food from which the alcohol is made (for example, wheat in the case of whisky, or corn in the case of bourbon).

Many of the cases of late onset allergies that I have treated have developed in adults who were never troubled by allergies as children. Invariably these adults can trace the beginnings of their allergy symptoms to a severe cold, 'flu, attack of glandular fever, hepatitis, tonsillitis or severe bacterial throat infection. Invariably this bout of illness is due to a period of overdoing it coupled with skipped meals, rushed meals and a diet comprising too many processed, tinned and frozen packaged foods. Such a lifestyle and diet strains the immune system to the point where resident viruses lower immune vitality. When the more obvious symptoms of the infection have abated the symptoms of the allergy remain and linger until the immune vitality is once more raised by the appropriate diet and lifestyle. The Metabolism-Balancing Program has been formulated for this purpose. It is an immune vitality raiser *par excellence*.

SLOW DEVELOPING ALLERGIES

Although many over-exposure allergies can develop from a sudden massive exposure to a given substance (for example, by being overcome by fumes during an industrial accident, or getting smashed on a particular alcoholic beverage while tired or suffering from a cold or 'flu), over-exposure allergies can develop slowly over a longer period of time. The continual eating of a given food, especially if it is a refined food such as white bread, can give us an allergy to wheat. In this case eating the white bread day in, day out, wears out the digestive enzymes in the wall of the small intestine and the liver, causing the semi-digested food to be absorbed into the blood. A semi-digested food is a foreign body and is recognised by an over-sensitive immune system as an allergen.

Because the digestive enzymes are made from vitamins and minerals, the cells need vitamins and minerals to replace enzymes that are wearing out. Refined foods (white bread, canned and frozen foods, processed meats, take-away foods) don't carry the nutrients they need to build replacement enzymes. Thus malnutrition contributes significantly to over-exposure allergies. It is significant that stress and malnutrition go together—most highly stressed people skip meals altogether and so completely miss out on their vitamins and minerals.

The slow drip-feeding into the blood of the toxic waste products, particularly acetaldehyde, from the yeast *Candida albicans*, can produce over-exposure to this chemical over a long period of time. Allergic reactions thus ensue.

OVER-EXPOSURE IN INFANCY

For many of us, our first massive over-exposure to an allergenic substance comes when we are babies. The substance is usually food. Up until the age of ten months the cells lining the wall of our intestines are still so under-developed that they are not able to absorb foods selectively. As a result, all foods are absorbed rapidly. This is the way nature has planned it. Up until that age we are supposed to be on mother's milk exclusively and absorbing from it, not only nutrients, but her antibodies as well.

As antibodies are whole proteins and very large in size it is important that the intestinal cells be under-developed. Otherwise the antibodies would be too large to pass from the digestive tract into the blood. The passage of the mother's antibodies to the child in this way is called passive immunity and is important for the development of the child's resistance to disease.

Problems begin when solid foods such as eggs, meat, fish, chicken, cows milk and cheese are eaten before the cells of the intestine are fully developed. Because the baby's intestinal cells are under-developed, proteins from these foods are absorbed into the blood. The proteins are not broken down into amino acids because the baby's pancreas is not yet sufficiently developed to produce the digestive enzymes needed to do this.

Amino acids are the result of fully digested protein and don't elicit allergic reactions in the blood. Whole proteins, on the other hand, are undigested foods and do bring about allergic reactions. Undigested food proteins are allergens.

Unfortunately, many babies won't accept their mother's milk. There are a number of reasons for this:

1. The mother's diet is vitamin and mineral deficient and therefore so is her milk. In such cases, the baby has to drink so much of it she/he becomes overloaded and brings it all back up. Not a nice experience and if repeated often enough will put the baby off mother's milk completely. Some mothers eat a nutritionally balanced diet but burn up so much of it working, exercising or socialising there isn't enough nutrition left for the baby.
2. Some mothers smoke or drink too much or eat too many exotic spices. This ruins the taste of the milk as do flavourings, preservatives and colourings in refined foods. Often these find their way into the baby's blood and cause reactions too.
3. The mother's food allergies may be carried in the milk and passed to the baby. This can be prevented if the mother has the foods she's allergic to removed from her diet (see Chapter 5, 'How

to cure your allergies') and breastfeeds her baby for the first ten months, introducing solid foods after this time.

BREAST MILK COLITIS

This condition can develop when babies drink allergen-containing breast milk. These babies become very colicky and often pass blood through the bowel and whereas the amount passed is seldom ever a threat to the baby it is an accurate barometer of just how inflamed and painful the lining of the baby's bowel is.

Some authorities claim that milk and wheat are the only causes of breast milk colitis. My experience is that this isn't so. Any food can do it. It all depends what the mother is specifically allergic to and not all mothers are allergic to milk and wheat. Don't take yourself off these foods unless allergy tests have proved your sensitivity to them. They are nutritious foods and going off them could reduce the nutritional value of your milk. For the same reason don't attempt to test for allergies by the elimination diet method. Go to an allergist and have the blood and skin tests.

The only exception to this rule is for those people of Mediterranean, Asian and African extraction. These people lack the enzymes needed to digest cow's milk properly and invariably have a sensitivity to it. This sensitivity is often carried through their breast milk to the baby. If you belong to one of these ethnic groups and your baby's breast milk colitis isn't responding to treatment go off milk for a trial period. Milk could be the culprit. Going off milk means going off all those foods that are made from milk or contain milk in their manufacture. (See the section on milk in the 'Food tables' at the back of the book.)

BABY FORMULAS

Breast milk colitis is a strong case for giving baby formulas a try. Many a paediatrician and parent has witnessed an improvement in a baby's allergies (often hives, eczema, asthma, nappy rash and breast milk colitis) when the baby is taken off the breast and put on a formula. This is because that particular formula didn't contain the specific allergens carried in that particular mother's milk. Unfortunately the erroneous conclusion that all formulas are good for all babies all of the time is drawn from this.

The facts are that not all babies improve on formulas. Some babies are allergic to the cow's and soymilk they're made from. Some are allergic to the malt and other inclusions and because of these sensitivities don't improve when taken off the.breast. If the baby has contracted a candida yeast infection from the mother, thc sugar in the formula will so aggravate the candida infection that the symptoms will become worse. If the candida infection is only mild it will take time for the symptoms to flare. Because an initial improvement was witnessed on the formula the emerging symptoms of a developing candida problem (see Chapter 4, 'Candida albicans') are not attributed to the formula and the baby is invariably kept on it with no cause ever found for its suffering.

Formulas are not the answer. The solution is to clean up the mother's breast milk by having her allergies treated in the manner described in Chapter 5, 'How to cure your allergies'. By doing this the baby will lose his/her allergies, won't need formulas and won't need to be on solid food before the age of ten months.

BREAST FED IS BEST FED

Breast feeding so effectively boosts the baby's immunity as to reduce the incidence of allergy by 25 per cent. This fact was discovered by research doctors in Finland who followed the lives of babies born in 1975 through to the present day. Eczema, asthma and food allergies had developed in 65 per cent of 17 year olds who had received little or no breast feeding. In those breast fed to six months the incidence was 40 per cent. These findings received such acclaim in the scientific world they were written up in the prestigious *Lancet* medical journal.

ALLERGIC TO OURSELVES

Auto-immune disease is the name given to the process whereby the body begins to produce antibodies against its own tissues. This constitutes over-sensitivity and erratic behaviour of the immune system taken to the nth degree, as under normal conditions the immune system recognises the body's own tissues as OK and not a threat.

This antigen–antibody reaction usually attacks the joints (rheumatoid arthritis), the joints and heart combined (rheumatic fever), the skin and blood vessels (systemic lupus erythematosis) or the muscles and joints of the lower back (ankylosing spondylitis). Sometimes it attacks the thyroid gland (acute thyroiditis), causing it to be either over- or under-active. A disrupted thyroid gland further unbalances the metabolism.

In my experience the great majority of people with an auto-immune disease have either an allergy, a yeast infection or both. In most cases the treatment program laid out in Chapter 5, 'How to cure your allergies', brings about complete remission of these diseases.

FIXED ALLERGIES

A fixed allergy, to a food, chemical, gas, dust, pollen, grass or mould, is one that you are born with and will have till the day you die. It's something you have inherited a propensity for. Sometimes it can be controlled so that its effects are minimised. This is particularly so in the case of inhalant allergens, such as dust, grasses and moulds, where vaccines can be administered to desensitise the sufferer to the allergen. In the case of a fixed allergy to a food (for example, strawberries, tomatoes) the best treatment is to avoid the food completely. Fortunately, only 5 per cent of allergic people suffer from a fixed allergy.

GUT-MEDIATED ALLERGIES

Not everybody experiences their allergic reactions in the blood. Some allergic reactions are confined to the intestines and make up any or all of those symptoms listed under 'Gastro-intestinal' later in this chapter. Blood tests are of little use to these people as the foods causing the problem are seldom absorbed through the intestinal wall into the blood to register their presence there. However, the mechanism of the gut-mediated allergic reaction is the same as that of the blood-mediated one, except that in this case it is the white blood cells lining the intestinal wall that have become over-sensitive rather than those floating in the blood. Celiac disease (massive gluten sensitivity) and Crohn's disease are extreme examples of gut-mediated allergies.

The trial and error removal and reintroduction of foods—one at a time—is the only way to test for the offending gut-mediated allergies. However, this can't be done until the stress levels have been reduced and any existing candida yeast infections in the intestines (see Chapter 4, 'Candida albicans') have been contained. Stress and candida yeast infections give rise to the same symptoms as gut-mediated food allergies.

MIGRATING ALLERGY SYNDROME

Because allergies are carried in the blood they can, and often do, migrate around the body. The random coming and going of symptoms that is so confusing to both patient and physician can be caused by this. Many people are deluded into thinking they have outgrown their allergies when their symptoms disappear in this way. They seldom equate the development of new symptoms with the allergy that caused their old symptoms. As whacky and variable as this process is there are some common patterns.

Those who mysteriously lose (grow out of) their asthma frequently develop eczema and those who had itchy skin and hayfever as children frequently develop acne as adults. Don't be lulled into a false sense of security if, without treatment, your symptoms suddenly disappear. The probability of your untreated allergy emerging somewhere else, as something else, is very high.

ALLERGIES SPOIL YOUR APPEARANCE

The ways in which an untreated allergy can eventually alter the shape and appearance of the body are numerous and may include:

1. Fluid retention
- Thickening of the ankle and lower leg.
- Swollen fingers.
- Puffy (often black) bags under the eyes.
- Puffiness at the sides of the nose.
- Puffiness over the cheekbones.

The puffiness about the face may be permanent, or it may come and go for no apparent reason and have no apparent pattern.

The fluid may be spread about the whole body, and possibly mistaken for fat, or localised about the legs, thighs and buttocks as cellulite.

2. Skin disfigurement
- It may become hot and flushed for no apparent reason, at any time and without warning.
- It may perspire excessively, causing make-up to run.
- It may itch so that you scratch it and cause scarring.
- There may be isolated patches of redness that either come and go or remain permanently.
- The complexion may have the ghostly white, china doll appearance of anaemia, despite the fact that it doesn't show up in blood tests.
- It may become dry and flaky, or you may have dandruff.
- Acne, acne rosacea, hives, eczema, dermatitis, canker sores, boils and psoriasis can all be allergy based.
- Blushing, whether because of stress or not.
- Black rings under the eyes (allergic shiners)—a classic sign of allergy.
- Sensitivity to sunlight and inability to tan.
- Small white spots over the face, neck, legs and body.

3. Eye problems
Bloodshot eyes (conjunctivitis) itching, burning, pain, running eyes, heavy, puffy eyelids (upper, lower or both).

4. The mouth
The mouth is often open and gaping. The upper lip is often shortened and pulled up and back to the nose. The lower lip is often bulbous and drooping. This is frequently the result of breathing through the mouth because of a nasal blockage. Bad breath that persists despite the use of mouthwash is frequently the result of food allergy. The allergic food is putrefying in the intestine instead of being digested and absorbed.

5. *The nose*
   It will often have puffy skin, sometimes red, sometimes pale. A transverse crease frequently found on the nose of the chronically allergic, giving it the appearance of a boxer's broken nose.

6. *The hair*
   This can be dry and lifeless, or oily and lifeless. Frequently it is lighter in colour than would normally be. Often it is blonde because of nutritional deficiencies.

7. *The nails*
   These are frequently brittle, creviced and have white spots (nutritional deficiencies).

8. *Facial expression*
   Allergy often causes a sad, anxious expression. This is particularly so if the allergy is affecting the tissues of the brain. Chronically allergic people often look older than their years.

There are other symptoms too. Frequently the head is tilted to one side because of allergy-based spasms in the neck muscles; the joints of fingers, elbows and knees can be swollen, stiff or gnarled.

The torso often loses or fails to develop a good shape in the chronically allergic—particularly in cases of allergies in the nose, bronchial tubes and lungs (sinusitis, bronchitis and asthma). A narrow, thin chest with grooves below the nipples, prominent breastbone and collarbones are common. This results from a lifetime of impaired breathing and frequently from nutritional deficiencies as well.

DO I HAVE AN ALLERGY?

You should consider yourself a strong candidate if you have one or more of the signs mentioned above. Most people have a combination of two or more signs and some have as many as a dozen. Read carefully the list of symptoms below and tick any that apply to you. If you have one or more symptoms and have not been able to get rid of them with standard treatments, you may well have an allergy. If you have any of the symptoms listed below but as yet have none of the conditions that cause degenerating appearance listed above, then seek treatment for your allergies anyway. Although you may have been lucky enough to have escaped skin, hair, nail and fluid problems until now, this will not last.

The official statistics put the incidence of allergy among Australians at 45 per cent of the population. My experience based on twenty-two years of taking care of sick people puts it closer to 60 per cent. This is because many people are suffering from allergies without knowing it. The lists below illustrate just how varied the manifestations of allergy can be.

CLASSIC ALLERGY SYMPTOMS

1. *Headaches*
   Various kinds, including migraine.
2. *Eye conditions*
   Conjunctivitis, eye pain, periods of blurred vision, sensitivity to light, tearing, temporary refractive changes.
3. *Ear conditions*
   Hearing loss, infections, inflammation, Menier's syndrome, noises in the ear, repeated ear trouble.
4. *Cardiovascular*
   Angina, high blood pressure, irregular heartbeat, low blood pressure, rapid pulse.
5. *Gastro-intestinal*
   Constipation, diarrhoea, gall bladder pains, gas, gastric ulcer, gastro-intestinal bleeding, heartburn, haemorrhoids, indigestion, mucous colitis, nausea, nervous stomach, pains or cramps, spastic colon, vomiting.
6. *Respiratory*
   Asthma, chronic rhinitis, coughing, frequent colds, hayfever, mouth breathing, nosebleeds, post-nasal discharge, sinusitis, stuffy nose, wheezing.
7. *Urological*
   Bed wetting, frequent night urination, frequent urination, painful or difficult urination.
8. *Musculo-skeletal*
   Arthritis, joint pains, muscle cramps, muscle pains and aches, muscle spasms, muscle weakness.
9. *Mental and behavioural*
   Anxiety, delusions, depression (including psychotic), dizzy spells, drowsiness, epilepsy, floating sensation, general fatigue, hallucination, hyperactivity, insomnia, irritability, learning disorders, minimal brain dysfunction, nervousness, periods of confusion, phobias, poor concentration, poor memory, poor muscle co-ordination, restlessness, schizophrenia, falling asleep at inappropriate times, sleeping too little or too much, chronic fatigue syndrome, unsteadiness.
10. *Miscellaneous*
    Abnormal body odour, diabetes, excessive sweating, hypoglycaemia, general weakness, night sweating, over-weight, under-weight, virus infections, bad breath.

The following are examples of combinations of allergic symptoms that I have treated:

Woman, 33: Acne on face, dark rings under eyes, cramping pains and constipation, periodic puffing of eyelids unrelated to seasonal changes. Allergic to wheat, corn, milk, mould and house dust.

Woman, 23: Stubborn cellulite at backs of legs, bloating of stomach, periodic puffing of face, cheekbones and under eyes, periodic dark bags under eyes. Allergic to asbestos, after-shave sprays, dust mites, milk, brewer's yeast.

Woman, 37: Periodic breakouts of dermatitis on the face, inability to lose weight, constipation, erratic mood swings, depression without warning and without reason. Allergic to moulds, grasses, wheat, milk, beef, eggs and peanuts.

Girl, 17: Acne on face, puffiness over cheekbones, dark rings under the eyes, shortened upper lip, sinus blockage, mouth breathing, sad appearance. Allergic to potatoes, tomatoes, beef, corn, milk, moulds, pollens and house dust.

SUMMARY

The tendency to react allergically is passed on in the genes from parent to child. In some children this tendency is obvious right from birth. These kids are born with such typical allergy symptoms as asthma, allergic rhinitis, colic, hayfever, hives, rosacea, infantile eczema, runny nose or glue ear.

In others the tendency remains dormant only to be activated some time in childhood or adult life due to:

- the over-consumption of refined junk food, such as lollies, cakes, tinned foods, ice-cream, soft drinks, biscuits, white bread, chocolates, alcohol, etc.;
- stress—the major one being a deficiency in the essential nutrients;
- the consumption of solid foods before the age of ten months;
- *Candida albicans* yeast infection;
- over-exposure to environmental factors—mainly pollutants.

Because you probably won't know whether you have a genetic predisposition to allergy it won't pay to press your luck by eating junk foods. Junk foods are themselves a major stress to the body and also feed candida yeast infections (see Chapter 4, '*Candida albicans*'). Junk food consumption should be kept to a minimum, no more than 3–5 per cent of the total food intake.

A complete multi-vitamin and mineral supplement (one which contains the six essential minerals—calcium, magnesium, potassium, iron, manganese and zinc) should be taken once per day before the main meal to ensure optimum nutrition.

There are those people who eat a lot of junk food all their lives, don't supplement their diet with vitamins and minerals and yet don't develop allergies. These individuals don't carry the predisposition to allergy in their genes. They are usually symptom free (thought often tired and lethargic) until later in life, when such degenerative diseases as heart attacks, ME, multiple sclerosis and cancer catch up with them. In a way, the allergy sufferers are luckier as they get early warning symptoms that something is wrong and have the chance to balance their metabolism before a serious disease develops.

Finally there is no such thing as a specific allergen always causing a specific reaction. For example, strawberries causing hives only or eggs causing migraines only. Any allergen can cause any of the symptoms listed in this chapter.

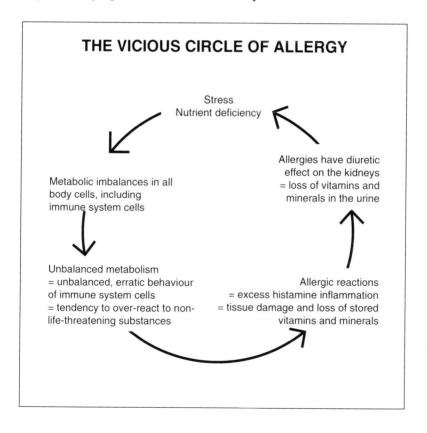

THE VICIOUS CIRCLE OF ALLERGY

Stress
Nutrient deficiency

Allergies have diuretic effect on the kidneys = loss of vitamins and minerals in the urine

Metabolic imbalances in all body cells, including immune system cells

Unbalanced metabolism = unbalanced, erratic behaviour of immune system cells = tendency to over-react to non-life-threatening substances

Allergic reactions = excess histamine inflammation = tissue damage and loss of stored vitamins and minerals

3.
Allergy addiction

'There are certain persons who cannot readily change their diet with impunity; and if they make any alteration in it for one day, or even part of a day, are greatly injured thereby.'

Hippocrates, 500 BC

Not everybody suffers from the usual, immediate allergic reaction to a given substance or food. Some suffer delayed reactions, making it difficult to associate their symptoms with a given allergen. These 'hidden' or 'masked' allergies can dog the unsuspecting sufferer for a lifetime as he or she travels from doctor to doctor looking for an answer to his or her particular pot-pourri of symptoms. Unlike the easily recognised cause and effect allergy such as hives after eating strawberries, swollen mouth after eating lobster, migraine after eating a Chinese meal with MSG, the allergy-addicted people actually feel better after eating the food they are allergic to and ill when away from it for too long.

WHY IS THIS SO?

The answer lies in the very nature of the addictive process. If we make repeated contact with a substance that disagrees with us we can, in time, get used to it and learn to live with it. So used to it can we get that if we no longer make contact with it we start to experience withdrawal symptoms. These withdrawal or hangover symptoms are usually the same symptoms we experienced on first contact with the substance and can be stopped immediately we make contact with it again.

Former smokers (and drug addicts) are familiar with this

pattern. As beginner smokers, many of them found their first cigarette unpleasant and even disagreeable. Peer pressure forced them to continue smoking and in time cigarettes started to agree with them, indeed they found they needed them to cope with life's daily stresses and to relax. When they finally decided to give them up they went through withdrawal symptoms that often left them tired, cranky, irritable and depressed.

Over-exposure to any substance, even those that don't give us an initial bad reaction, can give rise to an eventual addiction to that substance. This happens as readily to foods and common environmental and food chemicals as to cigarettes and other drugs.

As explained in the last chapter, certain people come into the world with a genetic predisposition to allergy. Lowered resistance due to stress and insufficient nutrients in the diet triggers the tendency to react allergically to things we are over-exposed to. (It's important to note that those who don't carry this genetic predisposition can expose themselves to foods and chemicals with impunity for many years—even a lifetime.)

Frequently the first over-exposure to a given substance is encountered in the womb where the substances the mother is allergic to floats through the baby's blood as well. Later these substances are taken into the baby's body in the breast milk. Eating solid foods before the age of ten months further aggravates the problem of over-exposure (see Chapter 2, 'Allergies').

As a result of this, many kids come into the world with allergies (asthma, eczema, colic, nappy rash, stuffy, runny nose, etc.) to certain foods and chemicals which in time they grow out of—or so everybody thinks. What has happened, in fact, is they have become used to these foods and aren't reacting as overtly as before. Their bodies have adapted to these allergenic foods or to the chemical flavourings, colours and preservatives in them. This happens because the allergenic food is spooned into the baby whether he/she wants it or not. As babies are not able to communicate that a given food doesn't agree with them, the parent continues to give it, even when the baby repeatedly spits it out.

Often, from about two years of age, children are ordered to eat foods they dislike because those foods are considered 'good for them'. Even though they instinctively know these foods disagree with them, they continue to eat them (1) because there is nothing else to eat and (2) because they are under orders to do so. In time Mum's stance is vindicated because they are growing well and are no longer afflicted by those childhood complaints. It is concluded that they have outgrown their allergies. In fact they have simply become used to the presence of those foods in their systems, so marvellous is the body's ability to adapt to undesirable situations.

In fairness to the well-meaning parent there is no way out of this dilemma as babies and little children are in a rapid growth spurt and need to eat as broad a spectrum of nutritious foods and as much of it as possible. The withholding of foods at that age could do more harm than good as malnutrition, and the impaired growth and development it gives rise to, is more serious than allergy. Besides, nature has coped with the situation by giving the body the powers of adaptation.

During this period of adaptation everything is fine and the allergic person is often symptom free so long as the foods or chemical flavourings, colours and preservatives that used to cause the allergy symptoms are regularly consumed. If they are not, unpleasant withdrawal symptoms start. When this happens, eating that food makes one feel immediately better, which is why so many allergy foods turn out to be favourite foods. Not surprisingly, allergy-addicted people believe these foods are good for them.

As time goes by the body becomes tired of having to cope with this allergenic substance and its powers of adaptation begin to wane. At this point, the withdrawal symptoms (which are a repeat of the original allergy symptoms and can be any of a number of those listed in Chapter 2) begin to appear, and eating the allergic food does nothing to stop them. The body has now passed from the phase of adaptation to the phase of exhaustion and the symptoms that used to appear only on contact with, and later withdrawal from, the offending food are now there day in, and day out. The acute cause and effect allergy has become the chronic hidden or masked allergy.

It is at this point that most people seek treatment for their allergy symptoms. Because these symptoms are never attributed to the foods they have eaten all their lives and especially not to those that have in the past given them a pick-up, they are usually suppressed by drug medication or treated by surgery. Not surprisingly, some people baulk at the idea that symptoms which have appeared out of the blue in adulthood could be caused by foods that have been their favourites since childhood. That symptom free period in their life makes them hard to convince.

Sometimes the scenario is slightly different, and instead of the child going through a symptom free period that lasts all the way to adolescence or to well into adulthood, he or she experiences a series of changing symptoms that are never attributed to allergy. These people don't have the same powers of adaptation as those who experience a symptom free period in their lives. The scenario

40

of the less well-adapted person goes something like this, though subject to variation from person to person.

The colicky infant becomes the chronically sick toddler with fevers, cold, runny nose and ear infections. The chronically sick toddler becomes the hyperactive, slow-learning child who grows to become the moody (sometimes delinquent) teenager with learning and adjustment problems. From adolescence the allergy sufferer moves into the low energy twenties. The physical symptoms of fat, fluid retention and skin problems become apparent and there is often much absenteeism from work. The chronically tired syndrome of the thirties follows and leads into the functional sickness of the forties, often attributed to menopause in women. By the fifties the years of allergic inflammation within the body have so damaged the tissues as to give rise to diseases such as stage 3 arthritis, diabetes, benign and malignant tumours, kidney, heart and artery problems.

VARYING SCENARIOS

To further complicate the picture, not all those in the 'less well-adapted' category experience the low energy phase of the early twenties. Some have adrenal glands that are strong enough to continue their allergy-based hyperactivity well into adulthood (see Chapter 16, 'Scientific explanations—Stress'). This hyperactivity is the driving force behind some, but not all, of the hard-charger personality types described in Chapter 11, 'Stress'. Unfortunately, not all young people choose to channel their hyperactivity into hard work. Others try to ameliorate it by smoking marijuana and/or drinking too much alcohol, which soon makes them dopey, disorganised, undisciplined and unproductive.

Some kids don't have allergic mothers and escape all the childhood trials previously described. They remain perfectly well until adulthood when the combined effect of the mounting stresses of life, vitamin and mineral deficiencies, and over-exposure to a certain substance for the first time starts off the allergy addiction process. These people carry a genetic predisposition to allergy handed down from either the father or a grandparent on either side of the family. Repeated contact with a given food, beverage or chemical can start the process off.

Here's an example by way of explanation. For some people the first contact with alcohol can be an harassing one. After a few drinks they can feel headachy, groggy, nauseous, tired, spaced out and even incoherent. In more severe cases those afflicted have to periodically excuse themselves to vomit the beverage out of their stomach. Peer pressure, a desire not to be left out or appear a piker, or the need for company, keeps the alcohol sensitive person drinking with the group. In time they find that alcohol starts to agree with them and they learn, as seasoned drinkers would say, 'to hold their liquor'.

Finding that alcohol agrees with them, these people often develop reputations as hard-headed drinkers, much to the delight of the friends, workmates, bosses, clients, spouses or relatives, they've always so wanted to please. Alcohol is now being experienced as a delightful pick-me-up and is consumed more and more often for the feeling of buoyant well-being it gives. Imperceptibly a dependency on alcohol is now developing and the one in question is now drinking more and more often to maintain the liveliness which comes with each drink and to avoid the hangover symptoms that accompany abstinence.

Eventually the body's powers of adaption weaken and our now compulsive drinker finds that each drink can make him/her groggy, ill, headachy and nauseous once again. As the experts on alcoholism would say, 'He/she has lost his/her tolerance for drink.' This is a well-known stage in the alcoholic's sad path to decline. Not all alcoholics are created by this exact route but the great majority are. By now a full-blown, hidden allergy has developed to one or more of the foods and/or chemicals in the beverage habitually consumed and total abstinence is the only thing that will heal the body.

Some drinkers find alcohol agrees with them from the outset and although it takes longer for them to develop an allergy addiction to their favourite drink, in time they do if they over-indulge.

Some heavy drinkers elect to stop drinking before the stage of exhaustion is reached and anyone who knows a reformed alcoholic will be aware of the compulsive food or nicotine cravings they develop in lieu of the alcohol. Wheat (bread, pasta, etc.) is craved by the former whisky drinker. Sweets and refined, processed and savoury biscuit foods are craved by the former beer and wine drinker and corn products by the former bourbon drinker.

Many compulsive drinkers become compulsive eaters and an over-weight condition, if it wasn't a problem before, certainly becomes a problem after giving it up, as withdrawal symptoms are allayed by the constant eating of the allergenic food. I remember one lady who had developed such a dependency on brewer's yeast she 'would kill for Vegemite' and ate Vegemite sandwiches all day long. Not surprisingly she consulted me for her over-weight problem. She recalled how one day she was just about to leave for the corner store to buy a loaf of bread and a jar of Vegemite when a girlfriend phoned and kept her on the phone for some time. By the time my patient got off the phone she was in such a state she nearly crashed the car in her haste to get to the store and, on procuring her bread and Vegemite, sat in the car and 'had to literally scoff it down there and then before I could drive away'. It was at this point that she realised she had a problem and needed help. Like many over-weight, compulsive eaters she didn't understand her problem and was depressed that she was so weak willed when it came to food.

Treating alcoholism by the cold turkey, food and cigarette substitution method never completely restores the former drinker to complete health. The adaptation phase is still being sustained by eating the food the favourite alcoholic beverage was made from and the adaptation phase still comes to an end with the symptoms of exhaustion, eventually manifesting as any of the allergy symptoms listed in Chapter 2. If untreated, eventually it will manifest as any of the chronic degenerative diseases mentioned earlier.

FOOD CRAVINGS

Compulsive eating can develop in those non-drinkers who developed their particular food sensitivity as children or young adults. Many young people when they leave home to live with friends are too busy socialising and having fun in their out of work hours to take the time to cook balanced meals with a good variation of foods. Eating on the go becomes the thing and the diet is usually made up of refined takeaway foods and TV dinners which are (1) vitamin and mineral deficient and (2) made up basically of the same things—white sugar and white flour. Chemical flavourings, colourings and preservatives give this monotonous diet its variety. Ambitious young high achievers fall into this food category as well. They're too busy working to cook balanced meals.

Many of the over-weight compulsive eaters I've treated developed their food cravings as a result of over-exposure to a given food as a child (in the manner previously described) or as a young person who left the nest and Mum's home cooking. These food cravings can manifest in one of two ways. Either as a craving for the food in question or as a craving for sugar. Allergic hypoglycaemia is the term used to describe this latter phenomenon. Hypoglycaemia means a sudden dropping in the levels of glucose in the blood. When this happens, a message is sent to the brain that glucose levels must be restored immediately, and a craving for sugar results. Those people whose allergy withdrawal symptoms trigger hypoglycaemia are driven by an unbelievable compulsion to eat sweets or white flour foods, lots of them and often. Uncontrollable over-weight soon becomes a problem for them. The treatment program laid down in Chapter 5, 'How to cure your allergies', is of great benefit to people with allergic hypoglycaemia.

CHEMICAL SENSITIVITIES

Often it's the chemical additives in the food that are causing the hidden allergy rather than the food itself. Many of the chemical flavourings, colourings and preservatives in processed, refined foods (white bread, cakes, biscuits, frozen and tinned food, processed meats, TV dinners) are derivatives of chemical pollutants in our environment. Over-exposure to these airborne chemicals can both perpetrate and perpetuate hidden food allergies. For instance, one of the most prominent chemicals used in strong smelling paint strippers is also used as part of the chemical make-up of vanilla-flavoured ice-cream.

GARRY

Garry graduated from university as a solicitor believing he had found his chosen vocation. Before going away for an after-exam holiday, he secured a junior position with a large firm of solicitors in the city. Returning from his break, tanned, relaxed and fresh he couldn't believe how badly he felt after his first week's work. Putting it down to a readjustment to work syndrome, he didn't pay much attention to it, believing it would soon abate as he settled in. This settling in period took about nine months and he was beginning to doubt whether law was really what he wanted to spend his life doing. On arriving at work he'd feel tired, make silly mistakes, experience erratic mood swings, forget things, get depressed, have trouble paying attention to what clients were saying and feel sleepy all afternoon if he had wine at business lunches. He thought it must be the job that was the problem because on the weekends he felt great. Stacks of energy, mentally on the ball, no headaches and no drowsiness after alcohol.

In time the long awaited settling in process was over. He found he was coping much better at work. So much so, in fact, he didn't mind working back at night and even popping in on Saturday or Sunday morning to do a bit more. Working was now giving him a buzz; it was mentally stimulating. After a few years he realised he had become a workaholic, when during his summer vacation he kept wanting to go into work. The fact was he couldn't relax at home. Home made him edgy, headachy, tired, bored, listless. Even escaping to his parent's beach house with his girlfriend didn't help. Being at work gave him mental stimulation, it gave him energy and enthusiasm, he felt optimistic and confident while there. Being away from work made him feel as bad as when he first started going to the office.

Although Garry felt much better at work, there was one thing that bothered him. Since starting work he had developed a stuffy, itchy nose and regular sore throats which, although not as bad as when he first started work, were still persisting. His girlfriend persuaded him to see me. That summer he had trouble relaxing as his nose was so blocked not even swimming in the surf would clear it.

To cut a long story short, I eventually persuaded Garry to take me into his office one weekend and sure enough, one whiff of the place said it all. That suffocating smell of synthetic carpet, synthetic upholstery, synthetic curtains, plastic-covered and synthetic-wood desks pervaded the place. The synthetic carpet still smelt as new as the day it was laid as the air in the building was recycled through the air-conditioner. All the windows were sealed. Hardly a breath of fresh air had been through that room since the building was completed. In short, the building was sick. And smelt it.

Garry's plight was obvious. He'd started off reacting vigorously to the chemically toxic environment, had adapted to it and then went into withdrawals while away from it on weekends and vacations.

Going on the Metabolism-Balancing Program reduced the intensity of his withdrawal symptoms on the weekend. He didn't show up allergic to any foods which was fortunate as many people in his position show up allergic to those foods with preservatives, flavourings and colourings that are chemically related to the environmental toxins they are inhaling. I don't doubt that if he had stayed in his place of work long enough, spin-off food sensitivities would have developed from the over-exposure to the ambient air chemicals he was breathing each day.

Garry saw the light immediately and sorted out his priorities very quickly. He is now working in his own small practice in one of the northern beach suburbs of Sydney where he can open the window of his office to fresh air. His office has slate floors and is lined with wood panels (real wood). All upholstery is leather, and wool and cotton covered in some cases. The office is not air-conditioned and plastic has been limited to pens and a few other essentials.

After going through the initial withdrawal symptoms, which knocked him around for a short while, Garry hasn't looked back. He claims he hasn't had a day's illness since he moved and he's happy working a forty hour week.

MARY

Every morning Mary would wake up with black puffy eyes, and red lumpy acne under her skin's surface. She had trouble fitting into her high heels as her feet and ankles were swollen. She felt tired, cranky, was mentally disorientated and very clumsy. By mid-morning she was looking and feeling better and by mid-afternoon she had noticed a marked reduction in all the symptoms. She was making less mistakes, thinking more clearly (though not perfectly), had lost most of the puffiness around the eyes and the ankles and had only a mild ruddy complexion instead of the red bumps.

After exhaustive tests Mary's allergy turned out to be her favourite perfume. She adored the perfume, indeed, she craved it and was most upset when I told her she had to give it up. During the day she would get periodic urges to dab some more on herself, just to experience that gorgeous scent again. As the day went on and she became more exposed to the perfume, her symptoms would lessen in intensity, and she would begin to feel almost human again. Towards the end of the day, as the effects of the perfume wore off, the first signs of withdrawal would begin. She would feel tired and slightly more swollen than at work. After eight hours of going cold turkey in her sleep she would awaken feeling and looking like death. It took five days of sheer hell to withdraw. She was so mentally distraught she had to take a day off work. For most of that day she was depressed and weeping. By the fifth day she was picking up and by the tenth day the swelling had gone from under her eyes and from her feet and ankles. Within five weeks her skin had completely cleared and the dark rings around her eyes had faded by 75 per cent.

She never used that perfume again and when going out in a group would phone her friends to see if they were wearing it.

Mary had developed her allergy by using the same, highly chemical perfume over a long period of time. Had she alternated between a number of perfumes, preferably ones made from flower extracts, the chances of her developing an allergy addiction would have been far less.

Mary was lucky in that she was only addicted to one thing. Some of my patients are allergic to perfume, the gas from the cooker, sugar, insect sprays and wheat—all in one go. Withdrawing from so many allergens can be extremely difficult, and avoiding them takes a lot of organisation. Because so many people feel worse when coming off their allergenic food or chemical they naturally believe the allergen to be necessary for their well-being and they become confused and frightened when advised to go off it.

ANNETTE

Annette had an addictive allergy to corn. At first she refused to believe this because she only ate cornflakes and she did not have a craving for corn.

However, when her lifestyle and diet were fully analysed it was found that she was eating corn every day. She regularly licked stamps and envelopes (the glue contains corn resin), ate bacon (corn-cured), took aspirin, used baking powder, drank bourbon and instant coffee, used bottled French dressing on food and a spray-on starch when ironing. All of these contain corn. All day, every day, Annette was bombarding her liver enzyme chains with corn and because much of her diet was refined junk foods (containing corn) she was not getting vitamins and minerals needed to rebuild the enzymes as they wore out.

Annette's overt allergy was to the eggflip she had every morning for breakfast. It was the only thing she felt she had the slightest craving for. On rising each morning she felt and looked terrible. Thirty minutes after the eggflip she began to come to life. However, taking her off milk and eggs did not give her withdrawal symptoms, nor did it ease her fluid retention problem. It turned out that the brand of glucose she used to sweeten her eggflip was manufactured from corn, and it was the glucose that took her out of her withdrawal each morning. Because Annette's routine brought her into contact with corn so frequently she was able to keep her addiction topped up throughout the day. It was only during her eight hours of sleep that withdrawals set in and she developed a craving. By the time all the corn had been removed from her diet, she was left with a simple regimen. She was only to eat fresh fruit and vegetables (nothing canned or frozen), freshly killed meat or chicken, fresh fish (nothing tinned, frozen or cured), fresh eggs, homemade bread (using flour, water and yeast only), fresh bottled milk, butter and cheese. Look familiar? Sure it does, it is simple, wholesome food on which our grandparents fared so well.

At first Annette baulked at the idea of living on such basic foods but eventually gave it a go. Once she had gone through the withdrawal, 6.5 kg (14 lb) of fluid and fat dropped from her body. The ruddiness went from her acne and the pimples began to shrink. Within two months she began enjoying the foods she was eating. At restaurants she chose simple meat, fish, chicken and vegetable dishes. She came to realise just how much of a useless habit her old eating pattern was.

The hardest thing for her was giving up her gourmet club activities because most of her life revolved around drinking and eating. But her new shape, appearance and well-being made her want to make the change. She took up golf and joined a hiking club where she made lots of new friends and met her husband.

At last contact with her she was very happy. Her new lifestyle was meeting all her needs instead of just some of them. She had two new interests, new companions who did not pressure her back into junk foods and a social life that revolved around fresh air and exercise rather than food and wine. But her love of food was not lost and she learned to create delicious meals with simple food. They kept her looking and feeling good. Today, when Annette and her family eat chicken it's not the fast-food version. Annette can tolerate chicken but not chicken with chemical flavourings and colourings.

ARE YOU AN ALLERGY ADDICT?

1. Do you often yearn for a particular food, to wear a particular perfume or to smoke a cigarette?
2. Do you feel dissatisfied unless you eat that food, wear that perfume or smoke that cigarette?
3. Do you feel any of the following symptoms before eating that food, wearing that perfume or smoking? Weakness, tiredness, headaches, restlessness, depression, irritability?
4. Do the above symptoms disappear after indulging in that particular craving?
5. Will you go out of your way to find a food or perfume or cigarette brand that you crave?
6. Do you daydream about eating a certain food, the smell of a certain perfume or cigarette?
7. Do you stock up on this food, perfume, cigarette to make sure that you have a good supply?
8. Do you regularly cook a certain food, or buy books on how to prepare it?
9. Do you feel dissatisfied unless you finish a meal with something sweet?
10. Are you well-known among your friends for a certain recipe?
11. Do you keep your favourite chocolate bar in your purse or pocket so that you may munch on it through the day?
12. Do you go on eating binges?
13. Do you wake up and raid the fridge at night?
14. Do you need to have a snack (always containing the same food) before you can sleep at night?

If you have any of the allergy symptoms listed in Chapter 2, have tried unsuccessfully to cure them through conventional medicine and answer 'yes' to five or more of the above questions then you have an allergy addiction.

Because most addictive allergies are to food or the chemicals in a given food, it is very likely that you will be over-weight—as a result of both fat and fluid increase. If you have trouble reducing your weight or keeping it down and can answer 'yes' to three or more of the above questions then you are most certainly suffering from an addictive allergy to a given food.

CHEMICAL SENSITIVITIES

In my twenty-two years of clinical practice, I've noticed that chemical contaminants of food, air and water are the most potent contributors to allergic reactions and in particular the masked reactions of allergy addiction. Petrol fumes and the gas from gas cookers, heaters, hot water systems and gas refrigerators are major problems. The most pervasive gas of all is the odourless, colourless formaldehyde found in all plastic and synthetic products (see Chapter 5, 'How to cure your allergies', for details of formaldehyde). The outgassing of formaldehyde from paint, carpets, curtains, upholstery, insulation and plastic products when the heating is turned on in winter raises the level of this gas to toxic levels in both home and workplace. The combined and cumulative effects of formaldehyde, gas from home appliances, chemicals in drinking water and processed foods, places a tremendous strain on the immune system. In time it becomes so agitated by this chemical assault, it starts over-reacting in its attempt to protect the body from it.

This over-reaction, which was initially to the chemicals, does in time carry over to the less noxious allergenic substances of moulds, pollens, grasses, dust, dust mites and animal dander. Eventually it carries over to the foods we eat. At first we react to the processed, packaged, tinned, frozen and refined foods, as they contain colourings, flavourings and preservatives that are chemically related to formaldehyde and the hydrocarbon gases. In time this sensitivity can spill over to the whole fresh foods that still have some residual herbicide spray on them.

The successful treatment of allergies relies on lowering our contact load with chemicals. We can do this by using only electrical appliances, having 100 per cent wool carpet and cotton, wool or leather upholstery, and opening windows in lieu of air-conditioning. The ideal house for allergic people has a slate floor, sandstone or natural wood-panelled walls (not synthetic plywood or chipboard), a tiled roof lined with natural wood, all electrical appliances and no insulation. Leather upholstery, natural wood furniture, and stainless steel cooking utensils complete the chemical free house. Fresh spring or mineral water is used for cooking and drinking and tinned, frozen, processed and packaged (particularly in plastic) foods are kept to a minimum. All fruits must be peeled (unfortunately chemicals sit under the skins of apples, pears, peaches and apricots where most of the vitamins reside) and only the inner leaves of lettuce, cabbage, brussels sprouts and all other leafy vegetables are to be eaten; the outer chemical-contaminated ones being discarded. All vegetables, even those growing below the surface, must be thoroughly washed in warm water.

By lowering the overall chemical load in this manner, and by adhering to a nutritionally sound diet that includes supplementary vitamins and minerals, the immune system will settle down and allergy symptoms will begin to abate.

For some people the greatest source of chemical exposure is to the chemicals their own bodies can produce on a day-to-day basis. Acetaldehyde is a chemical that is closely related to formaldehyde. Acetaldehyde is the major waste product produced by a certain fungus called *Candida albicans*. *Candida albicans* lives in the intestines of many allergy sufferers. If our sensitivities to chemicals and the air, water and foods that contain them are to be overcome, any *Candida albicans* colonies in our gut must be thoroughly contained. The process by which this is achieved is described in detail in the next chapter, '*Candida albicans*', and in Chapter 5, 'How to cure your allergies'.

SUMMARY

Allergy addiction is a curious phenomenon that affects many unsuspecting allergy sufferers. It differs from acute allergic reactions that manifest every time contact is made with a given substance, in that its symptoms manifest when contact is *not* made with the allergenic substance. And whereas the acutely allergic person feels better on withdrawing from contact with the allergenic substance, the allergy-addicted person feels worse. The complete process of allergy addiction passes through three distinct phases.

Phase 1

Known as the *alarm phase*, it is not unlike the normal acute allergic reaction (which could include any of those symptoms listed in Chapter 2) every time they make contact with the substances (food, drink, chemical, grass, mould, etc.) that they are allergic to.

Phase 2

This is known as the *adaptation phase*. Here is where the difference begins. Instead of continuing to react allergically every time they make contact with the allergenic substance the body seems to get used to, or accepts, the substance and stops reacting to it. The body is now addicted to that substance and, in the true addictive way, only displays its symptoms if that food is withheld from it. The withdrawal symptoms of the adaptation phase are the same acute allergy symptoms of the alarm phase. The victims remain symptom free so long as they keep topping up with their specific allergenic (harmful) substance (most often foods, drinks, chemicals). Most victims know instinctively when to top up to prevent withdrawals and so go for years without experiencing any noticeable or worrisome symptoms.

Phase 3

This is known as the *exhaustion phase*. It develops progressively as the body's adaptive capacity wanes. The time span varies from person to person and can take years—in some cases, many years. This can be a problem for the diagnosing physician as, over time, people tend to forget they ever experienced an alarm phase— especially if they did so as children.

The tiring body is no longer coping as well with the on-going allergenic contact and the victim has to resort to ever-increasing doses over shorter periods of time to keep the withdrawal symptoms at bay. And yet the symptoms continue to appear more and more often and last longer and longer. As time goes by and the powers of adaptation continue to run out, the victim spends more and more time in the hangover zone as withdrawal symptoms follow closely behind each exposure. For the first time in memory the victim begins to feel noticeably 'ill'.

The foodaholic is getting up to raid the fridge at night or has chocolate or biscuits beside the bed instead. The 'cigaholic' hoards cigarettes in case he or she runs out and the alcoholic is having a drink before breakfast to get rid of the headache he woke up with. By this time, if they're perceptive enough, allergy addiction victims seek help but don't usually get well as both they and the doctors believe this is the beginning of the disease and settle for treatment of the many different symptoms with drugs (see Chapter 2). Its hard to convince these people that their *melange* of symptoms is the result of a lifetime's eating of their favourite food or wearing their favourite perfume (or working in a given office).

Why some people remain acutely allergic all their lives and others become allergy addicted is hard to say. It is possible to have a strong constitution and genetic predisposition to allergy and it is generally felt that those with a stronger constitution (despite being genetically predisposed to allergy) are more inclined to develop allergy addictions. Strong cells are better able to adapt to toxins entering them than tired weaker (undernourished) cells. However, even strong constitutions have their limits, as evidenced when adaptation breaks down.

The treatment for both vehicles of allergy is that outlined in Chapter 5, 'How to cure your allergies'.

4.
Candida albicans
(The allergy–yeast connection)

'Things sweet to taste prove in digestion sour.'

Shakespeare, *King Richard II*

GUT-BORNE CANDIDA INFECTIONS CAUSE BLOOD-BORNE ALLERGIES

Candida yeast infection has been dubbed the twentieth-century disease and during my twenty-two years in practice I have found it to be widespread. Up until recently its most common manifestation, the vaginal thrush that plagues many women, was brushed off as a minor women's ailment and treated locally with fungicide creams, often unsuccessfully. It is now recognised that candida can cause a range of symptoms, including headaches, fluid retention, skin complaints, bloating of the abdomen, mental disorientation and, in extreme cases, schizoid behaviour and paranoia.

More importantly, it can both mimic all the symptoms of allergy as well as cause allergic reactions. Because of this, the containment of a candida yeast infection is the secret to the successful containment and ultimately the cure of most allergies. The discovery of this allergy–candida connection offers new hope to those many disillusioned allergy sufferers who've tried every available treatment regimen and still have their allergies. Containment of a candida infection has its greatest effect on reducing allergic reactions to the chemicals in our food, air and water.

Candida albicans yeast lives in the intestines of at least 90–98 per cent of human beings (not normally in over-growth proportions though). In women it migrates from the large intestine to the vagina through the practice of wiping the bottom in a forward motion towards the vagina and through the wearing of tight jeans and nylon underwear.

Yeasts, like their cousins the moulds and fungi, are small plants that prefer to live in a warm, dark and moist environment. The crevices in the mucous membranes that line the walls of the vagina and intestines provide an excellent habitat for yeast of the candida family. Like all plants, yeasts have a root system, a stem and foliage on top. The *Candida albicans* yeast sinks its roots into the mucous membranes of the body, which to it are fertile soil (see Fig. 4.1 and Fig. 4.2).

Most plants use their roots to draw nutrients from the soil they live in. These nutrients travel up the stem of the plant and into the branches, leaves and flowers where they contribute to the normal metabolism of the cells. The waste products of this metabolism are then released into the atmosphere. Fortunately for us, the major waste product released from plants is oxygen.

With *Candida albicans* the reverse process takes place. Nutrients are taken in through the foliage on top and the waste products are released out through the bottom. *Candida albicans* feeds on sugar and white flour. When either of these food types make contact with the yeast, the enzymes in the foliage of *Candida albicans* quickly convert them to the chemicals it needs to sustain life. The waste product of this enzyme conversion process is a toxic chemical called acetaldehyde (CH_3CHO), which is a general narcotic of the alcohol family of chemicals (also known as acetic

Fig. 4.1: A candida colony growing on the wall of the large intestine. Candida overgrowth of this proportion constitutes an infection.

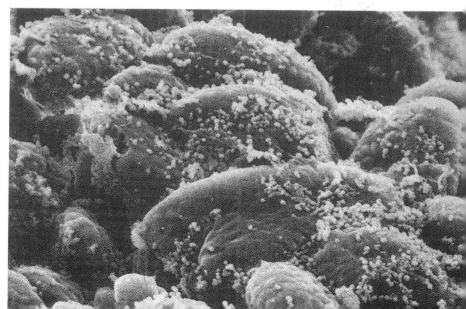

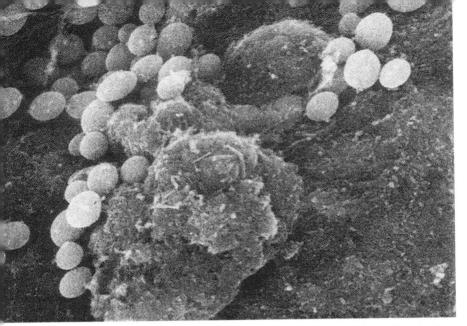

Fig. 4.2: Close-up of a candida colony showing the mushroom-like structure of the individual plants.

aldehyde ethanol). Acetaldehyde travels down the stem and into the roots from which it is liberated into the mucous membranes.

Because the mucous membranes are so richly supplied with blood vessels it doesn't take long for the acetaldehyde to find its way into the bloodstream. Once in the bloodstream it acts as a typical allergen and is capable of creating typical allergic reactions. In this way, the seemingly harmless little yeast that grows in the intestines and vagina can cause all the symptoms listed in Chapter 2, 'Allergies'. People who are not responding to treatment for their allergies, despite sticking faithfully to their Anti-Allergy Program, getting adequate rest and religiously taking their anti-allergy vaccine and vitamin/mineral supplements, usually have a candida yeast infection.

Because acetaldehyde is at the narcotic end of the alcohol spectrum, special symptoms set its action apart. These symptoms help us to recognise whether the problem is simple allergy or allergy plus candida overgrowth. The narcotic effect of acetaldehyde is recognised as a typical narcosis. A fuzzy, foggy, spaced-out, off-the-planet feeling in the head, where the head sometimes feels out of kilter with the body, is the give-away sign. The flow-on from this 'unreal' feeling in the head is periodic loss of memory, concentration and an inability to clearly articulate one's thoughts and feelings. This inability tends to manifest as emotional volatility with overt crankiness and irritability in women. In men, it tends to manifest as a sullen, silent moodiness accompanied by introversion and withdrawal.

Losing the drift of what is being said halfway through a sentence, whether we're speaking or listening, forgetting what we read at the top of the page when we're only halfway down it, or walking into a room and forgetting why we are there, are all symptoms of the narcotic effect of acetaldehyde. Acetaldehyde causes allergic reactions in the tissues it affects as well as a separate narcotic reaction in the cells of those tissues.

Although the mental symptoms just described can be caused by stress, they are recognised as candida symptoms if they go hand-in-glove with consumption of sugar, white flour and alcohol. Feeling spaced-out, faint, or drunk on only one or two glasses of alcohol invariably confirms a candida problem as these one or two glasses top up already high levels of alcohol (acetaldehyde) in the blood.

Sudden bloating or distension of the abdomen or sudden onset of allergic reactions (for example, arthritis, acne, headaches, fluid retention or psoriasis) when only small amounts of sweets or alcohol are consumed usually indicates candida. The sugar in sweets and alcohol feeds the candida plants so effectively that there is a sudden spurt of metabolic activity in the existing plants and growth in newly forming plants. This means the sudden dumping of more acetaldehyde in the blood with a consequent exacerbation of any existing allergic reactions.

ALLERGIES AND CANDIDA GO TOGETHER

Not everyone with a candida yeast infection has allergies, though most do. Allergic sensitivities to other members of the yeast, mould and fungi family frequently develop in those with a candida yeast infection. For this reason, a reaction to alcohol can be a result of both candida and an allergy to the yeast used to ferment the alcoholic beverage if wines, beers and ciders are being consumed.

If the reaction is a response to the unfermented alcohol (whisky, vodka or gin), then candida alone is often the culprit (though sometimes the food the alcohol is made from is involved). Other fermented foods such as breads, cheeses, yoghurts, vinegars and mould foods such as mushrooms and leftovers that have mould growing on them must also be avoided.

Acetaldehyde invariably creates sensitivities to other chemicals. Candida sufferers characteristically become sensitive to perfumes, anti-perspirants, household cleansers, aerosol sprays and gas from cookers and heaters. Sometimes gas from home cookers and heaters is such a problem to these people that complete containment of their symptoms is impossible until gas appliances are removed and electrical ones installed.

WHAT CAUSES CANDIDA YEAST INFECTION?

Most often we are born with it, contracting it from our mothers as we pass through the birth canal. The majority of women suffer from some degree of vaginal thrush (monilia) during pregnancy but may not know that they have it if the symptoms are mild, with only a slight vaginal itching now and then. In severe cases symptoms are unmistakable with excruciating itching, discharge and odour.

It has been observed that the female sex hormone progesterone promotes the growth of *Candida albicans*. Small colonies of the plant can rapidly grow to large colonies when the levels of progesterone in the blood are high. Although the mechanism is not clearly understood, it is believed that progesterone changes the chemistry of the mucous membranes making them exceptionally fertile to the growth of candida.

As pregnancy is sustained by high levels of progesterone for nine months it is not surprising that existing colonies of candida in the vagina should increase in size. This is particularly so for women who have been on the contraceptive pill (high in progesterone) for extended periods of time and have lived on a diet high in white flour and sugar. (The pill prevents conception by chemically simulating pregnancy.)

At birth, as the baby's head passes through the vagina, the pressure of the vaginal walls against its face causes it to scoop up a mouthful of candida plants with its bottom lip. The candida in the baby's mouth is pushed down to the intestine with its first few mouthfuls of milk. If large quantities of candida are ingested at birth the baby contracts oral thrush. If smaller quantities are ingested oral thrush won't show, though the baby will usually be colicky and discontented. If it is one of those babies who look unhappy and seems to spend its first twelve months crying and screaming for no diagnosable reason, and if it develops a rash around its anus soon after birth, it is bound to have a candida infection.

The degree of discomfort a baby (and adult) experiences from candida infection is determined by the size of the colony in the intestines. Although the colony may be small at birth it will grow as time goes by if the diet is too high in sugar and white flour. The formulas that many babies are put on in lieu of mother's milk are high in sugar content and are major culprits in instigating the growth from a small candida colony into a troublesome large colony.

A huge candida colony can grow on the walls of the digestive tract all the way from the rectum to the mouth. It can be recognised in the mouth as a white coating on the tongue, and in the back of and on the walls of the mouth. Under high magnification this white coating can be seen to be made up of lots of little mushroom-like plants. Huge candida colonies not only mean large quantities of acetaldehyde in the blood, they can also mean a bad breath problem that no mouth wash can cure.

ANTIBIOTICS

Constant runny nose, recurrent colds and 'flu that develop into viral and bacterial infections, especially streptococci throat infections, are common afflictions experienced by young candida sufferers. Worried mothers usually have these children in and out of doctors' surgeries and there is still a body of doctors who readily prescribe high potency, broad spectrum antibiotics, despite the fact that these kill not only the malevolent bacteria but also the friendly bacteria in the intestine.

Lactobacillus acidophilus is one such bacterium killed by antibiotics. It is a normal resident of the intestines and lives quite happily on the bowel wall where, among other things, it breaks up proteins and carbohydrates into lactic acid to help maintain an acid medium in the bowel. Because it takes up space on the wall it limits, by its presence, the spread of candida colonies. When lactobacillus is killed by antibiotics clear spaces are left on the intestinal wall for candida colonies to grow on.

By killing lactobacillus, antibiotics in the long-run aggravate the very symptoms they are called upon to contain. Although they kill the bacteria causing ear, nose and throat infections they don't remove the excess mucus accumulation that enabled the infection to take hold in the first place. The excess mucus is produced by an allergic reaction in the mucous membranes of the nose and throat caused by acetaldehyde.

As more lactobacillus dies off more candida plants grow in the unoccupied spaces and more acetaldehyde is produced. More acetaldehyde in the blood means more mucus in the nose, throat and ears. Because mucus provides such a favourable breeding ground for bacteria their numbers soon begin to build up to infection proportions again after each course of antibiotics. This is because there are always a few bugs that get away and live to propagate a new generation.

Each new generation is a little bit more antibiotic-resistant than the last and for this reason each successive course of antibiotics has to be a bit longer. So more and more antibiotics are needed to kill off stronger and stronger bugs. This ends up giving us more and more mucus to facilitate the breeding of more and more bugs. A vicious cycle develops which can only be broken by treating the *Candida albicans* infection.

Killing off the yeast reduces the blood acetaldehyde levels and mucus in the upper respiratory tract. The removal of the mucus makes it very hard for bacteria to proliferate, especially if the body is well fed and rested. Sound nutrition and adequate rest ensure that the white blood cells are capable of keeping bacteria numbers down.

CORTISONE DRUGS

As described in Chapter 11, 'Stress', cortisone suppresses the power of the white blood cells to kill viruses, fungi and bacteria. The white blood cells are the mainstays of the body's defence against infection. They swim through the bloodstream and into the tissue spaces like tiny amoeba, killing foreign bodies on contact. They also produce protein antibodies to neutralise foreign substances.

White blood cells work against the attempts of progesterone to change the chemistry of the mucous membranes to favour candida growth, by producing and sending protein antibodies to the membranes. The increased number of protein antibodies in the membranes changes their chemistry, yet again, rendering them infertile for candida growth.

Because candida yeast infections can produce inflammatory conditions such as eczema, psoriasis, asthma, arthritis and systemic lupus, cortisone creams and pills are often prescribed to candida sufferers. Like antibiotics, they only treat the symptoms. As a potent anti-inflammatory agent cortisone does this very efficiently, but it also suppresses the white blood cells' ability to produce antibodies to line the wall of the intestine. Ultimately cortisone, like antibiotics, increases the size of the candida colony. (See Chapter 12, 'Dangers of allergy drugs'.)

WHEN CANDIDA COLONIES ENTER THE BLOODSTREAM

As individual candida plants grow in size and number their roots put down deeper into the bowel wall. In time, the roots can be so deep, numerous and large in circumference that they can cause splits in the bowel wall. This splitting effect is analogous to the splitting of the pavements by trees whose roots are growing too big, a phenomenon often witnessed by those of us who live in cities that have trees growing out of the footpaths.

The crevices formed by this splitting effect allow the spores that bud off from the top of the candida plant to fall through into the bloodstream. Carried along in the bloodstream the spores settle out in various body tissues (for example, joints, skin, brain, mucous membranes of the nose and throat) to grow to maturity and set up new colonies. These colonies, known as internal colonies, live on glucose that is carried in the blood each day and if they grow large enough can cause the blood glucose levels to drop seriously, giving rise to hypoglycaemia.

In my experience, few candida sufferers have internal colonies. Those who do can take a number of internally absorbed preparations such as garlic and Nizoral (prescribed by a physician). Blood-borne candida infections are diagnosed by blood tests or by the lack of response to treatment for a gut-borne candida yeast infection.

HOW DO I KNOW IF I HAVE A CANDIDA PROBLEM?

If you have any of the symptoms listed in Chapter 2, 'Allergies', and can answer 'yes' to three of the questions below you should be treating yourself for candida infection as well as for allergy.

1. Have you ever taken any type of cortisone drug for more than two weeks at any time in your life?
2. Does exposure to perfumes, tobacco smoke, insecticides, household cleansers or fabric shop odours (some fabrics are treated with fire retardants) aggravate your symptoms?
3. Have you taken any antibiotics for acne for a month or longer?
4. Have you ever taken broad spectrum antibiotics for throat, respiratory, urinary or ear infections for two months or longer or in shorter courses four or more times per year?
5. Are you on the contraceptive pill or have you ever taken it?
6. Do you crave sugar, white bread or alcoholic beverages?
7. Do sugar-containing foods (sweets, cakes, biscuits, soft drinks), white bread or alcoholic beverages cause your abdomen to distend and/or give you wind?
8. Do these foods give you a foggy, spaced-out, detached, off-the-planet feeling in the head?
9. Do you suffer from premenstrual tension, vaginitis, menstrual problems or lack of sex drive?
10. Are your symptoms worse on a damp day or in a mouldy environment?
11. Are your symptoms worse on a cloudy (dry) day and disappear on a sunny day? (Cloudy days hold in city pollution and most candida victims are chemically sensitive.)
12. Does walking into new buildings (such as office blocks and department stores) make your symptoms worse (formaldehyde)?
13. Does the smell of newly laid carpet make your symptoms worse (formaldehyde)?

14. Does getting into a new car aggravate your symptoms (formaldehyde)?
15. Did you have oral thrush as a baby or did your mother have vaginal thrush while carrying you?

BEATING CANDIDA

Successful treatment of yeast infections is not much different from successful treatment of bacterial infections. Seven basic ingredients are needed:

1. The candida must be starved of the food it normally lives on.
2. A substance must be used to kill the candida.
3. Adequate rest must be taken during the time of treatment to give the white blood cells the time and strength they need to do their share of the organism killing.
4. A nutritious diet with supplementary vitamins and minerals to boost energy levels, white blood cell vitality and resistance must be strictly adhered to.
5. Stress levels must be reduced.
6. A positive attitude needs to be adopted.
7. As many chemicals as possible must be removed from your living and working environment and from the food and water you consume.

THE PROGRAM

Because most people with candida yeast infections also have allergies and because the symptoms of these conditions are identical, I send all my candida suspects for the full battery of allergy tests if after four to five weeks on the Anti-Candida Program they're not showing significant improvement.

Having written a program which takes their food allergies into account I also exclude all sugars, white flour, alcohol and foods containing them. This includes fruit and milk products which contain natural sugars. The naturally occurring sugar in fruit (fructose) and in milk (lactose) are capable of sustaining *Candida albicans* even though white sugar, white flour and alcohol have been removed from the diet. In most cases, however, fruit need only be removed from the diet for about four weeks and milk for about six to eight weeks (providing there is no allergy to it) while the killing effect of the anti-fungal treatment takes place.

NYSTATIN

Nystatin is the anti-fungal drug that I favour to kill off candida plants. Used in combination with the program it is very effective; used on its own it is not nearly as effective. This is because candida, like all noxious weeds, is a hardy little plant. Like all weeds, it at first yields to the use of a herbicide but tends to grow back after the effects of this herbicide have worn off. The only way to kill a weed is to first spray it with a powerful herbicide and then starve it of the food it lives on. Candida is no different. By removing sugars, white flour and alcohol from the diet the plant becomes malnourished and very run down. In its weakened state the Nystatin (herbicide) is able to kill it off right down to its roots.

Nystatin is a very safe drug in so much as it is not absorbed from the digestive tract into the body. It passes through the digestive tract killing the yeast on contact. Its passage is on-going and it passes out of the bowel with each bowel movement. For this reason, it must be taken two to three times per day for at least three months and in a few cases for up to a year before the colony is successfully killed. Because it is not absorbed into the body proper and has fairly rapid passage through the digestive tract, Nystatin is an effective 'pipe cleaner' and does much to relieve even the most stubborn of constipation problems. Raw garlic is nearly as effective at killing off candida colonies. It takes a little longer for results and most of my patients prefer not to use it because of the breath and body odour it leaves. Even the 'odourless' varieties, if used for about eight weeks or more, will give off a garlic odour from the body.

If, at any time, it becomes absolutely necessary to take antibiotics take them with Nystatin powder and *Lactobacillus acidophilus* to negate their detrimental effects on the body.

VIRTUES OF REST

Although starving candida plants and killing them with Nystatin is essential for the containment of the yeast, the real action lies with the white blood cells. It is the white blood cells that go after and kill candida spores that get into the bloodstream as well as producing the protein antibodies that make the mucous membranes infertile for candida growth.

If the white blood cells are tired they cannot perform at full capacity. They are not able to swim as far, which means they have trouble reaching candida colonies in remote tissues. Even if they manage to make contact with the yeast they often lack the strength to kill it and sometimes end up being killed by it. Tired white blood cells produce far less antibodies than energetic ones.

Rest is as essential for the successful treatment of candida infections, as it is in the treatment of other common infections such as 'flu. Unfortunately, some people receiving treatment for candida problems fail to take this seriously and end up getting only mediocre results.

With adequate sleep and rest most people can completely contain their candida problem within three months. Without adequate sleep and rest they are usually still on the program and Nystatin nine months later, receiving only mediocre results. Some give up after four to five months and slip back to their original state of ill health, thoroughly disillusioned with the whole program. Some people refuse to heed the call to rest because they feel they are progressing well enough without it. Then, at the end of the three months, they stop taking the Nystatin and go off the program and their symptoms return.

STRESS

Stress causes the release of the hormones adrenalin and cortisone from the adrenal glands. Adrenalin speeds up the metabolism of the body causing the cells to burn more glucose than normal. Cortisone, as mentioned, suppresses the power of the white blood cells to kill fungi, bacteria and viruses (see Chapter 11, 'Stress', and Chapter 16, 'Scientific explanations—Stress').

Over-work, over-commitment, over-exercising and over-social-ising (with attendant late nights) are stresses sometimes encountered by candida sufferers. These people think that because they are regularly taking Nystatin and sticking to the program, they can continue life at its normal frenetic pace and that everything will be fine. Not so.

Paradoxically, one of the greatest stresses can be the very program that is designed to starve the candida. The big problem with the anti-allergy and anti-candida programs is that, by their very nature, they are food restrictive. By restricting the number of food types on a given program you restrict the quantity and the spectrum of nutrients in the diet.

Because white blood cells require an on-going and large supply of many different nutrients, their vitality can be lowered if restrictive programs are adhered to for too long. This is why a high potency broad spectrum vitamin and mineral formula (with the six essential minerals—calcium, magnesium, potassium, zinc, iron and manganese) must be taken in tablet form by those on an anti-candida program. However, a vitamin and mineral supplement is not fully absorbed by those who are stressed through over-work, over-exercise, over-socialising or negative attitudes. (See Chapter 11, 'Stress', and Chapter 16, 'Scientific explanations—Stress'.)

The initial Anti-Candida Program with its absence of natural sugars (fruit, honey, milk, yoghurt, etc.) is very food restrictive. Because a body under stress burns more glucose than normal, the foods eaten must provide that body with a ready source of glucose.

A shortage of glucose means the body becomes even more stressed and fatigue, light-headedness, depression and even fainting spells can develop. Depression and fainting spells usually lead to a craving for something sweet which invariably leads to a breaking of the program. This sometimes causes a flaring up of the condition being treated.

In any case, highly stressed people often show no improvement in their condition, despite the Nystatin and the program. When this happens they understandably become more stressed.

Highly stressed people have reduced digestive capacity. This means that the fresh, unrefined foods in the Anti-Candida Program, which are generally digested and converted to glucose more slowly than refined foods, take them even longer to digest and absorb. Yet rapid digestion and absorption of food, especially glucose, is what highly stressed people need the most.

The glucose depletion problem is aggravated in stressed people if some form of carbohydrate food (bread, brown rice or potato) is not eaten in the middle of the day. My experience with the over-worked, over-exercised, over-socialised types is that they are frequently too busy to organise a substantial meal in the middle of the day and usually grab a salad on the run. Most of these salads turn out to be only rabbit food, without a substantial protein (meat, fish, poultry, egg) or carbohydrate food. Consequently, by mid-afternoon, they are feeling weak, faint, depressed and crave something sweet.

Within eight weeks these people are complaining that they are still retaining fluid, their acne is only slightly better, as is their eczema, their headaches and their asthma. And as far as they are concerned *Candida albicans* is definitely not the root of their problem.

Once they realise that they have to cut down on their workload, social life and sporting activities they invariably get good results––their skin clears, fluid (weight) falls, and headaches and asthma attacks disappear. At this point I suggest you read Chapter 11, 'Stress', to find out if stress is a problem for you. This is important if you're one of those highly motivated, enthusiastic, hard-charger types who enjoy their work, work long hours and are always on the go. Often these types are under stress without realising it.

Anti-candida treatment gives across the board results. Meaning that when the candida infection is contained, *all* the symptoms disappear. If they don't then stress is frequently involved. For instance, if your sinusitis, skin complaint and asthma go but your abdomen remains distended and/or you're still tired or you catch a cold or 'flu while on the program, you're stressed and in need of rest.

ALL-IMPORTANT ATTITUDES

Even after cutting down on commitments and activities, adhering to the program and taking Nystatin, some people still fail to get optimum results. The reason for this can be summed up in three words: the wrong attitude.

There is no sense cutting back on workload and commitments if you are going to feel guilty, frustrated and annoyed about it. If your attitude is: 'This dammed candida program is restricting me and slowing me down,' then you are going to remain as stressed as you were when you were overdoing it. You're not going to receive the results you are looking for if you cannot adopt an attitude that is in line with your more relaxed workload. Because we all have the ability to change our attitudes there is no excuse for feeling annoyed and frustrated when we cut back our work and commitment loads (see Chapter 16, 'Scientific explanations—Stress').

Habitual whingers are as unsuccessful as the over-workers when it comes to getting optimum results on the anti-candida regimen. Adopting the attitude of 'Why me?', 'It's unfair!', 'I can't stand it!', 'Life shouldn't treat me this way!', 'It's awful!' is a guaranteed recipe for disappointment. That sort of self talk puts cortisone in the blood as quickly as over-work, over-exercising and over-commitment. (See Chapter 16, 'Scientific explanations—Stress'.)

If your first reaction to the thought of going on the program is a negative one read the program again. After reading and reflecting on it a few times you'll find there are more foods to eat than you at first realised. Some people take longer to adjust to change than others. You could be one of them. Be patient. Give yourself time to become familiar with the program and the thought of going on it. In your own time you'll be ready. It takes as long as it takes.

CANDIDA ALLERGIES AND NUTRITION

It is significant that the very foods that predispose us to allergies (refined, junk, tinned, frozen and packaged foods) are the very ones that favour the growth of candida yeast colonies. As Dr Weston G. Price in his book, *Nutrition and Physical Degeneration,* discovered: 'Nutrition is the key to preventing the onset and perpetuation of allergies.'

Candida sufferers like sweets. Some have profound cravings for sweets. This is because they have large colonies of the yeast growing in them that are calling out to be fed on sugar, honey, fruit and white flour. If you have a sweet tooth the thought of going on the Anti-Candida Program may daunt you. Don't let it. Resolve to go on the program and tough it out. Resolve not to let anything stand in the way of achieving your goal of optimum health. If you do this you'll be well rewarded for, after the program, you'll notice an amazing thing—your sweet tooth will have disappeared. Your taste for sweets won't go entirely as it's perfectly natural but you'll only be eating 10–20 per cent of the amount you were eating before. You won't be able to cope with any more. Your tastes will have changed so much that any more than 20 per cent will taste sickly. This lack of desire for sweet things is confirmation that the size of the candida colony is so small, it's having a negligible effect on you.

WHEN TO START THE PROGRAM

My advice to anyone wishing to go on the anti-candida regime is to get your attitude right first. Even if it takes a month or two to get yourself appropriately attuned to the task ahead and your work-loads down, so be it. Take whatever time is necessary, there's no rush. Experience has taught me that if it takes much more than three months to get results you may become disheartened and find it difficult to stay on the program, believing that you'll never get well. Results must be forthcoming early in the piece to keep enthusiasm up (see Chapter 16, 'Scientific explanations—Stress').

During this attitude attunement time it pays to be on the Metabolism-Balancing Program and taking a high dosage multi-vitamin and mineral supplement (containing the six essential minerals—calcium, potassium, magnesium, iron, zinc and manganese). The metabolism-balancing effect of the diet and supplements will boost the vitality of your white blood cells and ensure quick results when you commence the Anti-Candida Program outlined in this book.

Do not embark on the program if there is a major social event such as Christmas, New Year or an anniversary looming. Wait until you get a clear three month run and forewarn your friends and family that for the next three months you cannot eat the prohibited foods at dinner parties.

Some major stresses cannot be avoided. If you are grieving over a loved one, going through a traumatic relationship break-up, or have been retrenched from work, do not attempt to go on the program until things are back to normal. You will not get the results you are looking for.

Don't attempt the program if out of town visitors are coming to stay. Nothing interferes with the anti-candida regimen more than the demands of entertaining house guests. Don't attempt the program while renovating the house. The dust, fumes, draughts and stresses that accompany renovations negate results. Wait until renovations are completed and you're settled.

HOW TO START AND STAY ON THE PROGRAM

The best way to start and stay on the Anti-Candida/Anti-Allergy Program is to grasp the nettle and say emphatically to yourself: 'I'm going to go on this program, it's my personal project, I've made up my mind, nothing is going to dissuade me from it.' There is nothing more powerful on this earth than the human mind and when it's 'made up' it's unstoppable. If you think you lack the willpower to start and stay on any program you're wrong. All humans have willpower and those who exercise their faculty of will, develop and strengthen their will. The Anti-Candida Program is an excellent opportunity for you to increase your willpower and the spin-off effects of this increased willpower, will serve you well in other spheres of your life.

Having completed the program you'll be impressed with your achievements and will experience a significant increase in self-confidence and self-esteem as well as health. Many of those who complete the program go on to tackle and achieve things they previously thought were beyond their ability. I've witnessed this in many of my former candida patients and have no doubt that it can happen for you as well.

If while on the program you experience a waning of your resolve, the most effective way to counter it is to sit yourself down and give yourself a good talking to. Make sure you pose yourself the following question: 'Well what's the alternative? Feeling as grotty as I did before starting the program?'

There are a number of things you can do to maintain your willpower:

- Get adequate rest. Tired people get depressed easily and lose interest in everything—including themselves and their goals. Tired people can't be bothered doing the shopping, preparing balanced meals, organising themselves or disciplining them-selves. Learn to pace yourself so that you don't get tired. (See Chapter 11, 'Stress—Stress and the hard-charger'.)
- Don't skip meals, especially the midday meal. Skipping meals causes a drop in blood glucose levels (hypoglycaemia) which in turn causes a rebound craving for something sweet. Hypoglycaemia can also trigger allergies leading you to believe the program has stopped working. This could upset you to the point of giving up the whole thing.
- Don't smoke marijuana. They don't call that stuff 'dope' for nothing. It makes you dopey, disinterested and undisciplined. It also gives you the 'munchies'. It's a guaranteed recipe for breaking a program and failure to achieve any of your goals. Passive dope smoking is just as bad as taking speed, heroin,

crack or any other mood-altering, recreational drug. Keep away from those who smoke or take drugs; they'll undermine everything you are trying to achieve and will drag you down to their own level of low achievement.

- Don't skip your vitamins, minerals and other supplements; you will get tired if you do.
- Don't cut yourself off from the mainstream of life by staying at home for the duration of the program—keep socialising. We humans are tribal creatures. We need the emotional nourishment provided by close and regular communication with friends, kin and acquaintances. Without it we become tired and depressed and try to compensate by binge eating, drinking alcohol or taking drugs.
- Don't shun restaurants. Go to fish restaurants and steak houses while on the program, saving the other restaurants for when you are well. There will never be a menu that fits your program perfectly so order what you can from the menu and explain to the waiter/waitress that you are not to have sauces or gravies because you are on a strict program. You'll be amazed how many waiters are familiar with anti-candida programs. Don't be fazed when your meal comes with everything on it that you requested not be included. People are fallible, especially when they're rushed. Just push the forbidden foods to the side of your plate, it's an excellent opportunity to exercise your willpower.

LIFE ACCIDENTS

Bad luck is a mathematical probability for all of us during our passage through life and you may experience some while on the program. If your given life accident is severe you will probably have your routine so disrupted you will temporarily break the program. Don't be hard on yourself if this happens. Be patient and understanding. You're not weak. Bad luck is something that's beyond your control. There is nothing weak about breaking a program when you are immobilised in plaster after a car accident, or emotionally traumatised because your spouse ran off with someone else, or the bank foreclosed on your mortgage/overdraft, or you were sacked, or your business partner ripped you off, or you are a new mother who is having your first experience with a severely fevered child, or you contracted food poisoning from your favourite restaurant. These life accidents are real tests of our will to get well and are to be viewed as such. Just wait until everything has settled down and carry on from where you left off. It doesn't pay to go back to square one in these circumstances because (1) it can be unduly disheartening and (2) it's not always necessary. Often the gains you have made before your life accident are such that you can carry on from where you left off and still get the results you are looking for. *'C'est la vie'* is the attitude that will carry you through to a winning end when bad luck strikes.

Don't worry about whether or not you will have the ability to start the program again. If you've committed yourself to getting well the mental and emotional power generated by that commitment will get you started. The only thing you need to start and stay on a program is a good reason for doing so. If the reason is a good one it will impress your subconscious mind, from which you will draw great strength of will, and the successful completion of the program will be automatic—life accidents notwithstanding.

From my observations I've noticed that those who are motivated by the more profound reasons of wanting to elevate their disposition, such as to improve their capacity to think, work and achieve, to improve their emotional well-being so they can enjoy more harmonious relationships with others, to have the vitality and confidence to take on new challenges and broaden their horizons, to look and feel the best they can, are more motivated than those who go on a program because others are doing so. That is, to be trendy. If you don't let the desire to 'look right' to others usurp a personal commitment to your own growth and development, you will have no trouble going on and staying on a program. To be trendy is to be an also ran; to be committed to your personal goals is to be a winner.

Constantly reminding yourself of your goal is a sure way to achieve it. Writing down on paper that which you want to achieve helps greatly to develop the will to make that achievement a reality. The written word carries great power and is a potent reminder. Self talk is also a potent reminder. During the program keep telling yourself how much you are looking forward to feeling well, having energy, looking great, with nice skin and an ideal body weight. Take time out to picture yourself as you'll be when the program is completed and the goals have been achieved. This self talk and creative imagery will generate enthusiasm for the program. Enthusiasm is power.

WILL MY CANDIDA COME BACK?

No, not if you are sensible and go onto the Metabolism-Balancing Program and supplements for the rest of your life once the Anti-Candida Program has been completed. So long as you limit your in-take of junk food to 5 per cent of total food intake, you will be quite OK.

Yes, if you go back to your old ways of eating too many refined, processed foods containing sugar and white flour. If you over-indulge in alcohol, cigarettes and take drugs. If you over-extend yourself at work, play and exercise, you will so lower your immune vitality as to predispose yourself to candida infection again.

Some lifestyles include, by necessity, certain travel commitments, work commitments or social commitments connected to travel and work. The disruptions to everyday routine these commitments cause can mean periodic consumption of more junk food and alcohol than is desirable for keeping candida at bay. The cumulative effects of these breaks in routine can mount up over time and cause the candida symptoms to slowly return. If you are involved in this life mode make a point of going on the full Anti-Candida Program, with Nystatin, for one month every year. The best time to do it is at the beginning of each year, starting the week you return to work after the summer holidays. This will get you in good mental and physical shape for the year ahead and will give you the energy to take on all challenges. It will clean your system of any candida plants that have grown over the previous year and especially as a result of the Christmas celebrations. It will get rid of that taste for alcohol and sweets that is so often the legacy of Christmas. It will set you up for another year on the Metabolism-Balancing Program and minimal junk food.

VAGINAL THRUSH

Recurrent vaginal thrush is a significant problem for some women and is harder to treat than gut-mediated thrush (candida infection). Some authorities argue that vaginal thrush can't be cured. Where it's probably true that all candida plants could never be completely killed, it's equally true that the colony can be reduced to such a minuscule level that no symptoms ever manifest. To achieve this I've found the following steps must be taken.

1. Sex with a condom is a must. Many men have candida yeast infections in their penis and candida spores are carried out with the sperm. Some have blood candida infections which can give rise to candida in the sperm itself.
2. Sex with a partner with jock itch must not be engaged in. Jock itch results from candida plants growing in the pubic, scrotal and groin areas. Jock itch can be eliminated if the man goes on the program outlined in Chapter 5, 'How to cure your allergies', which, of course, includes the full Anti-Candida Program. Make sure he shaves the whole pubic area (base of the penis, groin and scrotum). Make sure he uses a safety razor and not a barber's razor. He must then apply the Nystatin cream (same as the ladies use) to the whole area every day for fourteen days—no sex during this time.
3. While your partner is doing this you must be doing the same.

69

Shave the pubic and vaginal area and apply Nystatin cream to it and inside the vagina for fourteen days. This is so you don't give him back the jock itch that he will give back to you as vaginal thrush—no sex during this time. Do this even if you have no symptoms of thrush. During this time make sure you are wearing only 100 per cent cotton knickers which must be zapped in the microwave after laundering (while still slightly damp) for five minutes. This will effectively kill the candida spores that survived the wash.

If you have suffered repeated severe bouts of vaginal thrush in the past and find the emotional stress of it overbearing, you won't want to be going through this treatment procedure too often. I suggest then you bring the big guns to bear on your vaginal thrush. Ask your doctor to put you on a course of Nizoral. Nizoral is very effective at killing blood-borne candida and those that are deep seated in the walls of the vagina. Make sure you have a liver function test first. If you suspect your partner may have blood-borne candida and if oral sex is a preference of yours he must definitely go on Nizoral too. The chances of you contracting gut-borne candida infection from oral sex are too great otherwise. Gut-borne candida infections give rise to vaginal thrush again in time. While taking Nizoral you must be on the full Anti-Candida Program and Nystatin under the supervision of your doctor or other health professional.

Vaginal thrush must be contained if the systemic allergies and candida infections are to be overcome. You won't get 100 per cent better if acetaldehyde is entering your blood system from *Candida albicans* plants that are deep seated in the walls of your vagina.

GUT-BORNE CANDIDA INFECTIONS AND ALLERGY: ANGELA AND JOHNNY

Angela and Johnny are typical examples of how a *Candida albicans* infection can sensitise the body to chemicals and produce spin-off allergic reactions to less noxious substances.

Angela

Angela (15) was brought to me by a distraught mother who was having trouble coping with her antisocial behaviour. As a child Angela was moderately, though not seriously, hyperactive. She was fairly clumsy and lacked the co-ordination needed to be good at ball-handling sports. Her concentration span was less than most of her peers and she had a low tolerance to frustration. She was below average in her schoolwork.

At puberty she became cranky, irritable, argumentative and aggressive. The bouts of aggression would alternate with bouts of depression which would see her become sullen and withdrawn to the point of spending hours at a time locked in her bedroom. She was a lover of junk food which she justified by her continuous craving for sweets. A craving for sweets is as much a symptom of candida infection as it is a symptom of allergy addiction. The candida plants live on sugar and white flour and call out for them when hungry.

The white spots on her fingernails indicated a definite zinc deficiency and she was immediately put on the Metabolism-Balancing Program for six weeks. She improved significantly on all levels but was by no means completely cured. Allergy tests revealed her to be allergic to malt, brewer's yeast, eggs, milk, MSG, dust mites, mould and a number of grasses. The appropriate Anti-Allergy Program (which was the Metabolism-Balancing Program minus the things she was allergic to) was prescribed and within six weeks there was a vast improvement.

Her schoolwork had improved so much she was pulling away from the middle pack and moving into the top ten bracket. Her concentration, memory, retention of details and sociability at school had improved out of sight. She had more energy than ever before and was experiencing such good physical co-ordination that her handwriting had become neat and legible without any concerted effort on her part. Her teachers and headmaster were thrilled.

Her parents were not so thrilled. They couldn't understand why, when she was sticking so rigidly to her program, she could be sociable every morning at home and all day at school yet so antisocial at home each evening. The problem seemed to hinge around Angela's allotted evening chore of washing the dishes. (Her younger brother dried them.) Dishwashing had always been the major hassle of the evening for the family as Angela would always throw a tantrum over it. At first, I tended to agree with Angela's mother, that she was just an intractable teenager, but after a long talk with Angela one day, I could see that she really did want to improve herself and was quite genuine when she said she didn't know why dishwashing made her so upset.

Further delving into her history revealed that Angela's mother had a mild case of thrush during her pregnancy with Angela. Angela had been born with a mild case of oral thrush. Her infancy had been marred by colic and a nappy rash which was focused mainly around her anus. The latter two were overt symptoms of a candida yeast infection situated in her gut. Clearly she still had the infection and the fact that her bloated tummy hadn't completely reduced following the Anti-Allergy Program was confirmation of this.

The sudden mood swings that assailed Angela when she reached puberty were at last explained. The sudden release of the hormone progesterone from her ovaries at puberty had encouraged the growth of the small yeast colony in her gut into a large yeast colony which was filling her system with the chemical acetaldehyde. Acetaldehyde, being a toxic chemical, had sensitised her to dishwashing chemicals which began to vaporise when put into hot water. Not only that, the heat from the sink caused the vaporisation of the dishwashing liquid in its container, as it was stored directly below the sink. The vaporised chemical released from the dishwashing liquid was formaldehyde, a close cousin of acetaldehyde.

Was it any wonder that by the time dishwashing was over Angela was cranky, aggressive and often crying? She would storm out of the kitchen and into her bedroom slamming the door so hard the house would reverberate. She would spend the rest of the evening sulking. Often in the dark.

Substituting soap for dishwashing liquids solved the problem. No more tantrums and no more withdrawing socially after dinner. What was most interesting though was that after three months on the Anti-Candida/Anti-Allergy Program, plus Nystatin powder, *Lactobacillus acidophilus* capsules and Formula Six multi-vitamin and mineral supplement, Angela was able to wash up with dishwashing liquid again without experiencing her usual massive mood swings and withdrawal from the family.

By removing the acetaldehyde from her blood the liver enzymes repaired themselves to the point where they could cope with limited exposure to formaldehyde. Evenings were no longer the bane of Angela's day and she made good use of the time to do some extra study which improved her position in class even more.

It is debatable whether Angela could have coped with exposure to large sustained quantities of formaldehyde but I was not prepared to risk the return of her symptoms in an effort to find out.

Johnny

Young Johnny's history is very similar to Angela's only he mucked up at school instead of home.

Despite sticking strictly to his program and seeing all his allergy and candida symptoms disappear and despite being able to do his homework easily and willingly he just couldn't settle down in class.

At first his parents, teacher and I thought it was an attention-seeking device as he still felt a bit neglected and inferior after years of being behind the other kids. We agreed that more individual tuition from his teacher would rectify this, yet to our shock and amazement it made him worse. The more attention she paid him the more hyperactive he seemed to become. Pencil throwing, hair pulling, teasing, incessant talking, fidgeting and backchat to the teacher increased. He just couldn't concentrate, lost interest very easily and just didn't seem to care.

On talking to him it was obvious he was interested in doing well at school and was genuinely sorry about upsetting his parents and teacher with his behaviour.

We eventually tracked the problem down to his teacher's perfume. Each time she bent over to help him with his work he got a potent whiff of it which sent him off. Naturally the more attention she gave him the worse his behaviour became.

Removal of the perfume completely removed the problem. Johnny settled down and became a model pupil. No more disruption to the class and no more backchat to the teacher. Not only that, his schoolwork and exam results improved dramatically.

After five months of his teacher not wearing the perfume and with Johnny sticking to the combined Anti-Candida/Anti-Allergy Program, everyone's happy. Johnny's doing well at school and can handle limited exposure to the perfume his teacher is now able to wear two to three days a week. We have not experimented to see if Johnny can cope with any greater exposure for fear of resensitising him again.

Both Angela and Johnny suffered from acute allergic reactions to chemicals. It's hard to say whether they would have remained acute reactors for the rest of their lives or if they would have drifted into phase 2 of allergy addiction if they had not been treated at a young age. (See Chapter 3, 'Allergy addiction'.)

5.
How to cure your allergies

'The aim of medicine is to prevent disease and prolong life; the ideal of medicine is to eliminate the need of a physician.'

William J. Mayo MD

No matter what your symptoms are, be they those of allergy, candida yeast infection, asthma or any one or more of the conditions mentioned in this book, the commencement of any treatment is always the Metabolism-Balancing Program.

RECOMMENDED TREATMENT PROGRAM

STEP 1

For an anti-candida or anti-allergy treatment program I recommend six to eight weeks on the Metabolism-Balancing Program first, for the following reasons:

- It removes all nutrient deficiencies. This is especially important for women who've had children, miscarriages and/or terminations of pregnancy. Significant mineral loss is incurred by the body during terminations and from the placenta at childbirth. Breastfeeding further drains the body of minerals. Many women who had mild allergies prior to miscarriage, termination or childbirth find they have full-blown allergies afterwards—this is due to mineral loss. Most of these women experience a significant reduction in allergy symptoms as the Metabolism-Balancing Program builds up their mineral and energy levels.

- It raises physical and mental energy, thus buoying the spirits and significantly alleviating depression. This enables one to cope with stress more effectively.
- It raises the resistance to allergies and candida yeast infections by boosting the vitality of the white blood cells, that is, the immune system. When immunity is up, sensitivities are down.
- It reduces the time it takes to overcome allergies and contain yeast infections by balancing the metabolism and boosting immunity as much as is possible while allergies and yeast infections exist.
- It improves the chances of total desensitisation to allergic foods after ninety days' avoidance of them.
- It significantly reduces the intensity of the withdrawal and yeast kill-off symptoms experienced during the first week on the combined Anti-Candida/Anti-Allergy Program.
- It reduces the number of things you are allergic to before you take the allergy tests. This is important as the less you're allergic to, the less restrictive and more nutritious and interesting your program will be. This of course makes it easier to stick to.
- In some cases of mild allergy, especially with kids, symptoms disappear completely on the Metabolism-Balancing Program.
- It ensures an adequate supply of nutrients to tissues that have been damaged by allergic inflammation. This enables a more rapid healing of the tissue when the allergens have been removed. Such quick results keep up enthusiasm for the program. Eczema, acne and psoriasis are examples of damaged skin tissue that heal quickly if the Metabolism-Balancing Program is first employed. Diverticulitis and Crohn's disease are examples of damaged intestinal tissues. Arthritis has damaged joint tissue, asthma has damaged lung and bronchial tissue and fluid retention has damaged the blood capillaries. All of these heal more rapidly if the Metabolism-Balancing Program is first employed. By balancing the metabolism of the body and brain, the program makes it easier to think more positively and to adopt self-enhancing attitudes.

After six to eight weeks on the Metabolism-Balancing Program you can begin the process of gradual withdrawal from cortisone and antihistamines. This is done only with your doctor's permission. During this time make sure you stay on Ventolin and any other non-cortisone/non-antihistamine drug your doctor has prescribed for asthma. If you are taking drug medications for any other condition don't withdraw them unless your doctor OKs it.

During this time make sure you have a dust mite cover (available from your chemist) on your mattress, doona (comforter) and pillow if you suffer from asthma or any skin complaint, hayfever, sinusitis, stuffy nose, post-nasal drip, glue ear or bloodshot eyes. If it is your children (and not you) who are suffering from these complaints make sure you have a dust mite cover on your mattress, pillow and doona if they like to get into your bed. If suffering from asthma, colds, 'flu, sore throat or glandular fever, follow closely the advice given in Chapter 6 on asthma. Read that chapter at this point. Remember the deep breathing exercises. They're part of the Metabolism-Balancing Program and are important for lowering the levels of histamine in the blood, which in turn reduces the intensity of your allergy.

Pace yourself. In fact do less than before. Certainly don't raise your work, exercise, social or commitment load as you feel your energy levels rise. Many people make this mistake and become tired again. If your energy doesn't rise your immunity won't rise, and if your immunity doesn't rise you won't get a good result on the Anti-Candida/Anti-Allergy Program. All things being equal your energy levels should be up after six to eight weeks on the Metabolism-Balancing Program. Don't go onto the Anti-Candida Program until they are. If you're getting plenty of sleep, not overdoing it and the doctor has cleared you of viral infection, diabetes, iron deficiency and thyroid/adrenal gland underactivity, and you're still tired, then allergy is the most likely cause. You can now proceed to step 2. If any of these factors are in evidence they must be corrected before moving on. Worm yourself and the rest of the family during the final week of the Metabolism-Balancing Program (Combantrin—over the counter from the chemist—is a good anti worm medication). This is particularly important for hyperactive, slow learning kids and those suffering from Chronic Fatigue Syndrome. If your allergy symptoms are significantly diminishing on the Metabolism-Balancing Diet, stay on it until this improvement has plateaued, even if it requires more than eight weeks. Chances are you could throw your allergies on this program alone.

STEP 2

If after six to eight weeks on the Metabolism-Balancing Program your symptoms haven't cleared go on the Anti-Candida Program minus all the foods on the monosodium glutamate, metabisulphite and food chemical lists in the back of the book. Delete also those foods from the very high, high and moderate amine and salicylate lists. Eat only from the low and negligible amine and salicylate lists and only those foods you're not allergic to. Do this even if you're still in the process of coming off antihistamines and cortisone. Expect to be on the Anti-Candida Program for three months.

If after four weeks you're feeling really good try introducing some amine and salicylate foods from the moderate and (possibly later) the high lists in the manner described on pages 363–8.

Remember: The Anti-Candida Program is a restrictive regime and for this reason you must never embark on it without having first built up a sound tissue reserve of vitamins and minerals on the Metabolism-Balancing Program.

STEP 3

If after four weeks on the Anti-Candida Program you're not seeing a steady improvement, keep off the amines and salicylates and check yourself out for allergies, both food and inhalant. There are two ways of doing this.

1. The preferred way is to ask your doctor or naturopath to refer you to an allergy specialist for the skin sensitivity test, cytotoxic food test and the RAST test. You can then ask for a suitable anti-allergy program, or you can go on the Anti-Candida Program in this book, minus the foods you're allergic to, if they're known. Having these tests will necessitate breaking the program by going off all the vitamins, antihistamines and cortisone. Stay on the Ventolin inhaler and any other non-cortisone/non-antihistamine drug your doctor has prescribed for you. Eat as wide a variety of foods as possible before the tests but not those you suspect are detrimental to your health. List them instead and delete them from the program along with those foods that you show up allergic to. Use cortisone puffers again after the tests. The cytotoxic food test is a very important one. Because it is a relatively new test not all allergists use it. If your allergist doesn't perform this test you'll have to go with the next option. The skin and RAST tests are not accurate for foods but must still be taken to determine the inhalant allergies (grasses, dust, pollens, moulds, animal dander, dust mites). During this time the elimination food allergy testing technique may be used in lieu of the cytotoxic food test. Get your doctor's or naturopath's advice on this and have them supervise the testing procedure.

2. To do the food elimination test, stay on the Anti-Candida Program and eliminate one food every four to five days. Eliminate first any food you suspect may be causing your symptoms. If removing them does not help then work your way through the foods listed below. Keep eliminating the foods one at a time every four to five days until your symptoms disappear (or, in the case of skin complaints, significantly improve). When you are satisfied that your symptoms have sufficiently abated, work your way back through the list, adding one each of the eliminated foods every four to five days to see if any symptoms return. This back check is very important. You may eliminate the foods in whatever order you feel is appropriate for you, though you must keep a record of those you have eliminated.

The Anti-Candida Program by its very nature includes a restrictive diet. Any diet that restricts the spectrum of foods eaten naturally restricts the number of nutrients available for absorption. For this reason a sound tissue reserve of vitamins and minerals is to be built up on the Metabolism-Balancing Program before commencing the

Anti-Candida/Anti-Allergy Program. Without this reserve you could become run down.

The popular misconception is that the Anti-Candida Program and Nystatin kills the yeasts. They don't—they only weaken the candida so that the white blood cells can easily kill them.

Here's the Catch 22. If you're tired and run down on the Anti-Candida Program it is because: (a) you didn't build up on the Metabolism-Balancing Program; or (b) you have overdone it workwise, exercisewise, socially or you have an infection, cold, or sore throat. Your white cells will be too tired to kill the weakened candida. It gets worse. If you're on the Anti-Candida Program while tired and overdoing it you'll become even more run down (the Anti-Candida is not a high energy program) and your white cells even less efficient at killing the yeast. You will end up feeling worse than when you started the diet and often with a larger yeast colony as well, especially if in your run-down state you caught an infection and took antibiotics. This can also happen if you stay on the Anti-Candida Program for more than three months. Detractors of the Anti-Candida Program are invariably those who have fallen into one or all of the above traps.

Some of those who break the build-up and rest rule manage to remain symptom-free for a while on this regime only to see their symptoms return soon after going off it. This is not supposed to happen and shouldn't if you're properly built up before, and sufficiently rested during, the ninety days of the candida-killing regime.

Do not confuse this with the elimination diet/challenge test regime used in some hospitals. This diagnostic procedure is potentially dangerous, for it places the patient on a very restrictive diet for four to six weeks. This lowers the immune vitality. Naturally, when the body, in this run down state, is challenged with concentrated food substances it reacts to practically all of them. The resultant diet is so restrictive that the body and immune system don't pick up and although patients will be symptom-free for a while, eventually they become so run down they begin reacting to the foods they are allowed to have. More foods are eliminated from the diet, malnutrition sets in, infections follow, as do the inevitable allergic reactions to the drug medications used to treat them. I've treated many refugees from this process. They're not a pretty sight and so allergic by the time they seek my help it's very hard to build/feed them back up to good health. Malnutrition is far more serious than allergy and is to be avoided all all costs.

Commonly found allergenic foods

These include malt, cow's milk, eggs, corn, rye, oats, wheat, cocoa, oranges, tomatoes, potatoes, peanuts and chicken.

Sometimes a strong allergy to a given food can make you mildly allergic to other members of its food family. Be on the look out for this. For instance, if you are allergic to onions and don't feel any better for having avoided them, experiment by going off chives, spring onions, garlic and leeks as well. Regularly consult the food family table in the back of the book. This is done as a last resort and only after all the commonly allergic foods and amines and salicylates have been tested for. Don't even consider doing it if you've broken the program.

If you show up allergic, go on your personal Anti-Allergy Program (which is the Anti-Candida Program minus the foods you are specifically allergic to) for a minimum of ninety days from the time of determining your allergic food(s). Those of you who have been on cortisone and antihistamines may find that once off cortisone, you still need antihistamines to keep your symptoms at bay. If this is the case you must still go off the antihistamines for seven days before the tests. (You must be completely off cortisone.) This could be uncomfortable as the symptoms may well flare up. I wish there was an easier way but unfortunately there is not. After the tests you can go straight back on to the antihistamines (but not cortisone tablets) while the program is starting to take effect and then wean yourself off them (under a doctor's supervision) as your symptoms abate. If suffering from asthma use a Ventolin inhaler during these seven days and any other non-cortisone/non-antihistamine drug your doctor recommends. If suffering from eczema or other skin rashes for which your doctor has recommended cortisone creams, keep using them. Cortisone creams won't interfere with the tests (cortisone puffers will). In fact cortisone creams help by keeping skin conditions at bay while the program is taking effect. Looking at a skin condition can be so distressing as to cause it to flare up (see the sections on eczema and acne in Chapter 6) and resist the healing effects of the program.

STEP 4

During these weeks you should be addressing all the stresses in your life and seeking to minimise them by:

- getting adequate sleep, rest and recreation;
- taking adequate (but not excessive) exercise in the fresh air;
- reading Chapter 11, 'Stress', and acting on the advice therein;
- driving the car within the speed limits;
- cutting back on work, social and sporting commitments—many of my allergy patients are so tired from playing squash two nights a week, tennis another and netball or football on the weekends that they can't get well;
- using cortisone creams and puffers to keep eczema and asthma at bay while the programs are taking effect (see page 189).

- avoiding lying on the carpet to read or watch TV. This is a significant stress to the mucous membranes of the nose, throat and windpipe due to the close proximity to dust, dust mite, wool fibre, nylon fibre and formaldehyde.

STEP 5

Stay on the combined Anti-Candida/Anti-Allergy Program for a minimum of three months—longer if under supervision and it's deemed necessary to do so. Then go back on the Metabolism-Balancing Program for the rest of your life. Those with acne should stay on the Anti-Candida/Anti-Allergy Program until no new pimples break out on the skin—however, if longer than three months your doctor or naturopath must OK it.

STEP 6

If after four or five weeks on the combined Anti-Candida/Anti-Allergy Program you are not showing steady improvements get your allergist to prescribe an oral desensitising vaccine. Make sure it has been made up specially for you and in accordance with test results. If it is a standard all-purpose vaccine, don't use it. If you feel worse on the vaccine, try licking the end of the dropper rather than taking the full drop. After licking, squeeze out the drop and wash the end of the dropper. That way you are licking a fresh drop each day. Some people respond better to homeopathic medicines than vaccines. So consider consulting a homeopath. Take a list of your allergens with you.

STEP 7

If you are allergic to dogs, cats or birds they must be kept out of your immediate environment for at least ninety days. Spraying them with a dust mite spray means that they can be kept in the house so long as you don't handle them. On no account are they to be allowed into the bedroom.

Pets that sit on pillows, doonas or blankets always drop some hair and leave some dust mites. It's no use having a dust mite cover to keep dust mites in if dust mites are sitting on top of the cover. Birds spread their dander when they flap their wings, so make sure they're kept on the verandah or in the laundry for ninety days. Make sure somebody else sprays the animals. You are to avoid all sprays at all times.

STEP 8

If you are using a densensitising vaccine make sure it is not an injectable one. The injection of any foreign substance through the skin and into the blood carries with it the risk of adverse (or if you like allergic) reactions. All substances are supposed to enter the blood via the digestive tract, that's why you should only take an oral vaccine. 'Anaphylaxis' is the name given to these adverse reactions which can vary from mild exacerbation of your existing symptoms to full-blown shock and possible death.

STEP 9

If after eight to nine weeks on the combined Anti-Candida/Anti-Allergy Program and vaccine you feel you're still not making sufficient progress (assuming you are not stressed and you are sticking to the program) it would pay to talk over with your doctor the possibility of a course of Nizoral. Make sure the doctor does a liver function test before you go on this drug.

Symptoms that get worse on cloudy days usually indicate the blood-borne candida colonies that Nizoral works so well against. Cloud prevents pollution escaping into the upper atmosphere causing it to concentrate at street level in greater than normal quantities. Chemical sensitivity is a give-away sign of blood-borne candida.

STEP 10

If at any time through this treatment program you suspect the slightest degree of vaginal thrush (symptoms—itching, burning, discharge, odour—however slight) go on a fourteen day course of Nystatin vaginal cream or pessaries. Three to seven days is not long enough. Persist for the fourteen days even if the symptoms have disappeared in five to six days. Vaginal colonies of *Candida albicans* can perpetuate all the symptoms of allergy even when the gut colonies have been eradicated (see Chapter 4, '*Candida albicans*', for full treatment program for vaginal thrush).

STEP 11

Be alert to gut-mediated allergies. If you still have any of the digestive tract symptoms of allergy after eight weeks on the combined Anti-Candida/Anti-Allergy Program and find that no food allergies show up on skin, blood or food elimination tests, then the foods that you are sensitive to are creating inflammation in the intestines. Because of this, they are not being absorbed and won't show up on the standard tests. Trial and error elimination of foods, one at a time, is the only way to treat a gut-mediated allergy. However, before eliminating any more foods from the diet, worm yourself again and have your doctor test you for giardia. Check your stress levels. Be more regular with the breathing and mental relaxation exercises. All of these factors can mimic gut-mediated food allergies.

APPROACHING THE DOCTOR

Medicine is a service industry. You, as a consumer, have the right to get the service you request and pay for. This should be your attitude when you approach your doctor. On your first visit tell your doctor:

- that you want to try a new approach in the treatment of your allergies and that you are on the Metabolism-Balancing Program;
- that you will be starting the Anti-Candida Program shortly and you want Nystatin powder;
- if you are on cortisone and antihistamine drugs, that you want him/her to supervise your gradual withdrawal from them so that you can take the skin sensitivity test, cytotoxic food test and RAST test;
- that you want to be referred to a competent allergist who does accurate work and who will, if required, mix up a desensitising vaccine to be taken orally.

If he/she does not agree to help, go to another doctor who is open-minded and willing to help you try a new approach. Shopping for a good doctor is no different to shopping around for a good plumber or painter. Unfortunately, some people seem to think they have no consumer rights in matters pertaining to doctors and must accept everything that is meted out to them. This is not so. Just as the plumber and painter are expected to provide the service requested, so is the doctor. Don't be intimidated. It is *your* health and it is *your* responsibility to take care of it. Experience has taught me that this assertive approach invariably ensures you find the type of doctor and the help you are looking for.

It is preferable that you consult a doctor who is familiar with the practice of clinical ecology. Many doctors are unfamiliar with this new science and will tell you that allergies have nothing to do with your symptoms. Don't fall for this one, but if your doctor wants to run additional tests, by all means go along with him/her. If you have not sought treatment for your symptoms, it is wise to let your doctor treat you conventionally at first. Remember, although allergy is the greatest mimicker of disease, there could well be some other reason for your condition.

THE ALLERGY TESTS

For the skin, RAST and cytotoxic food tests to be accurate you need to be off vitamin supplements (especially vitamin C), cortisone and antihistamine for five to seven days before the tests. These substances will block the reaction between the testing agent and the blood and skin, giving rise to inaccurate results. If you suspect any other medication you are on might affect the tests, check with your allergist first. It pays to be off as many drugs as possible (even the pill) before the tests, though the absolute no no's are the ones just mentioned. Other drugs will have only a minimal effect on test accuracy so don't go off them if its going to stress you in other ways. On no account should you ever go on or off any drug medication without your doctor's advice.

Seventy-two hours prior to the tests eat as wide a variety of foods as possible. The tests are more accurate if the blood has made contact with the food it's being tested for within a three day period. Don't eat any food you suspect will harm you. List those foods instead and take them into account when planning your personal Anti-Allergy Program. This procedure is applicable to all food tests including food elimination tests.

If your asthma symptoms flare up during this time use your Ventolin inhaler and/or any other non-cortisone/non-antihistamine drugs as often as your doctor deems appropriate to keep the symptoms and possible discomfort of food loading at bay. If your eczema flares up you may use cortisone creams during this time.

It's a waste of time taking any of these tests if you're on marijuana, speed, heroin or any other recreational drug.

Don't eat large quantities of each food: small amounts are quite sufficient. Use cortisone puffers (not pills) after the tests.

Having had the tests, remove from your diet those foods you are allergic to. Adhere to the Anti-Candida Program minus the foods you are allergic to. Use the Anti-Candida Program as your basis for treatment. Stick to it strictly for ninety days.

If you show up as having inhalant allergies to airborne moulds, yeast and fungi you must go off the mould foods listed at the back of the book. Some people make the mistake of thinking that because they have inhalant allergies only they don't need to go on a diet. Inhalant allergies cannot be cured if the foods they pertain to are not avoided totally for at least ninety days.

If you show up allergic to grasses stay off the herbal teas for ninety days and all foods pertaining to or containing that substance. For example, if you show up allergic to rye grass you must avoid all foods containing rye—rye bread, Ryvita, etc. If you are allergic to wheatgrass, then nothing containing wheat, and if you are allergic to common oats, then no porridge, oatmeal soap, muesli, oat bran or oatmeal.

EXERCISE

It is essential to exercise regularly to contain allergies. A strong blood flow moves the allergens through the body to the kidneys and the skin, where they are eliminated in both the urine and the sweat. A sluggish blood flow tends to hold the allergens in a fixed position so they become sedentary and begin to destroy the tissues around them. By continually moving the allergens through the blood they have far less time to inflame the tissues. Regular exercise expels allergens from the body.

Regular exercise does not mean you stress yourself by running marathons or play competition tennis or squash four to five times a week or do five aerobics classes per week. The best form of exercise to help you overcome allergies and candida yeast infections is walking. A forty to sixty minute walk four to five times a week is excellent. Walk at a steady pace. Don't try to up the pace too much. This will stress you.

Doing deep breathing exercises while walking (yogic walking) is an excellent way to speed the overcoming of your allergies. (See Chapter 11, 'Stress', for these exercises.) Make sure you're consuming adequate fluids. Fluid is needed to dilute the allergens so that their elimination from the body doesn't damage the liver and kidneys. Exercise causes extra fluid loss by evaporation, so make sure you up your intake before and after each walk. At this point you should read Chapter 10, 'The importance of water and oxygen', and you should check closely the fluid intake table listed in Chapter 13, 'The Metabolism-Balancing Program', to make sure you're getting enough.

Walking up stairs is the best exercise of all for toning the leg, bottom and back muscles. It improves posture and carriage. So, as a good form of regular exercise, avoid the lift—use the stairs wherever possible.

BREAKING THE PROGRAM

The object of breaking the Anti-Allergy Program is to get back onto the Metabolism-Balancing Program, or as close to it as your allergies allow, and to stay on it for the rest of your life.

After ninety days on the Anti-Candida/Anti-Allergy Program it's time to reintroduce the allergenic foods to see if you've lost your sensitivity to them. There's a 95 per cent chance that you will have. Start by getting your doctor or naturopath to supervise the reintroduction of foods. Have only one of your allergenic foods and wait for two or three days to see what happens. If you don't get a reaction in that time move onto another food from your no no list. If you do get an adverse reaction wait for the symptoms to abate before trying another food and stay off the food you reacted to for another month before trying it again.

If you're allergic to such foods as eggs, milk, malt, corn, beef or coconut try them first. These foods are used widely in manufac-tured–processed foods and your reaction to them in their whole form will determine whether or not you can eat the manufactured foods (manufactured foods should comprise no more than 5 per cent of food intake). At this point you should consult the food tables at the back of the book pertaining to eggs, milk, corn and malt, to see what other foods contain them.

Coconut oil is used widely in the frying of foods served in retail outlets (chips, etc.) and in confectionery. Read all labels carefully. Any product that contains palm oil or palmoline contains coconut. Beef emulsifiers are used in a wide range of commercially made biscuits, cakes, pies, savouries, etc., so read all these labels very carefully. Beef gelatin is used for making capsules. If you are taking anything in capsule form (even vitamins) assume the capsule to be made of beef until categorically proven otherwise. It pays to phone the capsule manufacturer if you're unsure.

By testing the whole food first you get an accurate idea of how you're going to react to anything that contains it. If you don't test them first you'll never really know what you're reacting to when you eat the other foods. It is most important that you never test yourself on a refined version of the whole food. The refined foods are quickly absorbed and rapid absorption can retrigger allergies. To explain: if you are allergic to wheat (very common) you should begin by eating only wholemeal bread, not cakes, biscuits or crackers. Remember, the more slowly it is absorbed, the less likely you are to develop a reaction to it. Also, the refined version of white flour is bound to have chemical additives and it could well have been the chemicals (flavourings, colourings and preservatives) that precipitated the sensitivity in the first place.

To further slow the absorption rate put butter or oil on the bread. If it is an unrefined food such as beef, fish, chicken or a vegetable that you were allergic to, stir fry it in a wok (Chinese style) to begin with. The fat will further slow the absorption of the food. On no account use tinned, cured or any form of processed meats. They are refined and full of chemicals. (The only exceptions are tinned tuna, salmon, sardines, herring and mackerel if you do not have an allergy to them).

It is essential not to start eating your former food allergens in a tired, depressed state, or after an illness of any sort. Especially after hepatitis or glandular fever. Should you come down with 'flu or a related illness and suddenly develop a craving for the once allergic food, resist it. Avoid it like the plague, drink water instead and keep drinking it until the craving abates.

ROTATION DIETS

Now that you're well you have to ensure that you stay well. This is achieved by making sure you don't over-expose yourself to any given substance. Rotating your foods is a good way of ensuring this. Singularly, the most important factor in the controlling of allergies is the three day rotation diet. Simply stated, it means you only eat any given food once in three days. This means all foods. Break away from your former monotonous eating patterns. Eat different foods every day. This way you will not wear down your enzyme chains. You will prevent your former food allergies from returning and prevent the accumulation of new ones. If this rotation diet requires that you put more time and effort into organising your eating patterns and lifestyle in general, so be it. To survive we simply must live in accordance with nature's laws.

Nature gave us four seasons and lots of different types of nutritious foods so that we don't overload on any one food. Nature's pantry is rich and varies with the seasons. Variety is not only the spice of life it's the stuff of life as well. Remember it was over-exposure to a given food that caused the problem in the first place and food allergies can recur if we fall back into old habits.

DESENSITISATION

If you want to be rid of an allergy, once and for all, you must stick religiously to your Anti-Allergy Program for at least three months. If you break the program in that time, even a tiny little bit, you'll resensitise yourself and have to start a new three month period from that point on. There are no shades of grey with the Anti-Allergy Program, it's very much a black and white situation. You're either on it or you're not.

Some patients find this three month mandatory time span hard to accept, especially if after a month or so all of their symptoms have disappeared. Some of them start to break the program a little bit at a time and if the symptoms don't return, feel sure they are well. Most often when the program is broken there is an immediate reaction, though sometimes there is sufficient desensitisation for a delayed reaction to occur. If after a few weeks there is still no sign of the symptoms, people who have broken a program are convinced they are fully desensitised and begin eating whatever they like. Without fail, a short time later, the symptoms begin to reappear and the dieter is back to square one.

A minority of my patients are actually happy to see-saw about like this. Choosing to stay on the program until their symptoms disappear then breaking it till they return again. At which point they go back on the program. Since this method will never cure your allergies I wouldn't recommend it. The choice is yours.

It is most important to remember that just because the symptoms have disappeared, it does not mean you're cured of the problem. Most people need at least three months to consolidate their desensitisation, even if their symptoms have disappeared in the first month. Some people, a minority, require six months and an even smaller percentage need twelve months to desensitise. People in this category need their treatment supervised and closely monitored by a doctor or naturopath to prevent vitamin and mineral deficiency developing.

Only 5 per cent of people don't desensitise and have to stay away from the allergenic food for the rest of their lives.

The advantage of desensitisation is that you can, after the period of total abstinence, go back on the foods you were once sensitive to. You win on two counts here:

1. You lose the symptoms that have been troubling you.
2. You are able to eat anything you like.

And all of this achieved with three short months of total abstinence from the offending food or foods. Some of these 5 per cent of people who don't fully desensitise after ninety days on the program, and who aren't prepared to continue strictly on the program for twelve months or more, find they can lead a very comfortable life if they stay strictly on the Anti-Candida/Anti-Allergy Program through the week and break it on the weekends only. Two days of breaking it in moderation is usually not enough to cause a flaring up of symptoms. In those who do experience a reaction the moment they eat a forbidden substance the symptoms are usually mild. The up side of being on the Anti Candida/Anti-Allergy Program is that after ninety days most people are so used to it that sticking to it five days per week and breaking it on weekends only is no problem to them. The discipline and routine of having to get up each day for work is conducive to staying on the program. Breaking it on the weekend when relaxed gives the body that feeling of *joie de vivre* that comes from a rest and a change. The balance thus struck between discipline and rest contributes to a balanced lifestyle and a balanced metabolism. Balanced metabolisms are less prone to reacting allergically to contact with foreign substances/allergens.

The combined effects of diet and rest are so successful because they raise the body's resistance to allergies. A raised resistance is the greatest desensitiser of all.

Holidays often see a disappearance of allergies even though allergens are still present. Holidays are potent healers because they mean a temporary release from commitment and a rest from everyday routine. Under these conditions the body's resistance soars. I've noticed that the further away from one's place of work one holidays the greater effect the holiday has. It never ceases to amaze me how well allergic people feel when they travel to the other side of the world. Even though the climate may be unfriendly and the environment polluted their allergies invariably disappear for the time they are away, proving the healing potency of rest. It's a pity that in our fast moving, achievement-orientated world rest is no longer taken seriously as a healing modality. Rest always has been and always will be the most potent healer of all. No matter how positive your attitude may be it's limited if not backed up with rest.

DESENSITISING VACCINES

Because allergies are such whacky and variable things it is impossible to describe a treatment that will work best for everyone. I have talked to people who became desensitised to all their inhalant allergies just by having the skin test and others who were worse on the vaccine.

If after the first week on the vaccine you are no better, stop taking it until you have thoroughly detoxified your body and built yourself up on sound, wholesome food. Then if you still have symptoms begin with the vaccine again. Take it every second day the first week and every day the following week. Be prepared to experiment. I have had patients that responded brilliantly and cleared all their symptoms when they took the vaccine every day for the first week, every second day for the second week, every third day for the third week, then went back to every day for later weeks. Different formulas work for different people. Be patient with yourself, give it time, work it out and you will get better. I have found the best results are achieved if the vaccine is not commenced until at least four to five weeks on the Anti-Allergy Program, if it is needed at all. Taking the vaccine too early in the program seems to put undue strain on the immune system and many people react adversely to it. Being off all allergenic foods for four to six weeks seems to reduce immune system strain and reactions to the vaccine become more favourable.

I have noticed cigarette and marijuana smokers take much longer to desensitise than non-smokers do, even though they may stick strictly to the diet. Why these two drugs suppress the normal desensitising process is hard to say, but they do. Taking other drugs, including prescription ones, has the same effect.

A WORD OF WARNING

Don't kid yourself you're still on the Anti-Allergy Program if you've broken it only once or twice in the three month period. Many people try to delude themselves they've stuck strictly to the program, arguing that one or two little bits of this or that over three months couldn't make much difference. Well, unfortunately a little bit of this and that, imbibed once or twice over a three month period is enough to make all the difference to the Anti-Allergy Program.

Around 95 per cent of people are able to overcome allergies by avoiding the allergenic food or substance for a three to six month period. The reason that this is able to happen is that the old departing generation of white cells after this period 'forget' to pass on to new generations of cells the fact that they were ever sensitive to the substance.

However, eating the food just once in that three months, even in minute quantities, is enough to jog the memory of the old white cells and re-establish the allergic sensitivity. Sometimes white cells can live and remember foreign substances for several years. It would seem that in those 5 per cent of people who don't desensitise after twelve months' abstinence, this mechanism is still intact. (See Chapter 2, 'Allergies'.)

A LITTLE JUNK FOOD?

For those on the Metabolism-Balancing Program who are enjoying good health and are free from allergies, candida yeast infections and heart problems the inclusion of up to 5 per cent of junk food into their diet won't do any harm. However, the inclusion of that amount of junk food into the Anti-Candida Program will slow results down by feeding the yeast. But provided the junk food amounts to only 5 per cent, or less, of the total diet, this will not be sufficient to allow the yeast colony to grow back to its original size. Unlike the Anti-Allergy Program where even small deviation means a return of full-blown symptoms and resensitisation, breaking the Anti-Candida Program means only a slowing of the healing momentum. At worst, there is a slight exacerbation of symptoms and at best there is no change at all. This can present a trap for the unwary, as lack of reaction to continuous breaking of the Anti-Candida Program can lead them to believe that they can get away with it. Where the folly of breaking the program shows up is six months later when they are still having to remain on it because they are not 100 per cent symptom free, even though they may be feeling better than they were before starting it.

My experience in treating people by way of an anti-allergy or anti-candida program is that they do best it they go for it right from the start and do not break it at all. If you stick to these programs 100 per cent, most allergies and candida infections are cured in three months. Breaking the program with 5 per cent or less of junk or allergenic food means it's going to take six to nine months to get well (if you do at all when you break an anti-allergy program). If the whole process goes on this long most people get disheartened, and feel cheated, as they had expected to get better in less time.

It's important to note that breaking the program does not just mean eating foods that are black listed. It also means skipping meals, eating below optimum quantities, selecting only a few foods on the menu (that is, making the program stricter than it is) and not rotating foods.

Not eating the prescribed unleavened bread gives rise to the same problems as skipped meals. The bread must be eaten whether you like the taste or not. Wheat contains too many important nutrients for it to be left out, notably the minerals selenium and chromium, which are needed to help the hormone insulin keep the levels of glucose in the blood balanced and thus preventing hypoglycaemia.

Not taking your vitamins every day, as prescribed, has the same effect as skipping meals and leaving out essential foods.

It must also be remembered that if a candida sufferer has allergies as well, and most do, then the rules that apply to breaking the allergy programs apply to the Anti-Candida Program too.

DUST ALLERGY

If you have a dust allergy you must not dust, vacuum or be in the house for at least three hours after it has been done. Get another member of your household to do this sort of housework. Keep carpets, curtains and cloth-covered furniture in your home to a minimum and discard fan heaters completely. Keep books behind a glass cover and spray the bedrooms and living rooms with dust seal about three times per year. Spray your pets with dust seal about once a month. If this doesn't work they must always be kept outside. Don't have ceiling fans, floor fans and air-conditioners going at home during the ninety days on the program and where possible avoid them at work. They raise a dust that never settles, as well as blowing around pollens from indoor flowers and moulds from indoor plants. You'll not desensitise in this type of environment. They further aggravate allergies by chilling sedentary bodies. (See Chapter 6 under 'Asthma' and 'Colds and 'flu'.) If it's not possible to get someone else to vacuum, do it yourself with an anti-dust mask and dust with a damp cloth only.

CROSS-LINKAGE OF ALLERGY

Around 90 per cent of people with dust allergies have food allergies. Continuous contact with dust can be the sole reason for a person not overcoming their food allergies. Reducing the level of dust in the home and workplace reduces one's sensitivity to chemicals and foods.

DUST MITES

Most people who are allergic to house dust are allergic to the dust mite as well. This little animal lives in the kapok or sponge rubber of the pillow and mattress and comes out at night to feed on the odd bits of skin that are flaking off the body. If you're allergic to its bite or the mucous coating around its faeces, it can greatly aggravate any other allergy you may have and undermine the effects of any program you may be on.

If your skin itches, you produce more mucus or your asthma gets worse when in bed, you are almost certainly allergic to the dust mite (given that the bedroom window is closed and you're not being

90

chilled). I have found the dust mite cover to be more effective than the dust mite sprays (sealants) at preventing allergic reactions to this microscopic creature. I recommend you get the dust mite cover (from your chemist) for the mattress, pillow and doona.

Change the sheets twice per week. Spray the blankets, curtains, carpets, books, stuffed toys, teddy bears and favourite arm chair. Its preferable that kids don't sleep with stuffed toys. Spray all pets, but don't let them into the bedroom and if possible keep them out of the house for ninety days.

It's a waste of time having dust mite covers if cats and dogs are going to be sitting on the bed and scratching themselves. Pets carry dust mites and the dust mite covers and sprays will obviously give no protection if the dust mites and their faeces are being dropped on top of them. Don't lie on the carpet to read or watch TV. If doing yoga on the carpet, spread out a towel or sheet, sprayed with dust mite spray, to lie on.

CLEANING THE ENVIRONMENT

If your skin tests have drawn a positive to moulds, grasses, pollens and chemicals there are a number of things you must do to ensure the effectiveness of the desensitising vaccine.

First you must remove all the food correlates from your diet; for example, rye bread and Ryvita if you show up allergies to rye grass. (See inhalant section later in this chapter). Second you must remove as many chemicals from your environment as possible. To achieve this you must first remove as many synthetic products from the house as possible. Air pollution studies have shown that the concentration of chemical contaminants is 400 times greater in the home than in the outside air. Synthetic fabrics, curtains and plastic furniture are made from hydrocarbon (coal and oil) bases. Aerosol sprays, of any sort, are also hydrocarbon based. In fact, if it has an odour, remove it. This includes perfumes, after-shave, body deodorants and perfumed vaginal douches. Hydrocarbons frequently trigger off inhalant allergies (with nose, throat, lung, eye, skin and fluid symptoms).

For those people who show up with allergies to moulds it's important to keep the immediate environment mould free. Check all internal pipes. Pipes leaking into brickwork in the walls or into concrete floors can create mould traps.

It is important to air the house regularly. Houses are more humid these days, as they are more usually built on concrete slabs, rather than the wooden floorboards and vented walls of yesteryear. Humidity allows the rapid breeding and build-up of dust mites and moulds, especially in wardrobes. People these days spend longer daytime hours away from the house, and they leave windows and doors closed. This shuts in steam from the morning hot showers and kettle boiling making a cosy environment for dust mites and moulds. In these conditions their levels rise so high that they trigger allergic reactions despite the best efforts of anti-allergy programs and desensitising vaccines. Only hot water will kill dust mites yet these days people launder their clothes and bed linen in cold water. All clothing and bed linen is to be washed in hot water.

Many asthma and nasal congestion sufferers are over-medicating themselves on cortisone drugs to counter the effects of inordinately high dust mite and mould levels in the home.

To lower humidity, open doors and windows for a while on returning home and for an extended period on weekends. This may present a problem on returning home from work on winter nights as cold draughts can cause chills. If it's very cold, use the dry heat of a bar heater to dry the home. Use a fan-forced heater to dry wardrobes and linen cupboards. Always open the bathroom window and turn on the extractor (if you have one) when showering and cooking.

The best environment for the inhalant prone person is a wood-panelled house with tiled floors, only a few woollen rugs and cotton curtains. Nylon and plastic products tend to give off a hydrocarbon vapour (formaldehyde) when in a warm environment. Hot days in summer or an over-heated house in winter can cause this vapour to be in the air twenty-four hours a day.

Indoor plants help to reduce the overall chemical load by absorbing and neutralising formaldehyde. So, have plenty of the non-flowering varieties at home and in the office. Keep their leaves well wiped to prevent dust and mould accumulating on them.

Remember that riding in a formaldehyde-filled car can so aggravate allergy symptoms as to undermine the effects of sticking to the diet.

Constant exposure to such a chemical-laden environment greatly taxes both the immune system and the enzyme chains of the liver, as they strive unceasingly to break these chemicals down into less toxic products. If you live and work in such a toxic environment, yet eat well, exercise regularly in the fresh air, do not over-work, do not have a candida yeast infection, get plenty of sleep, have a harmonious love life, a good self-image, do not smoke, drink moderately and stay off coffee, tea (in excess) and drugs, you could well get by without developing any inhalant allergies, and the disfiguring symptoms that they produce. If you do not, it is only a matter of time before you will develop inhalant sensitivities if you have a genetic predisposition to them. A dose of hepatitis, the 'flu, a marital break-up, or the loss of a loved one could be all that is needed to trigger off the process.

Chlorine is the second most common chemical and is found in drinking water, washing water, swimming pools, bleaches, anaesthetics and many drugs. It is used in the refining of both cooking oils and sugar. In its free state chlorine is a deadly poisonous gas. It readily binds with other chemicals to form compounds. Time and again I find people with the symptoms of food allergy and/or candida yeast infection are reacting to the chlorine in drinking water.

For this reason, all drinking water from the tap should be boiled for ten minutes to evaporate chlorine. Better still don't drink tap water at all. Drink only bottled mineral or spring water (make sure the mineral water is from a recognised spa and not commercially made—commercially made mineral water is derived from tap water, as is soda water). There are excellent delivery services of fresh, clean spring water to office and home.

Tank water can be a problem for country people. Properties whose agriculture requires significant spraying can lead, in time, to a build-up of chemical fall-out on the roof of the house. While the weather is fine that's not a problem but the first rain sees a washing of these chemicals into the water tank with a consequent flaring up of allergy symptoms. I've found this to be a major cause of unexplainable, sudden flaring of allergy symptoms in country patients who are sticking to their programs and progressing well. Even those who don't use sprays on their property can experience the chemical fall-out of aerial top-dressing of herbicides and fertiliser from up to 20 kilometres away.

It must be remembered that many of the chemicals found in the home, work environment and agricultural sprays are also found as chemical colourings, flavourings and preservatives in food.

Take formaldehyde, for instance. It is the most common chemical in the average household. It has little odour but is the component of car fumes, smog and natural gas combustion (home heaters and stoves) that causes burning of the eyes. Formaldehyde is found in concrete, plaster, home insulation materials, home antiseptics, toothpaste, disinfectants, waxes, polishes, adhesives, fire proofing compounds applied to fabrics, foods, insect and rodent repellents, nail polish, wall-boards and resins. It is a by-product of the processes that make natural and synthetic fabrics crease-resistant, dye-fast, shrink-proof and more elastic and is evaporated from plastic pencils and pens when they are put in the mouth. It constitutes a major portion of the pollutants in the air that now cover the earth.

To get completely away from the formaldehyde would be almost impossible. To reduce your contact with it by as much as 50 per cent is both possible and wise if you are to prevent the onset of allergy and more life-threatening diseases later in life.

The softer the plastic the more formaldehyde there is in it. Car upholstery contains significant concentrations of formaldehyde. That sticky clear substance that appears on the inside of the windscreen is formaldehyde that has vaporised from the upholstery under heat.

If you've ever wondered why the kids are ratty some times after you've picked them up from school it could well be the high levels of formaldehyde in the car. If you've parked the car outside with the windows up on a hot day the outgassing of formaldehyde from the upholstery will be so great it will have reached toxic levels by mid-afternoon. Open all the doors to air and cool the car before you pick the kids up and keep the windows down while your driving.

CLEANING PRODUCTS AND PERSONAL PRODUCTS

I recommend getting rid of all aerosols, harsh disinfectants, cleaners and phenol products. Instead I recommend the following:

- Soda bicarbonate mixed to a paste for cleaning.
- Mix it with cooking salt for heavy duty use.
- White vinegar for mould removal.
- Pure yellow laundry soap for personal washing, grated and pulped for laundry use (for machine or hand washing).
- Pure soap flakes are also a better alternative to laundry detergents and cheaper.
- Don't bath or shower using perfumed soaps.
- Use washing soda to soften water for laundry use.
- Buy shampoos, conditioners and cosmetics that are free of petrochemicals (try the Herbon range).
- Use an aluminium free roll-on deodorant (see the shopping list in Chapter 14, 'The Anti-Candida Program').
- Use the pump packs available in supermarkets instead of aerosol products.
- Use fresh herbs in the toilet instead of Bloo Loo and deodorisers.
- Plain sorbolene cream, with glycerine, makes a very good inexpensive body moisturiser.

This list was kindly supplied by a patient who once suffered from environmental sensitivities. She finally cured her husband's itchy rash by getting him to eliminate perfumed soaps.

INHALANT ALLERGIES

Diet is as important for the treatment of inhalant allergies as it is for food allergies. Diet raises the body's resistance to allergies by building up the immune system. Make sure that foods pertaining to a given inhalant allergen are not consumed for ninety days. The removal of food correlates speeds the process of desensitisation to inhalant allergens by helping to reduce overall contact with them.

COMMON INHALANTS THAT HAVE FOOD CORRELATIONS

Common oats is a grass, the spores of which are frequently in the air during spring and autumn, to which many people have inhalant allergies (sinusitis, hayfever, asthma, conjunctivitis). Sensitivity to common oats is lowered by removing all oats from the diet, and avoiding all contact with muesli, porridge, Guiness stout, oatmeal soap, oatmeal skin preparations, oat bran and oatmeal. With rye grass sensitivity avoid Ryvita, rye bread and rye flour.

Those with a sensitivity to a number of grasses and pollen do better if they stay off herbal teas, most of which are of grass and pollen origin. Although herbal teas are better for you than ordinary tea and coffee, if you're allergic to grasses and pollens they can do more harm than tea and coffee. Rosehip and peppermint are safe herbal teas for the grass allergic.

Sensitivities to airborne moulds, including those that live in air-conditioning systems of large offices (namely alternaria) can be lowered by staying off the foods listed under yeasts and moulds in the 'Food tables' at the back of this book. If you're allergic to the cephlasporium mould that lives in the soil you must wear a dust mask (obtainable along with your dust mite cover and dust mite spray from your chemist) while digging and weeding the garden or repotting the pot plants.

If you're allergic to grasses, wear long pants to golf and put your dust mask on while driving, chipping, putting and playing out off the rough. Don't attempt to walk too far with it, as it'll restrict your breathing and fatigue you. Don't bushwalk, cut the lawns or ride a cycle on or near freshly cut lawns or in the bush for ninety days. If you're an orchardist or commercial flower grower wear the dust mask while sedentary (for example, on the tractor) and try to get someone to do the heavy work for ninety days so that you're not forced to breathe deeply and inhale airborne allergens.

The best mask to wear is the one the spray painters use. Unfortunately, it can't be worn if physical activity is engaged in. It's ideal for wearing around the house while someone else is cutting yours or your neighbour's lawn. Also while sitting on a tractor, ploughing, sowing, fertilising or spraying. After ninety days of the program and avoidance of the inhalants you should be able to make contact with them again without your symptoms returning.

The best time for grass allergic people to go on the programs is winter when the pollen and spore count is at its lowest and the body is having a seasonal rest from these airborne allergens. By observing over the ninety days of winter, adequate rest, strict adherence to the program and minimal contact with the inhalants, spring should see you symptom free despite walking in the fields, digging the gardens, working in the glasshouse or cutting the lawns. Often the desensitising vaccine is also required to achieve this.

A COMMON MISTAKE TO AVOID

Some people, despite warnings to the contrary, start taking on greater responsibilities and work commitments after completing the program. Others start over-exercising and/or over-socialising. The new lease on life people experience when they've overcome their allergies can lead them into this 'doing too much' mode without their realising it. Because they feel so good, and because the human memory is so short when it comes to former pain and illness, they busily engage themselves without a thought that they might be overdoing it. After a while some of their former symptoms return and thinking that their allergies are returning they put themselves back on their Anti-Candida/Anti-Allergy Program only to find that this time it doesn't work. Thinking they have acquired new allergies they take themselves back to their allergist for allergy tests only to find that nothing shows up. This is when they start to panic and begin to suspect serious diseases like cancer, diabetes, brain tumours, TB, polio and meningitis. Invariably their symptoms are those of stress, stress being a great mimicker of allergy, and when they slow down the symptoms soon abate.

Now that you're well, be ever careful that this doesn't happen to you. Constantly monitor yourself to make sure insidious 'overdoing it' is not creeping up on you. Constantly monitor yourself to make sure you're adhering to the Metabolism-Balancing Program. It's the Metabolism-Balancing Program that will keep your vitality and resistance to allergies high for the rest of your life—if you stick to it and keep taking the dietary supplements.

REFLEXOLOGY

This is a foot massage technique that works well for those who have allergies that are not responding as quickly as they should to dietary treatment. If you're in that category buy a book on reflexology from the health store and practise massaging those parts on your feet that are applicable to your symptoms. Reflexology is simple, safe and effective.

SUMMARY

If you avoid the food to which you are sensitive for 90 days you are likely to lose your sensitivity to it. How successful you are depends on:

1. How rich your diet is in nutrients.
2. Whether or not you have been on drugs, cigarettes, coffee (in excess) or alcohol.
3. Whether you are over-worked, have over-exercised or burned the candle at both ends.
4. How relaxed you are.
5. Whether you are content and happy. (You would be surprised how many allergies disappear when you find contentment.)
6. Whether you are going through a marital break-up, financial crisis or other major stress.
7. Whether or not your attitude to life causes you to be stressed.

If your stress levels are low and you have taken good care of yourself there is a very good chance that your food and inhalant allergy will disappear completely in ninety days. Appropriate weaning off drug medication is also a determinant. This means you use the medication every time you get your symptoms. As the program and your reduced stress loads begin to take effect you'll find you'll automatically be using less of your medication. Remember, symptoms are a stress that slows the healing of the body.

Once healed the body will remain in good health if you spend the rest of your life on the Metabolism-Balancing Program and take appropriate dietary supplements. A lapse in this discipline could see the allergies return if significant stress is encountered.

6.
Asthma, skin problems, arthritis

'Now learn what and how great benefits a temperate diet will bring along with it. In the first place, you will enjoy good health.'

Horace, 65–08 BC

Diseases as diverse as asthma, acne, eczema, psoriasis and arthritis all have one thing in common—they are most often allergy based and usually respond to treatment when allergies have been eradicated. I've found that asthma and skin complaint treatment is aided by reflexology massage of the feet. Buy a book on reflexology from the health store and practise this effective massage on yourself. Or get a friend to do it for you.

ASTHMA

Asthma is an allergy-based condition that causes muscles of the windpipe to go into spasm. A muscle spasm is a tight contraction of muscle fibres that will not let go. When this happens to the muscles of the windpipe two complications result:

1. the windpipe is narrowed, meaning less air can get in and out of the lungs; and
2. the rhythmic contraction and expansion of the muscles that facilitate normal breathing are disrupted, making it very difficult to breath out. Wheezing and shortness of breath result.

98

The windpipe is lined with a membrane that produces mucus. This mucus is there to trap bacteria, dust, pollens, moulds, grasses, fungi and other foreign bodies that are inhaled and acts as an effective protector of the delicate lung tissues. In true allergic fashion the mucous membranes of the windpipe become over-active during an asthma attack and the excess mucus produced further blocks the already narrowed passageways. In this way asthma becomes an extension of those most common symptoms of allergy that occur further up the windpipe: hayfever, rhinitis, sinusitis, stuffy nose and post-nasal drip (mucus that drips from the back of the nose into the throat).

Asthma is a classic example of a migrating allergy and is proof of the fact that we don't grow out of allergies naturally. Bronchial asthma is relatively infrequent in infancy but common after the age of two. At least half of those infants that were born with allergic eczema (dermatitis or severe rash) will later develop asthma as the allergies migrate from the skin to the windpipe. Sometimes the skin clears up and sometimes it doesn't. Long standing eczema is fairly common among adult asthma sufferers. Sometimes the allergy moves up from the lungs as the child grows older. These children are often diagnosed as having outgrown their asthma. The repeated sore throats, inflamed tonsils, stuffy noses, hayfever and brain allergies that inevitably follow this migration are seldom ever linked to asthma.

Asthma is attributable to factors other than allergy and candida yeast infection:

FACTOR 1: KEEPING WARM

This relates to the basic law of physics regarding the expansion and contraction of materials due to heat and cold. Because asthma is primarily the result of muscles that are in a state of sustained contraction it makes sense that body warmth is necessary for the expansion needed to effect their release. My experience with treating asthma is that even though the allergens that initially caused the contraction have been removed from the diet and ambient air, the muscles will not let go if any part of the body is cold.

This chilling of the body factor is something that many of my asthma patients have never taken seriously. Most of them were victims of a perennial summer mentality that makes them wear shorts, open neck shirts and get around in bare feet all winter. These people are usually avid fresh air buffs who make good use of breezes to air-condition their homes in summer. What they fail to realise is that comfort-bringing summer breezes become dis-ease-bringing draughts in winter. Because, in most most parts of

Australia, summer can be so long (up to seven months during good years) they fall into the comfortable habit of wearing less and less and leaving doors and windows open all year round.

I've had asthma patients arrive in my office for their first consultation dressed in shorts, shirt and thongs in the middle of July, complaining that it's a cold day! In fairness to them it's usually one of those brilliantly sunny winter days that we often get. Unfortunately those sunny days usually have a cold south-westerly wind blowing off the Snowy Mountains. In sheltered pockets out of the wind the temperature can be as high as 21–22°C. Walking around the corner can bring you face to face with the cold south-westerly whose chill factor can suddenly reduce the ambient air temperature to 8–9°C. If the full force of this south-westerly is caught on bare neck and chest (open neck shirt) it will immediately chill it—and the muscles of the windpipe—sending them into spasm. This is despite the fact that the rest of the body may be sufficiently warm, which it would be if a cardigan was being worn.

Another thing that asthma sufferers have in common is that they tend to wear cardigans rather than crew or polo neck jumpers. Although heavy woollen cardigans may well raise their body temperatures to a comfortable level they do nothing to prevent local chilling of the neck, chest and windpipe muscles. Crew or polo neck jumpers and scarves are a must for asthma sufferers. Without them they just don't get better. They must be worn all winter long whether it's windy or not as southerlies can spring up at any time and without warning. The belief that one can't stand things up around one's neck has to be vehemently disputed, and then changed.

Gymnasiums are notorious for draughts. Don't work out at aerobics or weights unless you're wearing a crew or polo neck sweater, cotton in summer, wool in winter. Perspiring in a draught gives asthma attacks if the perspiration is not absorbed from the skin by a sweater.

Other erroneous beliefs that must be disputed and changed are:

1. *'I can't sleep without the bedroom window open.'* All my former asthma patients have learned to sleep with it closed during winter. Open windows cause significant chilling when our body temperature drops during sleep. Cold air coming into the room at this time causes your body temperature to drop just that little bit more and when the temperature drops that extra degree the body's resistance also drops. When this happens the bacteria and viruses that live naturally inside you (particularly the nose and throat area) gain the upper hand. They are able to multiply

100

and infect you. That is why colds are called colds. This chilling effect also causes muscular contraction, that is, asthma. Chills cause colds and coughs at night, and colds and coughs cause asthma. Even if your bedroom window is open only a little bit, enough cold air can enter the room in a six to eight hour period to cause the chilling of the body. This is especially so if the sleep is restless and the blankets are being thrown off. This restlessness could be caused by dust mites in the mattress and pillow or by having a warm bath or shower before bed. The latter causes a rise in body temperature, enough to kick the blankets off and predispose yourself to chills. Night sweats—a symptom of allergy—can also cause this.

2. 'I don't need to wear a warm dressing gown and slippers on rising.' This attitude will guarantee you will never lose your asthma. Sudden changes of temperature even for a minute or two duration will throw the windpipe muscles into spasm. Make sure you heat the whole house at night. Going from a warm room to a cold room causes windpipe spasm. You can leave windows and doors open through the day while you are out of the house but close them when you get home. Airing your bedroom in this way will ensure plenty of fresh air for the sleeping hours. Although the bedroom window must be closed at night, the bedroom door may be left open.

Don't sit over a heater to keep warm when you've got a window or a door open. Even though the front of you is warm your back is being chilled and this will give you asthma. Close all windows and doors in winter. Don't worry, there's ample air in the house. Use door socks, as most draughts are created by the gaps under doors.

By conscientiously avoiding draughts, sudden changes of temperature and dressing warmly you will notice, as so many of my patients do, that you will not only avoid asthma attacks over winter, you won't suffer from colds or 'flu either.

FACTOR 2: NUTRITION

Muscle cell metabolism is fairly complex and delicate. If it is properly balanced the muscles expand and contract rhythmically and effortlessly. A deficiency in vitamin B complex, C and E, and the minerals calcium, magnesium, potassium and sodium, cause metabolic imbalances that predispose us to muscle spasms, especially when demands are put on muscles. Cramping of muscles in athletes, tennis players and footballers are examples of this. Asthma sufferers have a predisposition to muscle cramping that is greatly aggravated by deficiencies in the above nutrients.

I have found time and again that intractable asthma cases that are not responding fully to the combined Anti-Candida/Anti-Allergy Program, rest, warmth and protection from winds and chills, respond when sufficient of the above nutrients are taken. However, it does require patience as the minerals calcium, magnesium, potassium and sodium are not easily absorbed. At best we can only absorb 10 per cent of what we eat of them and, if significantly stressed, only about 1–2 per cent.

Stress reduces the amount of hydrochloric acid secreted by the stomach and calcium, magnesium, potassium and sodium can't be absorbed unless they are mixed with hydrochloric acid. The caffeine from coffee, tea, chocolate and cola drinks prevents the coming together of these minerals and hydrochloric acid and for that reason should be consumed no earlier than three hours after a meal or one hour before. The oxalic acid from rhubarb, spinach and cocoa (chocolate and chocolate drinks) combines with these minerals to form insoluble salt that can't be absorbed. They should never be consumed. The common practice of giving chocolate-flavoured milk to children to ensure their daily calcium and magnesium intake is an exercise in futility. Even if not allergic to milk (and many are) an asthma sufferer will be so starved of calcium and magnesium by this habit as to prevent a cure of their condition.

Raw nuts (with the exception of peanuts), sunflower and sesame seeds and fish are far better sources of calcium, magnesium, potassium and sodium. Deep and cold water fish contain vitamins A and D in their oils which help normalise the metabolism of the mucous membranes, reducing the amount of mucus produced in the windpipe. Asthma sufferers should eat these foods regularly and have three fish meals per week. Make sure you don't have a chocolate-containing dessert or coffee after the meal though.

High fat meals should be avoided as excess fat combines with these minerals in the intestine to form a rancid soap that can't be absorbed. Moderate fat intake is fine.

I have found that asthma sufferers need to take a complete multi-vitamin formula with the six essential minerals twice per day for the first six months to build up their calcium, magnesium, potassium and sodium reserves. This requires patience and acceptance as there is no other way. Dropping back to once a day after that usually holds the mineral reserves at desirable levels. Salting of one's food with sea salt in crystal form rather than the commercial free flow packs is also important. Sea salt is the best form of natural sodium and many asthma sufferers have aggravated their condition by cutting out salt completely. Too little salt does more damage than too much. Have ¼–½ teaspoon per day. Check to make sure there are no chemicals in the salt.

FACTOR 3: STRESS

Stress makes us uptight as it causes the muscles of our body to contract. Some people focus their stress in the muscles of the shoulder and neck. Stiff necks and headaches are the result. Some focus their stress in the muscles of the lower back and get lumbago or sciatica. Asthma sufferers tend to focus their stress in the muscles of the windpipe.

Self-sabotaging attitudes are a major cause of uptight feelings experienced by asthma sufferers. A change of attitude is imperative if a complete cure is to be achieved. (See Chapter 16, 'Scientific explanations—Stress'.)

Most of the adult onset cases of asthma I have treated have been the result of stress. Over-work, over-exercising, over-commitment, over-socialising (with too much alcohol and cigarettes) or vitamin and mineral deficiency, or a combination of these factors, plus the self-sabotaging attitudes that give rise to these behaviour patterns, are major causes. Many hard-charging over-achievers have experienced their first asthma attacks while jogging in the rain or head-on into a cold south-westerly wind while wearing only a runner's singlet; or from a cold or 'flu that resulted from a stint of over-work or over-socialising combined with skipped meals and inadequate rest and sleep.

As was mentioned previously, stress inhibits the absorption of nutrients and nutrient deficiency is a major stress.

COLDS AND 'FLU

Colds and 'flu are viral infections that take hold when the body's resistance is low (see Chapter 16, 'Scientific explanations—Viral infections'). The body's resistance drops because we are tired due to over-work, over-exercise, over-socialising, restless, broken sleep, crash diets, skipping meals, and the lack of protein, vitamins and minerals in our diet. In other words, when we're stressed out. The most significant stress that can trigger viral infection is chilling of the body. Colds are so named because we get them when we're cold. Viral infections produce toxins and these toxins float through the bloodstream causing irritations in the body's tissues and aggravating irritations that already exist. In this way colds and 'flu can trigger allergies and exacerbate allergies that already exist. Asthma caused by colds is called 'hypersecretory viral asthma' and is very common in children.

Asthma, acne, eczema and arthritis are particularly affected by colds and 'flu. Head colds, sore throats and chest colds cause mucus to drip down the back of the throat (especially while asleep) causing irritation of the windpipe and asthma attacks. Low grade colds and 'flu can smoulder away for weeks and months

103

preventing asthma and other allergies from responding to treatment.

Colds and 'flu will not go unless the body is sufficiently rested, properly fed and kept at an even, warm temperature. If you feel an attack coming on take time out to rest in bed and take a complete multi-vitamin and mineral formula. It's better to nip it in the bud so you can be back at work fighting fit in a day or two. If you soldier on, as many do, you'll find it will drag on for weeks. This will reduce your productivity at work and start your allergy symptoms up again.

A return of your allergy symptoms when everything was going so well on the program and you were practically allergy free, can be so disheartening as to cause you to give up and break the program before you are properly desensitised. It's not worth it. Colds and 'flu are so easily prevented. The moment you feel one coming on, go to bed with one of the standard remedies available from the chemist. Get your doctor to recommend the right one for you. If taken early enough these remedies are fantastic at knocking out colds and 'flu before they take hold. If they have already taken hold, these remedies are not very effective. (See Chapter 16, 'Scientific explanations—Viral infections—Stress'.)

As with asthma you must keep the bedroom window closed while you are in bed. By all means leave the bedroom window and door open all day, in fact even up to the point of going to bed at night. Close the window just before turning in. You can leave the door open if you like. Don't have the window open if you are in bed all day with a cold.

Draughts at school cause many colds, 'flu and asthma attacks in kids. Talk to the teacher and get him or her to close the windows on one side of the classroom. Kids can work up a sweat from playing at recess. Asthma, sore throats, colds and 'flu can develop when a draught blows on a moist body. Nylon wind breakers must be worn by kids playing outside in cold winds. Cold winds cut right through woollen sweaters and chill a perspiring body.

Cracker night and winter barbecues can be another problem. Don't stand too close to smoking barbecues and bonfires. The smoke can cause asthma. Don't take off your jacket or sweater because the fire is making you hot. The back of you will chill even though the front of you is warm. Asthma, colds and 'flu will result.

Ceiling fans, floor fans and air-conditioners are out until such time as you've completely overcome your allergies. They create draughts that keep house dust, dust mites and the pollens and moulds growing in plants perpetually airborne, thus aggravating asthma and sinus problems. The mucus that results provides an excellent breeding ground for bacteria and viruses, giving rise to colds, 'flu and sore throats. The air-conditioners in cars, trains, coaches and planes are diabolical. Turn them off wherever possible or at least train the jet stream away from you. If positioned directly on the body this jet stream causes significant chilling and is one of the main reasons people don't overcome their asthma, colds, 'flu and sore throats.

Summer colds, 'flu and asthma attacks frequently develop as a result of swimming in the afternoon. Cool on-shore winds always blow in from the sea in the afternoon and those who don't thoroughly towel themselves dry the moment they come out of the water are prone to chills. Swim in the morning only (no on-shore winds—see Chapter 16, 'Scientific explanations—Viral infections') or in sheltered home swimming pools. All asthma sufferers should wear a wetsuit vest while swimming and should not stay in too long. Watch out for the afternoon southerlies, get out of the water the moment they hit.

The big problem with colds and 'flu is that they produce mucus which, in the horizontal position during sleep, drains down the back of the throat and into the windpipe causing asthma attacks. Broken sleep results and this in turn fatigues the body making it hard to get the body's resistance up to the point where it can kill the cold or 'flu virus. This is why colds or 'flu must be nipped in the bud with adequate bed rest, adequate wholesome food, a complete multi-vitamin and mineral supplement and a cold remedy recommended by your doctor.

Remember: Cold feet cause a reflex chill through the rest of the body. Wear socks to bed in winter so that your feet are kept warm when you get up. Don't wear open sandals or thongs on winter days.

Around 70 per cent of body heat is lost through the head (heat rises). Don't leave the house with damp hair. Wear a hat or beanie on cold days. Put on a thick dressing gown even if you shower first thing. The thirty to sixty seconds between getting out of bed and under the hot shower is enough to chill you. Chilling also reduces the white blood cells' candida-killing ability.

ASTHMA TREATMENT PROGRAM

On no account attempt to treat asthma by yourself. You must always seek the guidance of a doctor or other health professional. Use only the skin sensitivity test, RAST test and cytotoxic food test to determine the specific allergens that are causing your asthma. Although you must be off all cortisone and antihistamines for seven days before the tests, you must remain on a Ventolin inhaler and any of the other non-cortisone/non-antihistamine drugs the doctor chooses to put you on. Although you must eat as wide a variety of foods as possible before the tests you are not to eat any of those you suspect would harm you. Write them down instead and give the list to your doctor or naturopath. He or she will take these foods into account while preparing your anti-allergy program.

- Read and follow the instructions laid down in Chapter 5, 'How to cure your allergies'.
- Keep warm. In winter always wear woollen crew and polo neck jumpers whether you perspire in them or not. Always wear shoes and socks. Don't surf or swim in winter even in a wetsuit. In summer, dry off the moment you come out of the water. Sitting wet on the sand allows summer sea breezes to chill you. Many summer colds, 'flu, and asthma attacks develop this way. If going out at night in winter wear a fleecy lined vest under your shirt or blouse and button it up to the neck. Wear a coat and scarf to and from the function. In summer always carry a crew neck cotton pullover with you. Most southerly busters come through in the late afternoon or early evening. Don't jog, play tennis or train at sports such as football, karate or judo on cold nights unless you are in an adequately heated building. Study the section on colds and 'flu and act on the advice therein.
- Start taking draughts seriously. Close all windows and doors at night and through the day if you are sitting around in winter. Maintain an even body temperature. Heat all the rooms in the house. Hop out of bed straight into warm slippers and dressing gown. Don't hop in and out of a warm car without a pullover. Don't be fooled by sunny days in winter, they are invariably accompanied by cold winds. Wear a beanie to football matches.
- Regularly spray a section of the carpet with dust mite spray so the kids have a dust free area to play in and the adults a dust free area for exercising. No lying face down on the carpet to read or watch TV.
- Practise daily (for ten to fifteen minutes) the deep breathing exercises described in the chapter on stress. These are imperative if the windpipe spasms are to be permanently overcome.
- I have found that the wearing of magnetic necklaces and sleeping on magnetic pillows (available from most medical supply stores) has helped many of my asthma patients achieve a better night's sleep and experience a reduced intensity of asthma attacks. (See Chapter 16, 'Scientific explanations—Water'.)
- If you have the time try to do the mental relaxation exercises described in Chapter 11, 'Stress'. Try to do them once a day for ten minutes.
- See your osteopath or chiropractor for heat massage and ma-

nipulation to the vertebrae between your shoulderblades. Have this treatment on a regular basis while the programs are taking effect and any time in the future that you feel you are tightening up in that area.

- A good acupuncturist is invaluable for maintenance prevention of asthma when all other healing modalities are being adhered to. Often it can reduce an acute attack. Sitting reading or watching TV while leaning back against a hot water bottle (between the shoulderblades) is very effective. The heat stimulates acupuncture points on the back that are specifics for asthma. Use the hot water bottle every night for the time you are on the program.
- Hot water with a couple of drops of eucalyptus oil in it provides an excellent inhalant vapour during acute attacks but must be used in addition to your doctor-prescribed medication, not in place of it and only by those not allergic to salicylates.
- You must give up smoking and live in a smoke free environment if you are to cure yourself of asthma. Other people smoking in the house means you will only experience temporary relief at best. Contrary to popular belief smoking marijuana does not help asthma, it makes it worse.
- Although asthma is often the result of direct contact with airborne allergens such as moulds, pollens and grasses, the removal of mould and fermented foods as well as grass and pollen foods (Ryvita, porridge, muesli and bread, alfalfa, barley, herbal teas) from the program does much to reduce the sensitivity to direct contact with these substances. The vitamins and minerals taken in supplementary form strengthen the walls of the windpipe raising their resistance to airborne allergens.
- Never blow your nose on paper tissues or wipe your face or hands with paper towels. The chemicals in these products (mainly formaldehyde) are easily inhaled as are the flakes of paper. Both the chemicals and paper flakes are toxic and can perpetuate allergic reactions in the windpipe.
- Do not clean or scrub (particularly mould in the shower recess). The formaldehyde in the cleaning agents could give you an asthma attack. Dusting and vacuuming creates airborne mould and will further exacerbate your asthma. Have someone else do it while you are not in the house.
- Do not have flowers in the house. The pollen will cause your allergies to flare up.

Remember: Although asthma is not normally a life-threatening disease the imprudent withdrawal of asthma medication can, under certain circumstances, lead to suffocation and death. Don't withdraw from any medication without your doctor's permission and supervision. Although the majority of asthma sufferers are able to enjoy complete freedom from symptoms without the use of drugs, some aren't. Some still need to use some drugs to keep their symptoms 100 per cent at bay. As a safety precaution always keep a Ventolin puffer handy. Life is unpredictable and, even though you haven't had an attack for a while, a sudden chill or drenching, especially if you're overweight or have a cold or sore throat, could trigger one.

Frequent long-term use of asthma medication, especially the cortisone puffers, can see the body building a resistance to it. The dietary/natural treatment of asthma builds up the body's resistance to this condition which sees the need for medication significantly reduced. This ensures its efficacy, particularly in times of emergency. The records show that many of those who have died from asthma failed to respond to their medication during a time of stress that caused a more severe than normal attack. Over-medication, coupled with vitamin and mineral deficiencies, had lowered their immune vitality. However, in my experience, those in this category who stick strictly to the Anti-Candida/Anti-Allergy Program for ninety days are able to get by comfortably on significantly reduced quantities of asthma medication.

SKIN PROBLEMS

The common skin complaints of eczema, hives, rosacea, psoriasis and acne can all be caused by allergy and are amenable to the treatment program described in Chapter 5.

Of all skin conditions caused by allergy and candida, acne is the most likely to be complicated by bacterial infection. If the red acne bumps have yellow heads then they have been infected by the bacterium *Corynebacterium acnes*.

The best way to tackle *C. acnes* is to raise the bacteria-killing power of the white blood cells. You can do this by:

- eating three balanced meals per day as set out in the Metabolism-Balancing Program or, if applicable, the Anti-Candida Program or the combined Anti-Candida/Anti-Allergy Program;
- taking a good multi-vitamin and mineral formula that contains the six essential minerals (calcium, magnesium, potassium, zinc, iron and manganese, plus hydrochloric acid to facilitate absorption);
- significantly reducing stress levels by doing the deep breath-

ing exercises described in the chapter on stress and, if you have time, the mental relaxation exercises as well;
• getting adequate sleep—'beauty' sleep is no myth.

If *C. acnes* is proving to be very resistant to the white blood cells, nature's own antibiotic, garlic, can be used to help kill the bacterium. The odourless garlic capsules are just as effective as the raw garlic and five to six capsules should be taken directly after breakfast. (See the shopping list in Chapter 14.)

Antibiotics should be avoided, wherever possible, as they aggravate candida yeast infections (see Chapter 4, 'Candida albicans') which in turn aggravates the allergic condition that gives rise to acne. In the long-term antibiotics aggravate acne, even though initially they reduce the intensity of it.

The only exception to this rule is in those stubborn cases that have not responded to the combination Anti-Candida/Anti-Allergy Program. If, after six to seven months of sticking strictly to the program, and vitamin and mineral supplements, Nystatin or garlic as well as getting adequate rest and sleep and significantly reducing stress you are still experiencing outbreaks of red bumps with yellow (pussy) heads, antibiotics may be used. However, you must continue to take the vitamins, minerals, Nystatin/garlic and *Lactobacillus acidophilus* tablets to prevent aggravation of the yeast infection. At this point a short course of antibiotics is usually enough to get rid of the problem.

Don't confuse flat, red blotches under the skin with acne lesions. These are acne scars and will fade in time. If you are taking a good multi-vitamin and mineral formula containing the six essential minerals the scars will fade a lot more quickly. Be patient, scars can take up to twelve months to fade.

If after six to seven months of sticking strictly to everything, including the short course of antibiotics, you are still getting red bumps (minus the yellow heads) breaking out you are more than likely allergic to something you are eating or are significantly stressed. Check yourself for allergies again by going back to your allergist for a second lot of allergy tests and reassess your stress levels.

Squeezing acne pimples produces more of them. When you squeeze a pimple only a small portion of it emerges through the top of the bump. The rest is pushed down into the skin where it spreads out and causes new areas of inflammation. These new inflammations spring up as new acne bumps. Leave pimples alone. Remember, if you kill one by squeezing it, four or five will come to its funeral and despite sticking to your program and resting you will never get rid of your acne.

STRESS

Stress will significantly aggravate acne (see Chapter 11, 'Stress'). Inflammatory emotions and feelings such as anger, resentment, hostility, rage, fury, embarrassment and frustration, especially if they are bottled up and not expressed, will inflame the skin. If these feelings are intense they cause antidromic (aberrant and reverse) nerve impulses to pour down the sensory nerves from the brain to the skin. When these antidromic nerve impulses arrive at the skin they cause the ends of the sensory nerves to release a chemical called 'neurokinin'. Neurokinin is a potent inflamer of the skin. While it is in the skin, diets won't work. Any existing skin condition, be it acne, eczema, psoriasis, rosacea, hives, dermatitis, urticaria, itchiness or flushing will be aggravated by neurokinin. (See Chapter 16, 'Scientific explanations—Stress'.)

PUBERTY

Puberty sees the release of the male sex hormone testosterone into the blood. Testosterone can cause the sebaceous glands to become so over-active they swell and burst. Bursting sebaceous glands are a major cause of acne in teenage boys as they have much more testosterone in their blood than girls. As boys reach their twenties, their testosterone-producing glands begin to settle down and less testosterone is released into the blood. As a result, their acne begins to clear up.

Although excess testosterone is the main cause of acne in teenage boys, I have found they still respond well to anti-candida and anti-allergy treatment. The appropriate programs can reduce the acne by as much as 90 per cent and in some cases even clear it up completely before they reach their twenties. This indicates to me that allergy and candida factors must also be involved. A complete multi-vitamin and mineral tablet is imperative as the minerals (especially zinc) are needed to strengthen the walls of the sebaceous glands and reduce the chances of them bursting.

In adult males and females, allergy, candida yeast infection, stress and sometimes an over-active thyroid gland are the major causes of acne. Stress causes the release of testosterone from the adrenal glands. Prolonged stress (especially over-work, over-exercise, over-commitment, over-socialising and the anxiety of knowing one has acne) can produce sufficient testosterone in the blood of adults to activate acne by the sebaceous gland mode.

In girls, the female sex hormone progesterone is released from the ovaries into the blood at puberty. Progesterone encourages the growth of candida yeast infections, the root cause of most allergies. Acne in girls tends to respond faster to the anti-candida and anti-allergy treatment than it does in boys as their acne bumps tend to be caused by allergies and candida only and are not complicated by the bursting of sebaceous glands, unless they are significantly stressed. The contraceptive pill frequently aggravates acne in girls and adult women if the pill being used is high in progesterone. Make-up and skin care products can aggravate acne especially when applied over a pimple that is open or weeping. Open pimples allow direct passage of skin preparations into the blood of the skin where they cause allergic reactions. All skin care products are designed to make contact with the skin only. They are not designed to make contact with the blood.

HOW TO CURE SKIN PROBLEMS

- Read and follow the instructions listed in Chapter 5, 'How to cure your allergies'—read the whole chapter.
- Consult a competent beauty therapist, one who specialises in skin care rather than cosmetician work. She will advise you on what cleansers, toners and moisturisers are best for you. Inform her of the allergies you have (for example, yeast, tomato, etc.) and make sure these substances are not included in the skin preparations you use. The products she recommends will have the correct pH balance for your skin.
- It is preferable not to wash the affected areas with soap and water. Soap has an alkaline pH which neutralises the skin's natural acid pH. The acid pH exists to keep viral, fungal and bacterial colonies on the skin as small as possible, thus reducing skin infections. If the use of soap and water is absolutely unavoidable you must dab a mixture of apple cider vinegar and water on your skin straight after to restore the natural acidity. Don't dab the mixture on broken pimples.
- Use cortisone cream on eczema while the program is taking effect. Keeping the inflammation down this way will reduce stress and neurokinin. As time passes you'll find you're using less of it less frequently and eventually not at all.
- If after all of this your skin is still not 100 per cent better see a Chinese herbalist. Make sure you find a good one. Phone my office for a referral if you can't. Chinese herbs get the best results when the body is well nourished on vitamin/mineral supplements, is candida-free and allergy desensitised by the Anti Candida/Anti-Allergy Program. Using the herbs too early can cause allergic reactions in those sensitive to grasses and see a return of the skin complaint after discontinuation of the herbs.

Toddlers, who are too young to go on restrictive diets, are the exception. Keep them on the herbs and a broad spectrum of foods until they're old enough (age four up) and big enough to go on the Anti-Candida/Anti-Allergy Program.

ANNE—ECZEMA AND ACNE

Anne (15) is a typical example of how the combined effect of histamine and neurokinin can cause inflammation of the skin.

Anne came to see me about an itchy eczema and red bumps that had the appearance of small pimples. She had the puffy dark rings (fluid retention) under her eyes that so many allergy sufferers have and suffered from periodic itching and stuffy nose.

Anne had a serious, somewhat intense personality. She was a worrier and tended to exaggerate and 'awfulise' life situations. Her skin condition was an emotional trauma and she was desperate to get rid of it. She was depressed by the fact that so far nothing had worked—she felt let down by medical science.

I gleaned all this at the first consultation and as the school formal and end of year exams were close decided to hold off starting the combined Anti-Candida/Anti-Allergy Program until the stress of these events had abated. The end of the year formal was causing significant excitement and concern which would cause Anne's skin to flare up and down in accordance with her moods.

Within three weeks on the combined Anti-Candida/Anti-Allergy Program (she was allergic to malt, oats, peanuts, capsicum, tomato, rye and all fermented foods) her eczema was completely gone. Only the little nerve bumps remained, giving her skin a mildly clogged appearance.

As her attitude was contributing to her problem Anne began reading the necessary books to help change her attitude and lower her stress levels. Along with the mental relaxation exercises (see Chapter 11, 'Stress') the changes in attitude began to reduce the level of neurokinin in her skin and the acne type bumps began to reduce in size and number. So effective was this regimen that her skin remained 80 per cent clear even when she broke her program a couple of times while on school camp. Tiffs with her parents were the only thing that would now cause the skin to flare up. Anne was at that difficult stage in a young person's life where the need for closeness and support of parents conflicts with the growing need for some independence, space and distance from them. She would complain to me about parental restrictions and it was obvious they frustrated and angered her.

At this stage breaks away from her parents would see the skin clear up 100 per cent, only to return slightly when she made contact with them again.

By working on her attitude, tiffs with her mother have become less numerous and communication with her father has improved.

Although Anne periodically experiences outbreaks of the pimply bumps she has technically overcome her allergy. The rash has cleared up. Because neurokinin is a substance that is generated by intense emotions and not by allergenic substances floating in the blood the inflammatory reaction it produces is technically not an allergic one.

On last contact Anne was doing really well. The rash was no longer bothering her and the pimply bumps only appear when she is upset or sleeping on a mattress and pillow that does not have a dust mite cover (she's allergic to dust mites as well).

Anne is a good example of the power of the mind over the body and how thoughts and feelings can change the chemistry and metabolism of it.

Some allergic people find that eating the things they are allergic to while tired or under stress (tired adrenal glands—see Chapter 11, 'Stress') can cause them to react to their former allergenic foods and bring back the histamine rash. This has happened to Anne a number of times yet when having a fun time in restaurants relaxing with her friends she can eat what she likes and not experience a break-out of her skin.

ATTITUDE AND ITS AFFECT ON SKIN PROBLEMS

To successfully overcome the emotional stress caused by acne, eczema, psoriasis and hives, one's attitude must be right. The big problem with skin complaints is that their visibility is a constant reminder of their existence and most owners of the skin complaints are constantly worrying about what others think when they see their skin. This in turn leads to feelings of anxiety, frustration and resentment on the part of the owner who invariably adopts the attitude of 'Why me? It's not fair! Life shouldn't treat me like this.' Such self talk leads to feelings of anger which often progress to hostility and rage as time goes by. These emotions only exacerbate the acne, eczema, psoriasis and hives by causing the antidromic nerve impulses to pour down the sensory nerves and release neurokinin into the skin.

The great truth that owners of skin complaints have to accept is that fully 95 per cent of people who look at them don't even notice their skin. They probably see it but it doesn't register in their brain because they are too busy thinking about themselves. Those who are aware of the skin complaint's existence would be so for less than a few seconds because they're not interested enough in others and their afflictions to let it be an issue with them. Very few people care that much. Fact.

The fact is that most people hold themselves and their own well-being at the centre of their attention. They are the centre of their own little universe and most expect to be the centre of other people's attention and universe as well, which is one reason conflicts arise in human relationships. This attitude is held by all those who worry about the opinions others hold about their skin. They are so self-centred they automatically assume that everyone else is noticing and thinking about them when, in fact, they're not.

This begs the question: If no one else is getting upset because you have a skin complaint, why should you? The fact is, the happiest, healthiest and most relaxed people are those who realise they are not the centre of the universe, have accepted that, and are happy with less attention.

These people tend to be outer rather than inner centred, meaning their focus in life is on their studies, hobbies, sports, friends, work, pets, family, art, music, nature, science or whatever outside interest they have, rather than on themselves and how others perceive them. Their waking hours and a good measure of their sleeping hours are taken up with thinking about all those interesting things they are involved in and/or the pursuit of their own particular goal which, in their case, is not attention seeking. (See Chapter 16, 'Scientific explanations—Stress'.)

This attitude to life shows on their face and skin. They are of healthy colour with relaxed facial muscles, an easy relaxed smile and clear skin. The attention seekers, conversely, tend to be more uptight, highly strung and, if they are the dramatic type as well, possessed of acne, eczema, rosacea or psoriasis.

Anyone can learn to be more self-contained, self-reliant and independent of the opinions of others by regularly talking themselves out of it and by forcibly stopping their attention-seeking habits (boasting, pouting, comparing ourselves with others, ranting, raving are all attention-seeking habits). To help this process along it pays to get some interests (studies, hobbies or sports) to focus on.

If you are suffering from eczema or psoriasis it pays to use the cortisone cream while the program and change of attitude are taking effect. It is easier to get yourself off centre stage if you're not having to look at a complaining skin each day. While the inflammation is down, your anxiety levels are down and while they are down the neurokinin levels are down.

If you have acne talk to your doctor about taking the drug Roaccutane while your program and change of attitude are taking effect. Roaccutane helps to shrink over-excited sebaceous glands and is very effective at reducing acne.

Some women find the pill helps. The oestrogen negates the acne-producing testosterone that the stress of looking at acne has put in their blood each day. The pill only works if it's low in progesterone and candida infections have to be contained by ninety days on the Anti-Candida/Anti-Allergy Program.

By using the drugs and program together you are enjoying the best of what medicine and naturopathy have to offer and that is the way it should be. As the program and change of thinking begin to take effect you can begin to wean yourself off the drugs (under your doctor's supervision). For eczema, psoriasis, rosacea and acne sufferers this tends to be an automatic thing as you will find your skin is flaring up less and less and without realising it, the time span between cream applications is getting greater and greater.

The deep breathing exercises (see Chapter 11, 'Stress') are excellent for quietening down the skin, especially for the dramatic types who tend to over-react to all of life's little antagonisms in a fiery and vociferous way. The dramatic types tend to awfulise life situations more vigorously than others and must learn to moderate their reactions. They blow things out of all proportion, making mountains out of mole hills and creating storms in teacups. Nothing flares up the skin quicker than dramatic over-reaction to life's events or the things others say and do. And although dramatic types tend to flare up and forget quickly, the neurokinin lingers in the skin for some time after.

The smouldering resenters are at the other end of the spectrum. They are just as intense as the dramatic type but keep everything inside and just fume and boil quietly. A skin complaint is usually the only evidence of their inner turmoil. Learning to be more philosophical about life and the things people say and do is the big challenge for smouldering resenters. Learning to forgive will quieten their skin down more quickly than anything. (See Chapter 16, 'Scientific explanations—Stress'.)

Shy people can experience a flare-up of their skin complaint because shy people embarrass easily and blush when they do so. Embarrassment is the inability to retaliate or find an appropriate answer to a challenge be it real or imagined. Assertiveness classes are the answer for the easily embarrassed as well as making a concerted effort to expand their vocabulary and learn to use it. Joining a debating society has done wonders for many of my formerly shy patients. It was the practice of debating that took the famous playwright George Bernard Shaw from an inarticulate introvert to the very articulate and entertaining extrovert he came to be. Doing the things we fear is the best way of overcoming our fear and embarrassment.

The following books have helped many of my patients who once suffered from skin complaints:

Your Erroneous Zones, by Dr Wayne Dyer.
Pulling Your Own Strings, by Dr Wayne Dyer.
Staying Rational in an Irrational World, by Dr Michael E. Bernard.
A New Guide to Rational Living, by Albert Ellis and Robert Harper.
See 'Bibliography' for publication details.

AM I MISSING OUT BY SETTLING FOR LESS ATTENTION?

Certainly not. Inordinate attention is like heroin, cocaine, alcohol or dope. The more you get, the more you want, as the temporary lift it gives you becomes shorter each time. One only has to look at how many high profile sports people, business people and performing artists turn to drugs, alcohol and suicide when their popularity and recognition are on the wane. Is the going up worth the coming down? The sad, neurotic state of these people indicates great unhappiness with their lot—memories of the going up don't seem to be buoying their spirits now. Attention seekers are always insecure as they never know how long they can sustain the interest of others. Insecure people are anxious and anxiety flares up skin complaints.

Attention seekers seldom develop close, emotionally nourishing friendships and relationships because they are so busy seeking they don't have time to give. A lack of meaningful friendships adds to their loneliness and insecurity. All human beings need some attention. Wanting too much is being greedy and greed always comes back on us in the end. How much is too much? Worrying to the point of distress about the opinions others hold of us is an indication we are wanting too much.

WHAT ABOUT MALEVOLENCE AND SARCASM?

If somebody makes a hurtful and sarcastic remark about your skin take it as a compliment because that is what it actually is. To evoke such a remark from someone means you have evoked enough interest for them to put you at the centre of their attention, which means at that point in time they consider you to be more important than they are. So bad skin notwithstanding there is something about you that is appealing. The best way to handle these situations is to keep your dignity, ignore the remark and keep away from that person. These people are (1) attention seekers who are annoyed that they are not getting enough attention from you to boost their own ego, advance their career, justify their existence or whatever. They are not worth being around as they will sap your vitality over time. (2) They are poor communicators. People are poor communicators for many reasons which we won't go into. Suffice to say, it's heavy going being around them and you just don't need that. Poor communication is a sign of immaturity. Kids will often punch or insult someone they fancy as they lack the more sophisticated communication skills and confidence that comes with age and maturity.

Malicious gossip and rumours about you or your skin are also a tremendous compliment. You really must be an interesting person if people are going to that much trouble. Enjoy it while it lasts. Hollywood stars and starlets work over-time to keep rumours and gossip about them alive, so aware are they of its complimentary value.

If you are lucky enough to have someone question you or make a remark about your skin be careful of the way you interpret it. The majority of those who are outer centred enough to make an issue of your skin would be genuinely concerned. Don't interpret what they say negatively, this will only incite anger and aggravate the skin. Be thankful they have taken the time to notice, hear them out, answer their questions and thank them for their advice even if you know it's wrong. Be thankful that someone out there cares enough to actually say something to you about it. Such people are few and far between. A negative response to this type of overture indicates shyness and lack of confidence. Best you join toastmasters and/or a debating society now.

Remember: There's an up side and a down side to everything. The up side to having a skin problem is that you have had the issue of inordinate attention seeking brought to your notice and have been able to avoid falling into its trap forever. You have had the opportunity of recognising and removing malevolent, poor communicators from your life. You have learnt more about diet and health than you otherwise would have. The spin-off effects from this in terms of health and happiness will significantly raise your levels of well-being.

Humility will set you free. Most importantly you have embarked on this treatment regime to achieve optimum health for yourself and to take advantage of the wonderful opportunity for growth and development it offers. You have not embarked on it to win the approval of others.

My observation is that adversity causes personal growth. This is nowhere more clearly demonstrated than in those who cure themselves of skin complaints and other allergy symptoms. These people all have one thing in common. They view their problem as

117

a challenge rather than an affliction. Instead of bemoaning the fact that they have it, they get excited at the prospect of overcoming it. They make a project out of curing their skin complaint/allergy and work as diligently and patiently at it as they would any other project. They acknowledge the great truth that the best way out of a difficulty is through it. In my experience, the only people who fail to get well are those who give up. Those who persist will always win in the end. In the words of Honoré de Balzac: 'All human power is a compound of time and patience.' And Benjamin Disraeli said: 'Adversity makes a man wise. There is no education like adversity.'

THE IMPORTANCE OF FLUID

Nothing will aggravate any skin complaint more than a lack of fluid (see Chapter 10, 'The importance of water and oxygen' and Chapter 16, 'Scientific explanations—Water'). Eczema and psoriasis in particular become dry, irritable and angry when insufficient fluid is being consumed. The programs in this book, deep breathing exercises and mental relaxation exercises have little effect when there is insufficient fluid intake. Adequate water is needed to maintain a balanced metabolism of the skin cells. The skin is considered to be the least important organ of the body so when fluid intake is down the body withdraws fluid from the skin. It does this (1) to slow down fluid loss by evaporation and (2) to keep the essential organs of brain, liver, heart, lung, kidneys optimally hydrated and fully functional.

Make sure you are drinking enough fluid to feed the skin after the essential organs' needs are satisfied (see Chapter 13, 'The Metabolism-Balancing Program'). Remember, if you're inconsistent with your fluid intake your skin will flare up immediately as body fluid levels can drop easily and quickly from hour to hour. They need constant topping up. A skin that was looking good in the morning can be red, dry and angry by mid-afternoon if you have been too busy to drink through the day. This often happens to people who are out shopping or driving around (for example, company representatives) without air-conditioning, on a hot day. It happens to kids who don't take bottled water or fruit juice to school with them, with strict instructions to drink it all. Kids cannot be relied on to drink adequately from the bubblers at school.

REDUCING STRESS

All skin complaint owners must practise the deep breathing exercises described in the chapter on stress for at least ten minutes, though preferably fifteen to twenty minutes, each day. They can be done all at once or morning and afternoon. If you have time, do the mental relaxation exercises as well, though the deep breathing is priority one.

Some people like to do the deep breathing at one part of the day and the mental relaxation exercises at the other, rather than doing the mental relaxation exercises straight after the breathing. That's fine. Do whatever is most comfortable for you.

Follow closely all the stress-reducing instructions laid down in the chapter on stress. Chilling is a stress. Keep all affected areas warm and, where possible, covered in winter. Chilling causes the body to withdraw blood from the skin and hold it in the centre core to conserve body heat. You cannot heal skin without a good blood supply to it. Keep the body at an even, warm temperature. (See section on asthma, colds and 'flu earlier in this chapter.)

IS IT REALLY THAT BAD?

This section would not be complete if I were not to mention that the great majority of the acne, eczema, psoriasis, rosacea and itchy rash sufferers I have treated have had a girlfriend, boyfriend or spouse in the waiting room indicating there is no lack of love in their life. And when I look back on my own teenage (acne) years I have to admit that it was I who had trouble talking to the girls not the other way around. I allowed myself to be so immobilised by some pimples on my face, I could not respond to Marcia Green's overtures. Clearly my skin wasn't a problem to Marcia and if I'd had the wisdom to focus on my good points I would have been much happier.

Looking back, my acne-induced shyness was just a big waste of time and I'm sure Marcia would have told me so if only I'd given her the chance. As a result of my attitude, some other lucky bloke swooped on Marcia and I was left to ponder what I was missing.

PSORIASIS

Coachaline is a cream used by equestrians to condition their saddles and other leather riding gear. Rubbed in, it keeps the leather in excellent condition. Rubbing it on psoriasis helps too. Coachaline contains minerals and trace elements needed by the skin to help it heal itself and rebuild deteriorating tissue. The dry, scaly patches of psoriasis are the result of mineral-deficient dead and damaged tissue. Rubbing Coachaline on your psoriasis patches morning and night helps speed the healing effect of the program and is not as far fetched as it probably sounds. Leather, when all is said and done, is skin. Coachaline is available at any saddle shop but is not to be applied to open wounds, weeping wounds or cuts. Check with your doctor if in doubt.

Limited exposure to the sun stimulates new skin growth and speeds the healing of psoriasis but only if you drink extra fluid to offset that lost by the increased evaporation exposure to the sun causes. Too much sun makes psoriasis worse. If your doctor wants to send you to ultra-violet radiation treatment, go with it. Make sure you increase your fluid intake while under that treatment.

Although the main cause of psoriasis is allergy there is a definite vitamin and mineral deficiency factor involved. So in addition to the supplements recommended on the Anti-Candida and Metabolism-Balancing Programs, add the following:

1 × 20 mg beta-carotene tablet
1 × 500 mg L-cysteine tablet
2 × 1000 mg lecithin tablets
2 × 50 mcg selenium tablets (script from doctor, obtain from chemist)
Increase the evening primrose oil capsules to 6 × 1000 mg and the MaxEPA to 4 × 1000 mg and have 1 teaspoon of linseed oil (Melrose brand is best)

NAIL POLISH

Believe it or not, nail polish can be the reason your skin is breaking out randomly despite sticking to the programs, drinking sufficiently and doing the breathing and mental relaxation exercises. Nail polish contains many toxic chemicals, formaldehyde being the principal one. When we are busy concentrating we tend to hold our chin or put our fingers somewhere else near our mouth. The heat from our breath causes a liquefying and vaporising of the chemicals in the nail polish and when we touch the other areas of our face, as we frequently do while concentrating at work or studies, these liquefied chemicals cause a localised inflammation of the skin. Because face touching is such a subconscious thing, I recommend no nail polish until the skin is completely healed.

MAKE-UP

It goes without saying that you must be very careful with make-up, foundations and skin care ranges; also mascara and eyeshadow. Some people are so sensitive they have to stop using them completely during the period of treatment. Touching the eyes, as so many people do when concentrating, can cause mascara to run or to adhere to the finger. Touching the face with the mascara can cause the skin to flare up at the point of contact. Touching the eyes with vaporised nail polish can cause conjunctivitis in the eye touched (bloodshot, itching and weeping). All these symptoms occur at a time when all the other symptoms of allergy are disappearing in response to the program.

A LAST WORD ON NEUROKININ

Neurokinin can so effectively inflame the skin it can lead you to believe the program isn't working when in fact it is. Looking at your skin complaint can, if you let it, get you so upset and angry that the skin immediately reddens and can stay inflamed for as long as you allow yourself to remain angry. Even dwelling on your skin without even looking at it can perpetuate the reddening to the point that you feel the program simply isn't working for you and you give up on it. Don't fall into this trap. Be on your guard against it.

Similarly, if your skin oscillates randomly between good and bad despite sticking strictly to the program don't automatically assume you have suddenly developed an allergy to something in the diet and begin to eliminate food on a trial and error basis. Take a look at your attitude: Are you getting angry, frustrated or embarrassed about your skin?

Neurokinin is as powerful as histamine at inflaming the skin. One has only to look at the skin of those who do not have skin complaints to see evidence of this. The ruddiness of the angry person and the hot, prickly blush of the embarrassed person are the results of neurokinin. When this redness is added to the existing redness of histamine-based eczema, psoriasis, acne, hives, rosacea, these conditions are perpetuated long after the Anti-Candida/Anti-Allergy Program has removed all histamine from the skin.

The use of anti-inflammatory drugs (cortisone creams, Roaccutane, even antihistamines) can reduce the inflammation while the programs are working and, in so doing, reduce the stress that causes the release of the neurokinin. Don't let neurokinin beat you. Don't let it trick you into giving up your program.

ARTHRITIS

Arthritis means inflammation of the joints. It can be caused by physical and/or metabolic factors. The cumulative effects of wear and tear due to over-work, over-exercise and over-weight can inflame the joints in those who are over forty. Nature does her best to protect and strengthen over-worked joints by laying down extra fibrous tissue over and around them. Unfortunately, fibrous tissue has a tendency to contract over time leaving the joints concerned stiff and sore. Even an excess of immobility can cause this fibrosis of the joints. The best treatment for this type of arthritis is light exercise, such as yoga, Tai Chi, walking or swimming, and regular visits to the osteopath or chiropractor to have the joints gently mobilised and manipulated. This treatment stretches and breaks the fibrous tissue giving relief of pain and greater mobility to the joint. Because fibrous tissue joins up again at the point of severance, regular light exercise and periodic manipulations for the rest of your life are necessary to keep the condition at bay.

Painkillers and anti-inflammatory drugs are not very effective at reducing the pain and stiffness of this type of arthritis, which frequently affects housewives in the fingers, athletes in the knees and ankles, bricklayers in the lower back and sedentary people who carry a bit of weight.

Metabolic arthritis results from imbalances in the body's metabolism caused by poor nutrition, an under-active thyroid gland, allergies, Candida albicans infections, auto-immune aberrations, serious bacterial or viral infections or a combination of two or more of the above. Most metabolic arthritis has allergy or candida yeast infection as its principal cause.

I have found that 70 per cent of the people I treat for joint pain and stiffness and/or muscle pain have a sensitivity to the nightshade group of plants. This sensitivity can exist despite the fact that no definitive allergy to any of the nightshades shows up on the cytotoxic food test.

The only feasible explanation I can come up with is that the chemical solanine that occurs naturally in the nightshade plants irritates the tissues of the joints and muscles.

Solanine is a potent poison preservative which accounts for the long shelf life of the nightshade foods. Fungi and bacteria don't readily decompose them. They tend to stay away as too much contact with them causes their own poisoning.

Those who have a sluggish liver find that the chemical-neutralising effect of such a liver is somewhat limited and those chemicals that should normally be broken down by the liver have the opportunity to spill out into the general circulation and cause toxic inflammation. Solanine is one chemical that is often not neutralised when the liver is under-functioning.

The chemical-neutralising capacity of the liver is significantly reduced when there is an excess of fat and alcohol in the diet and a deficiency of vitamins, minerals and oxygen. I have found time and again that the chemical-neutralising capacity of the liver is significantly increased when the Metabolism-Balancing Program and regular exercise in the fresh air are taken up and the deep breathing exercises are practised daily.

The nightshades include: potatoes, tomatoes, tobacco (smoking must be given up), paprika, cayenne, chilli, red and green peppers, eggplants and belladonna. An important part of the treatment of arthritis is the removal of this food group from the diet.

NUTRITION

Nutrition is very important in the treatment of arthritis. It ensures the reconstruction of damaged joint tissue. In his book, *Nutrition Against Disease*, Dr R. J. Williams (University of Texas) notes that many arthritis sufferers are deficient in vitamins A, B3, B5, B6, folic acid, vitamins C and D and minerals zinc, manganese and sulfur proteins. (The best sources of sulfur proteins are red meats, fish, poultry and eggs. Milk, cheese and yoghurt have reasonable amounts and garlic and onions are the best vegetable sources, though yielding far less than animal sources.)

The metabolic imbalances that result from these deficiencies lead to a structural weakness in the soft tissues of the joints (cartilage, capsule, ligaments and blood vessels).

Structural weakness of tissue leads to the regular leaking of blood into the joint, so that even moderate use causes bleeding. Regular bleeding into the joint causes the levels of iron to build up in the joint, while at the same time the levels in the blood drop, predisposing you to anaemia.

Deficiencies in the mineral zinc cause the blood levels of copper to rise, the excess of which also spills into the arthritic joints. Copper and iron excesses cause as much joint irritation as allergens, acetaldehyde from candida infections and the night-shades.

The minerals zinc and manganese displace excess copper and iron in the joints while at the same time normalising their levels in the blood. Taking a high dosage multi-vitamin and mineral tablet has other advantages:

- The full spectrum of vitamins and minerals increases the effect of zinc and manganese.
- Structural damage in the joint is repaired.
- Structural weakness in the joints is overcome.
- 100 mg of vitamin B3 and 1000 mg of vitamin C taken three times per day with meals will increase joint mobility, decrease stiffness and relieve joint deformity and pain, according to Dr William Kaufman, who pioneered this treatment in 1941.
- Fish oils (cod liver, halibut, etc.) are not only rich in the vitamins A and D needed to repair damaged joints, they have a natural anti-inflammatory component that helps relieve joint pain.

REST AND RECREATION

Eating in a hurry, hurrying off after a meal or working hard after a meal will ensure you don't digest and absorb that meal properly. The joints will not receive the minerals they need in sufficient quantity to normalise their metabolism and repair themselves.

Sit down after the main meal of the day, put your feet up and listen to music, read a book, have a relaxing chat or watch some TV. Unwind, take it easy, let your food digest and give your joints a rest. Eight hours' sleep a night isn't enough to allow joint regeneration, you need rest and recreation as well. Recreation means exactly that—re-creation—a time to create new tissue out of old. (See Chapter 16, 'Scientific explanations—Stress'.)

If you are the hard-charger, over-achiever type that always has to be doing something constructive and sees sitting around as a waste of time just remember there is nothing more constructive than making new body tissues. This principal applies equally to sufferers of skin complaints and asthma.

HOW TO CURE ARTHRITIS

- Read and follow the instructions laid down in Chapter 5, 'How to cure your allergies'.
- Be patient. It takes up to twelve months to remove all excess copper and iron from arthritic joints and to completely repair tissue damage. However, you'll be progressing all the time and should feel significantly better in five or six months. If you are one of those people who get dramatic results in the first month or so make sure you continue with the program. To break it will only see the problem return.
- Wash your daily multi-vitamin and mineral supplements down with a small amount of juice or water with one level teaspoon of vitamin C powder in it. Add also, twice only per week, one drop only of Lugol's iodine solution, using an eye dropper. The iodine is available from your chemist. As it is an old remedy, the younger pharmacists don't usually know how to mix it up. Go to a mature age chemist. Iodine, along with vitamin C powder and the multi-vitamins and minerals will help normalise the action of the thyroid gland. This is important as thyroid gland under-activity can cause the formation of a thick jelly-like substance (mucin) in the joints. This causes the joints to swell and when they swell they become stiff and painful.
- If, after six months of sticking strictly to the program, resting and following all the other instructions in this section, your joints are not reducing in size, pain and stiffness you most likely have an under-active thyroid gland. The best way to test for this is to take your under-arm temperature first thing in the morning on waking. Put the thermometer under your arm and lie perfectly still for ten minutes. Do not sit up or move around prior to the test as this will raise your basal temperature. Shake the thermometer down the night before. On waking reach out for it

without sitting up. Ladies, take your temperature on the morning of the second and third days of your period only. Body temperature varies up and down through the cycle. If you have reached menopause, start testing any time of the month and continue it over a two-day period. If your temperature is below 36.6°C (97.8°F) you almost certainly have an under-active thyroid gland. Ask your doctor to prescribe 0.1 mg daily of Oroxine and if in six to seven weeks the joints are still not improving take another 0.1 mg per day. This will usually do the trick though sometimes it takes 0.3–0.4 mg per day. As the oroxine begins to improve the function of the gland you will be able to reduce the dosage. The standard blood tests for thyroid under-activity are no good for diagnosing arthritis or those glands that are mildly under-active.

- Keep your doctor or naturopath informed.
- Take at least one teaspoon of codliver or halibut oil per day.
- Consult a good osteopath or chiropractor to make sure there is no fibrous tissue component to your problem and if there is follow his advice.
- Make sure your fluid intake is adequate. The synovial fluid that lubricates joints is made from water. Joints can dry up and become stiff and sore when water intake is sub-optimum.
- Do the deep breathing exercises every day. Deep breathing feeds oxygen to the joints and muscles around the joints. The joints repair themselves faster and the muscles around the joints relax, reducing joint pain and stiffness.
- Pineapples and paw paw contain enzymes that have a natural anti-inflammatory affect on arthritic joints. Eat plenty of these if you are not allergic to them and you have completed the first four weeks of the Anti-Candida Program.
- The green-lipped mussel is a potent anti-inflammatory and pain-killer that is a specific for arthritis. It's available as an extract in Sea Tone tablets available from your health store.

7.

Heart attacks and high blood pressure

'Thy food shall be thy remedy.'

Hippocrates, 500 BC

There is little doubt that high levels of fat and cholesterol in the blood contribute to heart attacks. Fats (known technically as lipids) and cholesterol can build up on the walls of any given artery to the point where blood flow is stopped. If this happens to the arteries that feed the heart the heart stops beating and we die of a heart attack.

WHY DO CHOLESTEROL AND FAT STICK TO THE ARTERY WALLS?

Over the years a number of theories have gained acceptance only to be challenged by other theories. For the last twenty years the experts have agreed that the smooth inner lining of the artery becomes damaged and that passing fat, cholesterol and blood platelets stick to the damaged roughened section of artery lining forming a little bump. Over time more and more passing fat, cholesterol and blood platelets stick to the little bump that is growing on the artery wall and the bump continues to grow until it blocks the artery off.

There's no clear consensus on the exact causes of artery wall injury. Cigarette smoke, high levels of fat and haemodynamic stress have all been mooted and there's every possibility that all can be involved.

126

THE ALLERGY FACTOR

In my twenty-two years of clinical practice I've noticed a direct correlation between allergy, heart and circulatory impairment in most of the people I've treated for heart-related problems. The research of leading allergists corroborates my own observations.

The allergic reaction involves the release of histamine by the tiny red blood cells known as the blood platelets. Histamine makes the blood vessel walls more permeable which allows the leakage of fluid and protein substances from them into the surrounding tissue. This fluid in the tissues gives rise to the swelling that accompanies allergic reactions. Over time an excess of histamine can cause tissue damage if it's continually released into a given area. It's highly probable that in some people artery-lining damage is caused this way. (See Chapter 2, 'Allergies', for a full description of histamine's effect.)

The experts also agree that the artery walls, for some reason, become permeable to fat and cholesterol. Fat and cholesterol get in behind the artery lining pushing it out into the hollow centre of the artery. This little bump with its roughened (damaged) surface makes an ideal fat and cholesterol trap—catching more of both as they pass. The more fat and cholesterol there is in the blood the easier it is to catch some and so build the little bump up. The further the bump pushes out into the hollow of the artery the easier it is to trap passing fat and cholesterol. So the bigger the bump grows the faster it grows.

The little blood platelets that release the histamine are very sticky by nature and many of them collide with and stick to the bump as well. Platelets love to clump together. Indeed one of their roles is to form clots (clumps) to prevent bleeding from damaged blood vessel walls. Perceiving the artery lining as damaged they willingly form a clot around the roughened area (and/or developing bump) which only adds to the size and stickiness of it.

To lower the fat/cholesterol levels of the blood is only part of the story. Stopping blood platelets releasing histamine at a given area is the only thing that is going to stop those same platelets forming a clot around the area of roughened artery lining. By continuing to damage the tissue around it the bump continues to grow in length and width as well as depth.

As dramatic as this sounds it must be remembered that the body is very tough and its powers of regeneration excellent. For this reason it takes years for lumps (atheromas) to grow to artery-blocking proportions.

There's no doubt the allergy factor is the reason some people still die from heart attack despite being on strict anti-cholesterol diets.

THE METABOLISM-BALANCING PROGRAM

Balancing the metabolism with the Metabolism-Balancing Program, combined with deep breathing and mental relaxation exercises, is the best way to begin any treatment regime for heart attack. There are a number of reasons for this:

1. People with the typical Type A personality, who are ambitious, aggressive, bustling, impatient and short-tempered, have high cholesterol levels. (See Chapter 16, 'Scientific explanations—Cholesterol—Stress', and also Chapter 11, 'Stress—Stress and the hard-charger'.)
2. Those with late onset diabetes or the beginnings of it have higher cholesterol. (See Chapter 16, 'Scientific explanations—Cholesterol and salt'.)

The Type A personality can produce metabolic imbalances by the power of thought (attitudes). Diabetes is the result of a significantly unbalanced metabolism. Attempting to lower cholesterol with a drastically strict diet in either of those situations only adds to the stress levels and metabolic imbalance of the one in question. Results are mediocre to say the least.

HIGH BLOOD PRESSURE

Allergies can cause muscles to go into spasm. A muscle spasm (often referred to as a cramp) causes the muscle fibres to contract and remain in a contracted state. Muscles can remain in spasm for as long as an allergenic substance (food, chemical, drink, pollen, mould) is irritating them. The walls of all the arteries are made up of three layers of circular muscles and if they spasm (cramp) the shortening of their fibres causes the circumference of the artery to reduce. This causes the circumference of the hollow centre (called the lumen) of the artery to reduce. Because there's no concomitant reduction in the volume of the blood passing through the artery the narrowing of its hollow centre compresses the blood, thus raising the blood pressure in the artery.

Removing the offending allergens from the diet and environment sees an immediate relaxation (expansion) of the tight artery muscles and an increase in the size of the hollow. The blood pressure drops accordingly.

Blood pressure can return to normal quickly and dramatically when allergies are treated, which is why you must always treat them under a doctor's supervision. If you're on blood-pressure-lowering drugs the pressure can come down too quickly and even drop below normal if your doctor isn't monitoring your progress and reducing the drugs appropriately.

Don't take yourself off blood pressure drugs because artery muscle spasm may not be the only cause of your blood pressure problem. There may be atheromas, kidney problems, carbon dioxide excess and/or hardened arteries as well. If these exist you won't improve as quickly as I've indicated. It'll take longer and you'll need to keep taking the drugs, weaning yourself off them slowly as you improve.

The heart is a muscle and is as prone to spasm as any other muscle. Some cases of diagnosed angina are the result of the cramping pain of a heart muscle in spasm. Removing the allergens sees the disappearance of the pain as well as the return of a strong regular heartbeat. People with allergy-based high blood pressure usually have headaches as well. The tendency to focus their allergies into the muscles sees these people with tight back, neck and scalp muscles. Tension in these particular muscle groups produces tension headaches that can endure for prolonged periods of time. The recurrence of tension headaches in allergenic people occurs often if their allergies are not treated by the methods outlined in this book.

OXYGEN STARVATION

If the levels of oxygen in the muscles and blood drop too low, the muscles go into spasm. This includes the muscles of the artery walls and the heart. Muscle spasm occurs because a deficiency in oxygen significantly slows muscle cell metabolism. Shallow (clavicular) breathing is the main reason for oxygen deficiency/carbon dioxide build-up and is often caused by allergies that restrict breathing (asthma, hayfever, sinusitis). Like allergies, excess carbon dioxide irritates muscles, predisposing them to spasm.

Deep breathing helps relax all the muscles of the body including the heart and blood vessel muscles and is an integral part of any blood-pressure-lowering regime. (See Chapter 10, 'The Importance of water and oxygen'; Chapter 11, 'Stress—Deep breathing exercises'; the section on 'Deep breathing and the metabolism' in Chapter 16, 'Scientific explanations—The metabolism'; and Chapter 16, 'Scientific explanations—Oxygen and carbon dioxide—Stress'.)

TREATMENT

Read and act on the advice in Chapter 5, 'How to cure your allergies'. Don't go off any medication. Get your doctor to supervise the treatment program.

8.
Glue ear
(Slow learning and bad behaviour in children)

'No illness which can be treated by diet should be treated by any other means.'

Moses Maimonide
Great twelfth-century physician

Where there is a definite link between glue ear, slow learning and bad behaviour (especially in kids) it's usually not a clear cut one. Not all those who have glue ear are badly behaved or slow in learning and not all slow learners have glue ear—some are just bored witless with their studies and don't absorb them for that reason. Bad behaviour is, of course, a grey area. What is considered bad behaviour by one person is not necessarily considered bad by another. And what is considered bad behaviour one day is not necessarily considered bad the next, such are the vicissitudes of human perception. However there are certain parameters by which most people would measure bad behaviour and it is in this context that bad behaviour will be described in this text. It must be remembered that tiredness due to overdoing it, dehydration, insufficient rest and sleep can make kids so tired as to be very antisocial. Before looking for any other reasons for bad behaviour consider the possibility your child may simply be over-tired. A good way to determine this is to compare behaviour after a day at school to a day on the weekend when a drink and a rest were taken in the middle of the day.

GLUE EAR

Glue ear is becoming increasingly more common. So common that it has given rise to a slang name for novice surfers on the Northern

Beaches of Sydney. They are known as 'grommets', after the little plastic tubes so often inserted through the eardrums of sufferers to restore hearing. Dr George Shambough, Professor Emeritus of Otolaryngology at North Western University in the USA, claims the insertion of plastic ventilation tubes is the most frequent surgical procedure undertaken with anaesthesia today.

Glue ear results from a build-up of mucus and other fluid behind the eardrum. This warm, stagnant pool is a breeding ground for bugs and the ear infection otitis media often results. The effect of antibiotics on such infection is limited, with recurring infection being the big problem. As any parent knows the pain and tinnitus (constant ringing) of ear infections can contribute to irritability, headaches and fatigue from sleepless nights in both children and parents.

Whereas there's no denying that plastic tubes ease the discomfort by balancing the air pressure on either side of the eardrum there is a better way: a change of diet. My treatment of glue ear has been overwhelmingly successful—dietary treatment addresses the cause of the problem rather than the effect.

Glue ear results from a build-up of mucus in the nose and throat due to colds, 'flu, allergies and candida infections. Slowly the mucus drains from these areas down the eustacian tube to the inside of the ear where it dams up against the eardrum, reducing the ability to hear. Most of this draining takes place during sleep where the combined effects of prolonged mouth breathing (which tends to dilate the oral opening of the eustacian tube) and the side lying position favour the drainage of mucus to the eardrum.

The unfortunate thing is that many of the kids with glue ear are never diagnosed. This is because they have only low grade allergies and colds that go unnoticed. Because these kids are only mildly afflicted they tend not to exhibit the overt allergy, candida and cold symptoms of sneezing, runny or stuffy nose. The raised body temperature that accompanies daily activities dilates their nasal passages sufficiently to facilitate normal breathing. It's only at night when they're asleep and their body temperature drops do they commence the mouth breathing that aids the flow of mucus to the ear and dries out the throat, leaving it prone to infection.

These are the kids who fall behind in class because they can't hear properly. Because their glue ear has never been diagnosed they are often labelled 'a bit dumb' by the other kids and 'uncooperative, rebellious, lazy and given to dumb insolence' by the teachers. Kids with this level of glue ear who are lucky enough to sit at the front of the class tend to get by. It's the ones sitting further back who miss out. The introverts tend to cope by withdrawing further into themselves while the extroverts respond by venting their frustrations in the form of overt attention seeking, disruption of others in class and fighting in the playground. Because this low grade glue ear doesn't lead to headaches or noticeable ear infections the way full-blown glue ear does, these kids muddle their way through school in the the belief they are not as intelligent as the others.

They seldom mention to their parents the fact they're having trouble hearing in class because they don't realise they are. Because they know no different they think their level of hearing is perfectly normal. Unlike their counterparts who have all the symptoms of full-blown glue ear and receive help these kids/adults struggle through life never reaching their full potential and never really knowing why.

As parents, uncles, aunts, friends, teachers and godparents its our duty to keep our eyes open for these kids and to get them into treatment as soon as possible. Often the only give-away signs are below average intellectual performance at school (comprehension, maths, writing, English) associated with one or more of the following:

- dark rings under the eyes;
- below average physical co-ordination;
- below average ball-handling skills (they are the last to be chosen when picking sides for football, netball, cricket);
- the habit of rubbing the nose with the palm of the hand (nasal salute);
- complaining of an itchy nose (as opposed to a runny or stuffy nose);
- the tendency to fatigue easily (wants to lie down or sit and watch TV after school; often tired on waking);
- a transverse ridge or crease in the nose (due to constant nasal saluting);
- shy, quiet, daydreamy personality; seems to be in his/her own world; appears switched off and doesn't always respond when called or spoken to; has trouble getting started on things; gives up easily (introverts);
- aggressive, stroppy personality; low frustration tolerance; can't concentrate; loud; won't listen; often ignores (extroverts).

TREATMENT

Glue ear responds well to six to eight weeks on the Metabolism-Balancing Program and supplements (Formula Six, codliver oil, evening primrose oil, vitamin C). During this time the energy levels and resistance to disease rise to the point where low grade smouldering allergies, candida, colds and 'flu are often totally contained. (Low resistance to disease has vitamin/mineral deficiency as its main cause.) The demeanour changes, schoolwork improves and more often than not the under seventeens go into a growth spurt. With no more mucus being produced the ears soon clear themselves of the mucus that has accumulated as the little hairs (cilia) in the ears sweep it back down the eustacian tube from whence it came. Mucus arriving back in the throat can cause a short-lived mild healing crisis until it is all expectorated.

Because lowered resistance is the root cause of glue ear the sufferer must stay on the Metabolism-Balancing Program and supplements for the rest of his/her life with only a minimum (5 per cent or less) of junk food. Those who require the Anti-Candida/Anti-Allergy Program to cure their glue ear will return to the Metabolism-Balancing Program when the anti-allergy treatment is completed. It goes without saying that the normal procedures for keeping the body at an even warm body temperature must be followed if any of the programs are to work. The procedures are detailed in Chapter 6, 'Asthma, skin problems, arthritis'.

A sub-optimum fluid intake is one reason the programs won't work. Even borderline dehydration will keep the body's resistance low despite faithful adherence to the Metabolism-Balancing Program and the supplements. Make sure the full measure of fluid included in the program is consumed (see Chapter 10, 'The Importance of water and oxygen').

If either low-grade or full-blown glue ear is not showing signs of reducing after four to six weeks on the Metabolism-Balancing Program, Formula Six and other supplements you can be sure that allergies and/or candida infections are the principal causes. If this applies to you read Chapter 5 carefully and follow the step-by-step procedure for treating allergies and candida yeast infection. If after four to six weeks on the Metabolism-Balancing Program and supplements you are showing improvement keep the program going until the improvement level plateaus or the symptoms disappear completely.

As the case histories in this chapter reveal, most kids respond well to the Metabolism-Balancing Program and supplements alone. Those who have to progress to the full Anti-Candida/Anti-Allergy Program find that those last remaining symptoms are cleared away in ninety days. The disappearance of all the symptoms is associated with improved annunciation as well as a rapidly expanding vocabulary as hearing becomes unmuffled for the first time. I've received many phone calls and letters from excited parents who are witnessing these changes for the first time. Some call me on talkback radio to let as many people know as possible––such is their desire for others to have this rewarding experience.

133

BRAIN ALLERGIES

Not all slow learning and bad behaviour is the result of hearing that's distorted by glue ear. I've treated many young people for behavioural and learning problems who didn't have it, yet these kids were suffering from the same low resistance allergy and candida problems as their glue ear counterparts.

WHY IS THIS SO?

It's because we're all biochemically unique and express our allergies, candida infections and lowered resistance (vitamin and mineral deficiency) in different ways. In the case of glue ear sufferers the tissue targeted by the allergy or infection is the mucous membrane of the nose and throat. In those who have learning disorders but no behavioural or hearing problems the areas of the brain that facilitate learning are affected. In those cases where behaviour is bad but learning and hearing are not affected only those areas of the brain that govern the way we emote, act and react are affected. Sometimes the nose, throat, behavioural and learning centres of the brain are affected simultaneously.

HOW DOES THIS HAPPEN?

The exact biochemical processes have not as yet been detailed. What is known is that in the case of allergies, candida and viral and bacterial infections the target tissue is inflamed. Inflamed tissues anywhere in the body always function abnormally and often unpredictably. In the case of glue ear the mucous membranes of the nose become inflamed and function abnormally by producing more of their protective mucus covering than is needed.

Instead of the mucus draining forward (as it normally does) to give the predictable symptoms of a runny or stuffy nose that makes colds and allergies easy to diagnose, it drains backwards down the eustacian tube giving rise to a clutch of seemingly unrelated symptoms. The affected tissues in the brain also function abnormally.

In the case of learning and behavioural disorders the picture is further complicated by the fact that vitamin and mineral deficiencies often exist, affecting the production of special brain chemicals called *neurotransmitters*. These are vital for thought integration, physical co-ordination, verbal articulation and elevated mood. (See Chapter 16, 'Scientific explanations—Food and mood'.)

THE DISCOVERY

My introduction to the link between food, mood and learning came by way of treating kids for colds, 'flu and allergies. Time and again parents would remark to me that in addition to their colds and allergies clearing up their child was more sociable and was getting better marks in exams. This was supported by reports from teachers that the child was trying harder and had a better attitude to work. At first I explained this as the result of less time off school and less physical discomfort giving rise to less distraction. But still time and again parents would insist the changes were so profound there had to be more to it. In time I decided to find out for myself and advertised for parents to volunteer their children for an experiment to determine the link between food, mood and learning. Fifteen children took part in the experiment, the full details of which will appear in a future book.

THE EXPERIMENT

To summarise, all the children were slow learning under-achievers. Some of them were, to varying degrees antisocial. Some had definitive glue ear, some had suspected low-grade glue ear, some didn't appear to have any glue ear. All of the children commenced their treatment regime by remaining on their normal everyday diet with the addition of Formula Six multi-vitamin and mineral supplement. As the following case histories indicate some were able to overcome their problems by the addition of Formula Six to their program and some had to embark on the full Anti-Candida/Anti-Allergy regime to get a desirable result.

Space unfortunately precludes a detailed explanation of each child though the following notes will give you some idea of how successful the programs and Formula Six were.

Each child was subjected to before and after aptitude and intelligence tests by two independent educational psychologists––one tested language, writing skills and English comprehension, the other tested mathematics. Their progress was monitored by their parents and schoolteachers on a day-to-day basis, and by me once a month. Both psychologists submitted written reports on their findings.

DENA (10)

On vitamins only (Formula Six)—no anti-allergy treatment.
Dena's case is very interesting as she was found to be suffering from a low-grade glandular fever that had gone undiagnosed for some time. My experience with treating slow learners and under-achievers has taught me that the vitality-sapping effects of low-grade (your doctor will refer to it as sub-clinical) glandular fever is often the cause of slow learning and under-achieving. These low-grade glandular fevers can drag on for years undiagnosed. It's not surprising then that so many adults are suffering from chronic

fatigue syndrome (CFS). The Epstein Barr virus that is involved in many of the cases of CFS also causes glandular fever. The only way to beat glandular fever, as with any viral infection, is to rest, drink plenty of fluid, breathe deeply using the lower lobes of the lungs and take supplementary vitamins and minerals along with a well-balanced diet.

Dena was put on Formula Six only and responded quickly. Her immune vitality rose dramatically and in no time she had fought off the low-grade glandular fever. After four weeks her mother reported that her energy and inquisitiveness had increased significantly, she questioned things a lot more and surprised her mother by choosing to read the advanced and more detailed books her older (Grade 7) sister was reading. At her monthly spelling test she got only eight words wrong out of ninety-five, a major breakthrough. Her artistic skills had improved, with neater writing and better drawings.

Her before and after assessment by the educational psychologist were summarised as follows:

11 July 1988—age 9 years 3 months—Grade 5. Comments: 'Dena is currently functioning at a Grade 4 level in mathematics.'

Nine months later the same assessment which included the Wechsler Intelligence Scale for Children (Short Form), the Woodcock Johnson Mathematical Calculation Test and the Basic Arithmetic Screening Test, were summarised as follows: Comments: 'The mathematical tests indicate that Dena has made significant improvement over the last nine months, she is now functioning up to age and grade levels.'

Dena is a typical example of what modern-day diet and living habits are doing to so many. The borderline malnutrition Dena was suffering from lowered her resistance enough for her to contract a low grade glandular fever but not enough to catch a full-blown, easily diagnosed glandular fever. The addition of the Formula Six multi-vitamin and mineral tablet to her everyday diet got rid of her glandular fever, giving her the energy to cope with life. I shudder to think how many other borderline malnourished kids there are. Without the addition of dietary supplements these kids will struggle through life denied the chance to reach their full potential as human beings.

PETER (17–18)

Peter's case is particularly interesting as it illustrates what a sudden and dramatic effect allergy can have on brain and mind function.

Peter's before and after psychological assessments revealed him to be of above average intelligence. He was assessed with the

Webster Adult Intelligence Scale—Revised—Short Form, the ACER Higher Test (WQ) (Mathematical Reasoning) and the APU Arithmetic Test.

Peter's problem was that his performance at school and his test results waxed and waned erratically. Because of this he was labelled as 'having ability but lazy and erratic' by his teachers. This wasn't a surprising assessment as he could get 90 per cent in a maths test one day and 20 per cent the next. He could write a lucid and imaginative essay one day and nonsense the next. His maths tutor eventually told his mother (Jan) that she didn't believe he'd ever learn and that it was a waste of money having him coached as she just couldn't get through to him.

Jan was unconvinced, for her own observations had revealed a direct correlation between Peter's performance and food. Each night after the evening meal Peter's father would sit down to help him with his physics and maths and sure enough one night Peter could do the problems and another he couldn't. What was most exasperating for his father was that on an 'off' night he couldn't do the problems he was able to solve earlier on an 'on' night. Jan noticed that his 'off' nights coincided with the eating of spaghetti bolognese for the evening meal. She applied to enter Peter in the program and was accepted.

Peter's history revealed a lifetime of allergies. Asthma since age two. Glue ear, ear, nose and throat and adenoid infections, which required antibiotics, every six months. He'd been on antihistamine for his almost continuous stuffy nose.

As Peter had been on multi-vitamins for quite a while prior to seeing me, and as the case was so pressing, I sent him for allergy tests immediately. Sure enough he showed up allergic to beef, tomatoes, malt, milk, cocoa, mould, house dust, dust mites, mosquitoes and mixed grasses. Beef and tomatoes are the major ingredients of spaghetti bolognese and malt and milk were to be found in the particular pasta Jan used.

On the Anti-Candida/Anti-Allergy Program and Formula Six results came quickly. His energy levels rose, the acne on his skin began to clear, he felt he had greater clarity of thought and he was more relaxed before tests. After one month Nystatin powder was added and he made a further leap forward from that point going from 23 per cent for physics in his HSC trials to 54 per cent in the final exams. Such an improvement on Nystatin indicated a candida infection had resulted from his childhood and that this infection aggravated his allergies.

After ninety days Peter was allowed to break the program. This coincided with the Christmas holidays. In the new year Peter sat an entrance exam to engineering school and scored 94 per cent in technical drawing, which included mathematics and 82 per cent for physics, which also included maths.

The fact that Peter was able to score such a hitherto unobtainable result after three months' holiday, during which time he did not study, is exciting. It shows that ninety days on the program enabled him to completely desensitise himself to the foods he was previously allergic to and that his candida infection had remained under control.

Although Peter's allergies didn't affect (inflame) that part of his brain that alters mood he was still labelled unco-operative by his schoolteachers and tutors who interpreted his inability to maintain a consistent work performance as rebelliousness. Peter's nature, even during the height of his allergies, was easygoing and congenial, though at times he exhibited frustration at his inability to maintain an even work standard. Had he not received treatment he would have struggled through life as an intelligent yet frustrated under-achiever. A lack of self-confidence and poor self-esteem would have dogged him for the duration of an unfulfilling life.

Time and space does not permit a detailing of all the young people on the program. The testing procedures, treatment regimes and step-by-step progress reports of the students will be detailed in another publication some time in the future.

Comments from the parents, educational psychologists and teachers of other children on the program are as follows:

AARON (12)

Minimal brain dysfunction—on vitamins (Formula Six) and anti-allergy treatment.

Mother's report: 'Gets As and Bs for effort more instead of Cs and Ds. Can feel the difference when he misses taking the vitamins (Formula Six). Grown up and out—more mature, confident, happy, relaxed and settled. Can concentrate better and keep up with dictation.'

Teacher's report: 'Improved approach and application to schoolwork. Healthier; better appetite, colour, skin, hair and energy; more relaxed before exams and better marks than when on antihistamines (prescribed by doctor).'

BEN (12)

On vitamins (Formula Six) only—no anti-allergy treatment.

Comments on final Educational Report from consultant psychologist who assessed Ben via the Woodcock Johnson Mathematics Test and the Basic Number Screening Test (Form B): 'The standardised tests indicate that Ben has made significant improvement over the past nine months. He is now functioning above his age level.'

Mother's report: 'Coping better all round, more enthusiastic, doesn't have to be pushed to do homework. Doesn't get upset at the prospect of having to do it. Doesn't get as upset if he can't do it. Can sit for an hour or so without whingeing. Is more motivated and wants to try learning to spell more words at a time. Absorbing his work. Remembering his times tables for longer. He's trimmed down, lost puffiness and improved muscle tone. Maths test marks are up in sixties as opposed to forties previously. He's keen to attempt problem solving and is getting the problems right where as before he'd be too frustrated to attempt them.'

Ben was able to overcome his allergy by raising his resistance with the vitamins.

SOPHIE (12)

On vitamins (Formula Six) only—no anti-allergy treatment yet.
Mother's report: 'After four weeks appetite has improved and cravings for sweets has gone. Moods seem to have been improved.'

After twelve weeks: 'Has improved dramatically, has gone from being unconfident to someone who is really excelling. Test marks have improved significantly. Gone from middle of the pack to close to top of the class. Tried out for swimming team which is something she would never have tried before. Gone from being negative, niggly, irritable, unco-operative to a positive person.'

Sophie is still on the program and will be sent for allergy tests soon as she still has the allergic shiners around her eyes and a few symptoms of upper respiratory tract allergies. Sophie presented with a long history of ear, nose and throat infections which affected her hearing. She had her first antibiotic at age six weeks and had been off and on them ever since.

Sophie is a good example of how supplementing the program with vitamins and minerals can so raise the body's resistance to allergies and yeast infections that they can be significantly contained. As a result Sophie will test allergic to significantly less factors than she would had she gone for the tests at the onset. This means her Anti-Allergy Program will be far less restrictive. This is good because (1) it'll be easier to stick to and (2) it'll be more nutritious, which is what she needs given that she's entering the growth spurt.

VIMILA (13)

On vitamins only (Formula Six)—no anti-allergy treatment yet.
Like Sophie, Vimila is still on the program and, like Sophie, had made similar strides forward. However at the end of the twelfth

week which coincided with the end of term her mother reported that she had slipped back to being tired, disorganised and lacking concentration. Yet she hadn't stopped taking the vitamins. Careful questioning revealed that Vimila was feeling so confident, energetic and well within herself she not only applied herself more vigorously to her schoolwork but took on too many extra-curricula activities—swimming, piano and flute—and literally burnt herself out in one term. The symptoms that were originally caused by allergies and vitamin and mineral deficiency were now being perpetuated by fatigue.

Although Vimila suffers from night sweats (classic allergy symptom) I can't send her for allergy tests until her energy levels are back up to where they were. Low energy means low resistance which means she'll show up allergic to more things.

It's most important that new found energy not be spent as soon as it is attained. Many people, children and adults alike, make the mistake of burning up their new found energy as quickly as they get it. This temptation must be resisted otherwise the treatment program will fail. To achieve long-term good health we must build up an energy reserve. Energy is the currency of life, just as money is the currency of business. To have a healthy business you must keep some money in the bank. To have a healthy body you must keep some energy in reserve. Don't be an energy spendthrift.

Because my particular program was designed to help kids improve their lot in life it was not structured as an analytical measure of intelligence. There were no control groups to provide a comparison because I felt no slow learning, under-achieving child should be denied help and used as a guinea pig to prove or disprove some intellectual theory. Because of this it can be argued that my study is not a scientific measure of the link between diet and intelligence and I accept that. What it did prove though is the link between diet and improved performance on all levels and I'm happy to say all those young people on the program who were once headed for a life of under-achievement and all the spin-off frustrations and emotional problems that accompany it are now able to realise their full potential. Such an opportunity is the birthright of everyone and it's such a pity that modern day diet and living habits are denying so many this basic right.

It would seem however that in addition to raising our ability to perform, vitamin and mineral supplementation can also raise our intelligence *per se.* In the 23 January 1988 issue of the *Lancet* (one of the leading British medical journals) the results of a double blind study (using placebos) of the link between vitamin/mineral supplements and intelligence can be found. The procedure and conclusions of the study are explained on pages 140–3 and describe how ninety schoolchildren from Darland High School, Rossett, Wrexham, were tested by the Department of Psychology, University College, Swansea. The four page report concludes that the administration of a vitamin/mineral supplement to a group of children on a typically British diet resulted in an increase in their non-verbal intelligence and that the implication of this finding is that dietary deficiencies were hampering neural function in these children.

Since doing my own experiment I've discovered more and more scientific data detailing increases in intelligence by up to 35 points after supplementation with vitamins and minerals. I've also discovered many excellent books describing the link between allergies behaviour and learning. These may be found in the 'Bibliography'.

Despite the stunning improvements in schoolwork and exam results a change of diet can bring, it is not a panacea. Hard work is always needed. There's no substitute for it. Tutoring always has been and always will be a principal component of learning. I recommend the programs in this book as an adjunct to, not an alternative to, remedial tutoring. Sophie's case is a good example of what dietary change and remedial tutoring can achieve. Sophie was being tutored by the Linda Mood Method, a remedial tutoring method for children who've grown up with auditory problems and aren't able to pronounce their words properly. She amazed everybody by completing the twelve month course in four months. In the words of her tutor 'she was a model student'.

THE IMPORTANCE OF FLUID

The great variable in the link between food, mood and learning is the daily intake of fluid. (See Chapter 10, 'The importance of water and oxygen', and Chapter 16, 'Scientific explanations—Water').

The brain is 80 per cent water. All the chemical reactions required to facilitate brain function take place in water. A drop in brain water levels below 80 per cent interferes with the chemical reactions, disrupting our thinking and feeling processes. I've found in my involvement with problem kids that the majority of them don't drink enough or don't spread their fluid intake evenly over the day. Most of them go to school without having consumed any liquid other than the milk on their cereal. A few quick drinks at the bubblers through the day sees them tired, dull and thirsty when they get in from school. At this point they fluid load by drinking three to four glasses of whatever fluid they can get their hands on. The problem here is that they take in more fluid than their body can make use of at one time and although it picks them up its usually after the evening meal before they feel the good effects of it. The correct drinking habits outlined in Chapter 10, 'The importance of water and oxygen', and Chapter 13, 'The Metabolism-Balancing Program', will ensure that the brain is properly hydrated through the day at the time when it is most needed.

JESSICA AND PAUL

Jessica (13—allergic to soya beans, wheat, moulds, tomatoes, malt, honey, peanuts and grasses) and Paul (14—allergic to moulds and all fermented foods, grasses, dust, dust mites, eggs, milk, wheat, beef and almonds) are good examples of just how quickly the removal of allergenic substances from the diet and environment can alter behaviour and improve brain function.

Jessica, although very bright, couldn't concentrate, was the class clown, could be rude to the teachers and wasn't interested in applying herself. Paul was easily distracted and although keen enough complained of not being able to concentrate for more than a few minutes. He had limited assessment skills and had trouble coping with mathematical problems. Both of them suffered from hayfever, sinusitis, itchy red eyes and stuffy noses. Paul was almost a permanent mouth breather.

Within a week on the program Jessica's teachers and parents were reporting a dramatic change in her behaviour and attitude to work. She was interested and studious. Within a month or so she changed her friends and moved into a group who were work orientated. She became happier and started smiling more.

Paul's mother phoned me to say that within four days of being on the program Paul was for the first time able to understand what the teacher was saying. He was feeling more confident and positive about his future.

Both Jessica and Paul are currently on the combined Anti-Candida/Anti-Allergy Program and will be for a month or so yet. After that time their previously allergic foods will be reintroduced one by one. Their respiratory tract problems have improved significantly. Jessica no longer has the sniffs and Paul can breathe through his nose.

So impressed were Jessica's teachers they asked her to give a talk on her program to the fifth and sixth form students. By year's end her schoolwork had improved so dramatically she had moved into the top ten of her class and was doing brilliantly at science, a subject she just hadn't been able to cope with before.

As is often the case in these situations Jessica's family took longer than Jessica to adjust to the changes in her attitude and behaviour. It took some weeks for them to get out of the habit of 'walking on eggs' to use her mother's expression. For a while they were still bracing themselves for vitriolic retorts that were never delivered. Situations, things said, times of the month and questions that would normally cause Jessica to flare up, no longer did and it took some time for the family to get used to this. Most pleasing of all was the dramatic improvement in Jessica's relationship with her father—they stopped fighting.

Jessica is so impressed with the program and the changes she's experienced that she's afraid to go off it. The chances of her reverting back to her old self are highly unlikely as ninety days on the program will allow enough desensitisation to her former allergens to allow a moderate imbibing of them without a return of symptoms.

FINAL RECOMMENDATION

I recommend that all children with adjustment and behavioural problems study and memorise the eight self-enhancing attitudes listed in Chapter 16, 'Scientific explanations—Stress'. Adopting these attitudes as a standard code of behaviour does much to raise frustration tolerance levels and lower stress levels.

Many children who are tired, cranky and irritable after school are dehydrated and sometimes overcome by formaldehyde. (See Chapter 5, 'How to cure your allergies', pages 93–4.) Because everyone gets bad tempered when they are thirsty, parents should not jump to the conclusion that their child has a candida problem or allergies until the possibility of dehydration has been excluded.

Dehydration raises stress levels, particularly in children. If you are unsure whether your child is under-drinking at school, organise for him/her to take a 0.5–1 L (depending on the size of the child) bottle of water or fruit juice to school, with strict instructions to drink it all. I've found that teachers are very co-operative and will check to see that your child alone is consuming the prescribed drink and that it's not being passed around the group. Bottled drinks are necessary as kids get so involved with friends and games at recess that they forget to drink from the bubblers.

Remember: your child's behaviour can be influenced by those she/he mixes with. Hyperactive and aggressive playmates can incite similar behaviour patterns in non-hyperactive, non-agressive children. Pay close attention to who your child is mixing with.

By following the instructions in this chapter there's every chance your child can come off Ritalin or whatever other drug is being used to treat his or her hyperactivity and slow learning.

9.
Chronic fatigue syndrome
(Kids on drugs, broken marriages, reduced productivity)

'His food was glory,
Which was poison to his mind
And peril to his body.'

Sir Henry Taylor, 1800–86

As with any disease there are a number of factors contributing to chronic fatigue syndrome (CFS). CFS sufferers have one or more of the following factors afflicting them:

1. Stress (see Chapter 11, 'Stress').
2. Lack of water and oxygen in the cells (see Chapter 10, 'The importance of water and oxygen').
3. An under-active thyroid gland.
4. Lack of vitamins, minerals, essential fatty acids, protein or carbohydrate in the diet.
5. Candida yeast infection.
6. Allergy.
7. Crummy jobs and crummy relationships that are so unfulfilling they're significantly enervating.
8. Viral infections, hepatitis, glandular fever, AIDS.
9. Tropical and Third-World gut infections like Bali belly, Delhi belly, giardia (blocks absorption of nutrients) or hookworm (causes anaemia). Don't holiday in the tropics, the Third World,

Melanesia or Polynesia (Hawaii is OK as are the islands of the Barrier Reef).

There is no doubt however that candida yeast infection and allergy are the most common causes.

Those suffering from CFS must follow carefully the instructions laid down in Chapter 5, 'How to cure your allergies', and Chapter 11, 'Stress'. Whereas it's true that viruses are the great energy suckers of the body it is invariably allergy and candida infections that allow them to multiply to energy-sucking proportions (see Chapter 16, 'Scientific explanations—Viral infections—Stress'.

EPIDEMIC

CFS, or ME or Epstein Barr virus, as it is otherwise known, is spreading. More and more people are enduring the unrelenting tiredness, depression, muscle pain, joint pain and often headaches and symptoms of fever it brings. This is not surprising given the dramatic increase in allergies since the massive industrialisation that's taken place in the West since World War II. The consumption of sugar and white flour (both of which promote candida yeast infections) has risen dramatically and our air, water, and food has become significantly chemically polluted.

Candida infection promotes our sensitivity to these chemicals which in turn lowers our resistance to the more common allergies of dust, dust mite, moulds, pollens, grasses, cats, dogs, feathers and foods. Often its the chemicals in the foods we're reacting to rather than the foods *per se*. All the evidence suggests that CFS is on the increase in direct line with the increase in the number of allergy sufferers appearing in the statistics. The official allergy sufferer count is 45 per cent of the population, though most doctors and naturopaths agree its closer to 60 per cent.

Most of these allergy sufferers are suffering from varying degrees of CFS. Many of those with mild to moderate CFS didn't even know they had it until their allergies were treated and they experienced a sudden rise in energy levels. They were so used to feeling below par they thought it was normal. Many a time I've had a patient remark to me, 'I had no idea how tired I was,' or, 'Now I've got something to compare it to, I don't know how I got by on my previous energy levels.'

KIDS ON DRUGS

The thing that worries me is the number of allergic kids taking drugs. Getting these kids off drugs is next to impossible if the allergies aren't treated at the same time. I've treated many drug-addicted young people over the years and the usual case history is as follows. As children they had obvious symptoms of allergy but never had them diagnosed. They always felt sick, tired, unwell and often hyped up, though nothing showed up in tests. They spent their childhood being taken from doctor to doctor. Because none of these could hang a definitive diagnosis on them, they were accused of being attention-seeking malingerers looking for excuses to get out of school. Diagnosis is often supported by low achievement at school and varying degrees of antisocial behaviour. The children go through life in a state of quiet desperation, often suffering from depression, which frequently manifests as quarrelsomeness as it is combined with frustration. The children don't know whether the doctors are right or not but know they don't want to feel like this forever.

Feelings of lethargy, low self-esteem, disenchantment and inability to cope leads kids into mood-altering recreational drugs in an attempt to elevate their spirits and physical disposition. Drugs don't prove to be the full answer but do give them temporary respite for the time they're on them. Marijuana is usually the choice of the hyperactive young person (often described as 'hyped up' or 'hypertensive' by them or their parents). Heroin tends to be the choice of those suffering from 'the blues'.

The other scenario is the child who had enough of the commonly recognised symptoms of allergy (sinusitis, hayfever, skin rashes, eczema) for the doctor to prescribe antihistamines. Antihistamines aggravated the symptoms of mental and physical sluggishness which were never associated with allergy by the doctor. A childhood spent on antihistamines has the teenager feeling worse than ever before, not only do they still have their allergies, they have these foreign chemicals in them as well. Drugs are sought as the only way out as 'anything's got to be better than feeling like this'.

It's significant that among the most popular and widely abused drugs of young people are those of the amphetamine family. In these synthetic stimulants so many of today's kids are trying to find the innate vitality of youth that has been denied them by the allergies that afflict them—allergies that have either never been treated or worse than that have been suppressed by potent tranquillising drugs (antihistamines). Kids that have been raised to believe they need synthetic drugs to get through childhood can't be condemned for thinking they need still other synthetic drugs to get them through adulthood. They've been conditioned to think that drug taking is part of normal living and that's a crying shame. Some take amphetamines to boost their energy levels and marijuana to calm their hyperactivity (prolonged hyperactivity brings with it chronic fatigue).

BROKEN MARRIAGES

It's quite frightening just how many broken marriages have their roots in undiagnosed or inappropriately treated allergies. Low energy levels leads to lack of interest in life and inability to cope with the responsibility of raising kids—putting up with their demands, high spirits and noise, and organising them and supervising their school work and social development. Coupled with the erratic mood swings that so many brain allergic people suffer from and often a job which is a stress because the brain allergic person lacks the concentration, memory and organisational capacity to do it easily and you've got someone who's anything but easy to live with.

If both partners and the kids are allergic the situation at home can become intolerable to everyone before too long. The whacky, erratic behaviour of the immune system which causes the allergies is so often mirrored in the whacky, erratic behaviour of the person suffering from the allergies. Being irrational and unreasonable is par for the course for brain allergic people and most people with allergies have some degree of brain allergy. Irrational and unreasonable behaviour puts tremendous strain on any relationship be it familial, conjugal, companion or work related.

Twenty-two years' experience in taking care of allergy sufferers and witnessing the mess allergies have made of so many lives has convinced me that allergies are undermining the very fabric of society. Those who seek relief from their allergies in marijuana become more tired and vaguer than before, making them less able to contribute optimally to society. Those who seek the mood elevation, confidence and optimism boost that heroin provides contribute to the rising crime rate in their efforts to pay for it. They are a burden on both family and society when they are without it and often waste their precious youth in prison because of it.

Some would argue that to blame allergies alone for drug taking and marital breakdown is too simplistic and I agree there is more than one reason a person would turn to drugs or a marriage breaks up. However the major underlying cause in both cases is an inability to cope and if such a person has allergies and has them treated by the dietary method then they will experience a dramatic increase in their ability to cope. This makes it less likely that either condition will arise. (See Chapter 16, 'Scientific explanations—Stress'.)

Many argue that alcohol is a major cause of marital breakdown. I agree with that. Alcohol is the most abused drug of all by adults and is rapidly heading towards number one status with young people as well. Just as the diet of refined, processed, convenience foods created a biological thirst for alcohol in Dr William's rats (see Chapter 2, 'Allergies') the same diet promotes the same biological thirst in humans. Alcohol is a brain and nerve depressant. It greatly aggravates CFS and lowers our ability to cope by using up B vitamin reserves and damaging cells.

One of the great joys of my job is to watch the thirst for alcohol and the appetite for synthetic drugs reduce on the Metabolism-Balancing Program and Formula Six and to witness its complete disappearance after ninety days on the Anti-Candida/Anti-Allergy Program. I've witnessed the remarriage of divorced couples, the coming together of broken families and the launching of new careers when significant changes to diet were made and allergies were cured. Reformed alcoholics lose their cravings for sweets on the programs.

The whole issue of allergies and their effect on society and productivity must be brought out into the open and given serious consideration for it is a serious problem. It is hoped that you will use the information in this book to inform others who you recognise as being allergic and in need of help.

Lack of productivity is inextricably bound up with low energy levels. Tired people are less motivated, less disciplined, less conscientious and less interested than vital people. However, there's more to it than that. Allergies, candida infections and vitamin and mineral deficiencies can affect the brain chemistry in other ways that have far reaching effects on productivity.

Max was a classic example of allergy-based low productivity. Just recently married he felt under great pressure to do well at work and to achieve the promotions and pay increases needed to provide his intended family with the standard of living he desired for them. Max was employed to take orders over the phone for a medium-sized manufacturing firm. He was doing reasonably well until his marriage after which he started making mistakes. These simple mistakes frustrated him greatly and distracted his attention which led to more mistakes. He described to me with pain how he knew he was taking down the orders incorrectly but couldn't seem to do anything about it. His mind was in a muddle. He wrote numbers down backwards and out of sequence. He wrote down messages and orders out of context.

Max's employers had told him to shape up or ship out. I phoned Max's employer requesting a four week stay of dismissal on the promise that I would have Max fully functional in four weeks. The employer agreed. Max went for allergy tests immediately (we didn't have time to do the mandatory six to eight weeks on the Metabolism-Balancing Program first). He went onto the Anti-Candida/Anti-Allergy Program plus Formula Six and the other supplements. Within four weeks, much to his employer's relief and his joy, he had stopped making mistakes. He had acquired energy, good concentration and memory, clarity of thought, mental acuity and a capacity to organise himself he didn't think possible. Job security became assured and promotion a probability.

Max is a good example of how stress can exacerbate allergies. While he was plodding along as a single guy without too many responsibilities he was coping reasonably well. The moment the demands of marriage were upon him he couldn't cope. Many people experience this. They're unaware of their allergies until greater demands to perform are put on them. Max was lucky he gleaned this through marriage. Had he won a promotion the increased mental demands of the new job could well have triggered his mistake-making symptoms and he probably would've lost the job and suffered a significant blow to his self-confidence and self-esteem.

This happens to a lot of people and naturally enough they blame the job as they're unaware of their underlying allergies. Those who are aware they have allergies don't make the connection between their asthma or eczema, or conjunctivitis or sinusitis or acne and their inability to cope with the job. The stress of the new promotion often leads them into drinking, 'to relax'. Whereas alcohol affords some short-term relaxation it soon begins to undermine their performance further. Alcohol burns up precious B vitamins and mineral zinc in the brain, the very nutrients that are essential for effective thought integration. Furthermore alcohol and marijuana (even worse) reduce memory, concentration, organisation skills and the ability to think and plan ahead. They do this via the toxic effect they have on brain cells.

Those with jobs that don't require a lot of in-depth thinking, don't require one to hold many facts and figures in one's head or to be forever thinking of new concepts, are usually unaware of the effects alcohol, marijuana and allergies are having on them.

Some below par performers don't focus their allergies in the brain but are suffering the side effects of the medication they're taking for their sneezing, stuffy nose, asthma or eczema. Antihistamines have a tranquillising effect on the brain and potentiate the action of alcohol. Combined with alcohol, marijuana, speed or any other drug they can turn the taker into a zombie (see Chapter 12, 'Dangers of allergy drugs'). Many people struggle through their whole working life functioning well below their ability because they were never told that a change of diet could rid them of the need for those stupefying drugs.

Not everyone fails to measure up the moment they take on the new job or promotion. Some seem to cope quite well until a major stress such as a bad 'flu or glandular fever or surgical operation grounds them. They emerge from this illness with exacerbated or newly acquired allergies that see them functioning well below par for the rest of their working lives if dietary treatment is not sought.

I remember one very intelligent and imaginative young woman who was the whiz kid of the company think tanks. She enjoyed a drink and by all accounts could put it away. Being young her brain cells were still vital and there were no obvious signs of insidious alcohol damage. However on a trip through Asia she caught hepatitis B from which developed eczema (not a bad case) and a tendency to catch colds easily. What really worried her was that now, although she could still come up with brilliant ideas and hold them in her head while developing them, at the meetings, when under pressure to deliver, they would simply disappear and she couldn't recall them.

At the time of seeing me she was depressed. She was losing her pre-eminence as 'the brains in the place' and her self-confidence and self-esteem were suffering as well. She proved to be (among other things) allergy addicted to yeast and wheat and avoidance of all fermented foods, wheat products and alcohol and the taking of Formula Six saw her capacity to think under pressure return. Realising she was lucky to be young enough to get a second chance she resolved never to touch alcohol again for fear that she'd lose the razor edge of her thinking faculties again.

And there's every chance she would have, for alcohol, over the longer haul, will permanently damage the brain cells in a way that only marijuana can match. Although she liked the effect alcohol had on her and the fun and camaraderie associated with it she decided she wanted the mental stimulation of being good at her job and the rewards of her achievements more. Realising she couldn't have them both she chose what, for her, was the more desirable of the two.

Many people in her situation choose to return to alcohol when they're well and over time regain their allergy addiction to it. (See Chapter 3, 'Allergy addiction'). Some enter the allergy addictive state without experiencing a serious illness but rather through the regular practice of a few drinks after work to relax which eventually leads to the imperative drink at the business lunch and in time to that nip of whisky in their morning coffee that no one knows about. All the time there is an inexorable decline in their productivity which they, for a while, manage to disguise by a series of easily recognised ploys—buck passing being the major one. The problem with alcohol is that in time it damages the brain cells permanently so that the good results from anti-allergy programs are harder to achieve and the incentive to stay on them is reduced.

HOW MUCH IS SAFE?

See the alcohol tables in Chapter 13, 'The Metabolism-Balancing Program', for recommended maximum amounts. Remember that you kill 10 000 brain cells every time you get drunk.

10.
The importance of water and oxygen

'Life is largely a matter of chemistry and physics.'

Scientific axiom

WATER

The human body is made up predominantly of water. Loosely described, we humans are nothing more than hairy, animated bags of salt soup. All the chemical reactions needed to produce heat and energy, to enable us to think, feel, emote, express, see, hear and move, take place in this salty water.

Collectively these chemical reactions make up what's known as our metabolism. To interfere with the body's water levels is to interfere with the chemical reactions and thus unbalance the metabolism (see Chapter 16, 'Scientific explanations—The metabolism—Water').

Falling water levels (dehydration) unbalances the metabolism in three ways:

1. A lack of hydrostatic (water) pressure in the blood vessels means less nutrients (oxygen, vitamins, minerals, protein) are forced out of the blood and into the cells.
2. The cells rely on the water that carried the nutrients in to also flush their waste products out. If waste products lie around in the cell they interfere with normally occurring chemical reactions and so unbalance the metabolism.

151

3. The osmotic pulling power of the blood is reduced and less waste products are drawn from the cells to the blood for elimination through the kidneys.

Optimum fluid intake ensures the process of cell feeding and cell cleaning operate at full capacity. Bathing the cells with water also reduces the concentration of any allergens that may be present in them. Allergens are notorious for gate crashing resident chemical reactions and interfering with their outcome. Diluting allergens also dilute the intensity of the allergic reactions they cause. The chemicals found in polluted water readily invite themselves into chemical reactions that neither want nor need them. Alcohol does too, so effectively in fact that some people slur their words after only one or two drinks.

Drinking chemical free water is imperative for balancing the metabolism. Avoid tap water wherever possible, unless its thoroughly filtered. Country people, who live in areas of top dressing and pesticide spraying zones, should avoid tank water. Fresh spring water (home and office delivered), mineral water from a recognised spa (not the commercially made ones, or soda water) and freshly squeezed juices are ideal.

The programs and dietary supplements in this book cannot balance the metabolism if the water levels are below optimum. Next to oxygen water is the most important nutrient. It is frequently the missing link in an unbalanced metabolism.

A deficiency in water can cause the same vagueness, disorientation and confusion that allergies and candida yeast infections produce. This vagueness, disorientation and confusion is frequently evident in middle and long distance runners who on crossing the finish line can't answer questions coherently, stare blankly at the TV camera and say nothing; or walk off in the wrong direction after the race. These athletes illustrate just how precarious the body's fluid levels are and just how quickly they can fall. One hour of strenuous physical activity can see 1 L of water evaporate from the body.

Fluid must be taken into the body at regular intervals through the day. Busy people tend not to observe this important rule and have patches of vagueness, mistake making, irritability and confusion in the middle of a working day as a result. This can be most disconcerting for people who're on the Metabolism-Balancing Program and are expecting not to experience such things. Those on the Anti-Candida/Anti-Allergy Program tend to blame what they ate for breakfast when this happens and as time goes by take themselves off so many foods they become malnourished. Malnutrition of course can give the same symptoms as fluid deficiency.

There is no excuse for going without fluid through the day. We can all find time to drink fluid, no matter how busy we are. Busy people try to get around this by fluid loading in the morning and fluid loading in the evening. This doesn't work. The harder we work, the more heat we produce; the more heat we produce, the more fluid we evaporate. Fluid levels can drop below optimum within an hour, which is why the aforementioned symptoms can come on so quickly and why we have to keep topping our fluid levels up, all day long. Sip from a bottle at your desk.

BUT I DON'T GET THIRSTY!

Busy people get out of the habit of drinking because they're too involved with other things to be bothered with it. Humans are profound creatures of habit. Busy people (and indeed lazy people) get into the habit of denying the subtle messages of thirst the body sends to the brain. Habitual denial eventually takes them to the point where they no longer hear the messages and can't understand why their bodies are racked with the symptoms of dehydration. In the words of Ovid (90 BC): 'Nothing is stronger than habit.' Keep a full bottle of water on the front seat of the car.

To further aggravate the situation, zinc deficiencies develop in those who don't drink and zinc is needed to activate the appetite and thirst centres in the brain. (Water deficiency = hydrochloric acid in the stomach deficiency = poor zinc absorption = lack of thirst = water deficiency.)

Unfortunately bad drinking habits are often learned early in life. Toddlers who appear to be forever harping on about wanting a drink are frequently misread as being attention seeking. To break this demanding habit the parent will often tell the child to be quiet as they don't need a drink at all. Not surprisingly the child starts to believe this after a while and learns to get by on sub-optimum fluid intake. By the time they're big enough to reach the tap or pour their own drinks from the fridge they're well and truly in the habit of drinking less than they need.

To return to good health we must simply re-educate ourselves back into appropriate drinking habits. We must alter our lifestyle and work habits to accommodate these new drinking habits. Fortunately that doesn't take long and drinking more soon gives you a taste for it. In the words of Pythagorus: 'Choose what is best, habit will soon render it agreeable and easy.'

'But all I seem to do is run to the toilet more?' That's fine. That's the way it's meant to be. Busy and lazy people just have to integrate that into their lifestyle. More regular drinking means better nourishment of cells and better flushing out of waste products, including allergens. More regular visits to the toilet means more toxins are being removed from the body. As you progress with your greater fluid intake you'll notice your visits to the toilet will taper off a bit. This is because improved water intake (especially when combined with the improved vitamin and mineral intake from the programs in this book) raises the metabolic rate. Greater production of heat and energy results, with increased evaporation of water through the skin.

This makes the skin moist, soft and younger looking. Busy people should bear in mind that they're going to be more productive if their metabolic rate is raised and this will more than compensate for time spent visiting the toilet. They'll be making less mistakes and repeating less work.

But I suffer from fluid retention, surely drinking more water will make it worse? No it won't. If anything it might help reduce it.

There are many reasons for fluid retention. One of them is a reduced fluid intake. When fluid is regularly withheld from the body it starts to panic and fearing dehydration begins to release the fluid-retaining hormones. This is an attempt on the part of the body to keep what little fluid it's getting in the body. Building up a reserve of fluid is nature's way of coping with the uncertainty of irregular and inadequate supplies.

When we start drinking greater quantities and more regularly the body soon gets its confidence up. Perceiving a regular and adequate intake of water the body stops secreting the fluid-retaining hormones and stored excesses of fluid are released and pass out of the body as urine.

If you retain fluid (that is, put on weight) on hot days it's a sure sign that you're not drinking enough. Feeling tired, cranky, and unwell on hot days is another. Headaches on hot days is a classic sign of water deficiency and a dry skin is the most obvious of all.

OXYGEN

The air we breathe contains oxygen. Oxygen is the spark of life. Just as a fire can't burn without oxygen our cells can't produce heat and energy without oxygen. Oxygen is extracted from the air we breathe by the lungs. It passes into the blood vessels that surround the lungs and is carried to all the cells of the body by the blood. Most of the oxygen is carried by the red blood cells, though some of it is carried by the water in the blood. A deficiency of water means reduced oxygen delivery by the blood. So important is oxygen, that even where optimum water, protein, vitamin and mineral intake exists, ill health will still exist if there's an oxygen deficiency. Under-breathing is epidemic among adults.

The mechanics of breathing determine oxygen supply. Shallow chest breathing gives rise to oxygen deficiencies, as there are very few blood vessels surrounding the upper lobes of the lungs. Most of the blood vessels surround the lower lobes of the lung. Deep, abdominal breathing is the answer to optimum oxygen levels.

Unfortunately most people breathe shallowly. Tight clothing and a lifetime spent rushing, sitting hunched over desks doing paperwork, studying, working computers and getting stressed out produces the bad habits of shallow breathing. Babies don't chest breathe. Neither do drunks. They're both so relaxed they breathe easily and deeply and their tummies rise and fall to the rhythm of this breathing. Shallow chest breathing is a bad habit we develop as we move towards adulthood. It's a habit that can be easily unlearnt by practising the deep breathing exercises detailed in the chapter on stress and by slowing down.

These exercises are an integral part of the programs in this book and must be practised daily if the programs and increased fluid intake are to be of significant benefit to you.

HYPERVENTILATION

Don't confuse the deep breathing exercises (done slowly and rythmically) with hyperventilation. 'Hyperventilation' means many, rapid, shallow breaths. This often accompanies and frequently causes anxiety, panic attacks and angina. It results in oxygen starvation of the tissues by causing the blood to become too alkaline.

Reduced levels of oxygen trigger the reflex mechanisms of yawning and sighing. Yawning and sighing are nature's ways of forcing us to breathe deeply, in an attempt to raise the blood oxygen levels before they cause metabolic imbalances (see Chapter 16, 'Scientific explanations—The metabolism').

Hyperventilation is, in many ways, a misnomer, for although it draws in more air than normal breathing, the rapid in-out shallow-ness of its action means that less oxygen is taken up by the blood.

Also known as 'over-breathing', hyperventilation is, in fact, 'under-breathing'. It causes serious acid/alkaline imbalances in the blood (see Chapter 16, 'Scientific explanations—Oxygen and carbon dioxide').

Water is important because we are made of it (see Chapter 16, 'Scientific explanations—Water'). Oxygen is important because we run on it. Under-drinking and under-breathing are epidemic and create metabolic imbalances that are stresses to the body. Stress can inflame mild (even asymptomatic) allergies into full-blown, troublesome ones.

11.
Stress

Hans Selye MD, *The Stress of Life,* 1978

Stress can trigger allergies. Most people who develop allergies in adult life do so after a sudden, significant stress or a build-up of lesser stresses over a period of time. Allergies often develop after such stresses as a bad case of 'flu, glandular fever, hepatitis, a surgical operation, pregnancy or termination of pregnancy. Over-work, loss of one's job, divorce, death of a loved one, living with a drug addict or alcoholic, over-exercise, crummy jobs and bad relationships can also trigger allergies.

Not everybody subjected to these stresses develops allergies. Only those with a genetic predisposition to allergy or the existence of a low-grade allergy, develop the full-blown symptoms. Many people go through life with allergies that are so mild they exhibit no symptoms at all. These people are unaware of the low-grade (called subclinical by your doctor) allergies smouldering away inside of them, until the stresses of life begin to mount up. Accumulating stresses over time lower the body's resistance to the point where out-of-the-blue allergies begin to appear.

For this reason all effective allergy treatments begin with the Metabolism-Balancing Program, to build up the body nutritionally, and a concerted effort, wherever possible, to lower any environmental and situational stresses that may exist. The deep breathing and mental relaxation exercises in this chapter help greatly to alleviate the latter two. Changing one's attitude is singularly the most potent stress reducer of all.

If your stress levels are not reduced you will not receive a 100 per cent improvement on the allergy treatment regime outlined in this book. The only program to be on while under stress is the Metabolism-Balancing Program. Remain on this program until you have significantly reduced the stress. This will probably take longer than six to eight weeks if you are getting over the loss of a loved one, going through a divorce, settling into a new city or country, grappling with the problems of living in an undesirable relationship that you are unable to extricate yourself from. If you are in one or more of these situations, be patient. Just concentrate on getting as much rest as possible, doing the deep breathing exercises and the mental relaxation exercises.

Work also on developing a positive attitude by not saying such things as 'Why me?', 'It's not fair!'. In time, with constant practice, you will be pleasantly surprised to discover your stress levels and the intensity of your symptoms will be reducing. If you have put yourself on the Anti-Candida/Anti-Allergy Program first and are not experiencing a reduction of your symptoms, you are almost certainly stressed. Stress prevents allergy cure.

The grieving process is both erratic and time consuming. It can take up to two years to get over a divorce or the death of a loved one. During this time, good and bad days will come and go for no apparent reason and to no set pattern. Be patient. Don't lose heart if you go into a sudden erratic downswing at a time when you are feeling good. This is normal, just accept it. By not dwelling on the downswings, they will pass more quickly and in time will recur less frequently. Your symptoms might reappear during the down-swings. Don't lose heart and think the program is not working if this happens. Keep on persisting. Time will heal all.

ATTITUDE

Don't underestimate the power of a change of attitude to lower your stress levels—even if you are locked into one of the aforementioned stressful situations. The human mind is all powerful and the thoughts we choose to think, for the main part, determine our levels of well-being. All the great thinkers in history have recognised this fact.

As the Greek philosopher Epicetus said 2000 years ago: 'It's never the things that happen to us that upset us. It's our view of these things.'

Shakespeare also captured this viewpoint in Hamlet: 'There's nothing either good or bad but thinking makes it so.' The Bible makes reference to the same idea: 'For as a man thinketh so it is.' And: 'As he thinketh in his heart so is he.'

By taking a more philosophical and tolerant view of the things people say and do to us, it's amazing how well we begin to cope. Any change of view takes time to manifest in lowered stress levels and requires regular, diligent practice. Those who keep at it surprise themselves with the levels of well-being they have been able to achieve. The deep breathing and mental relaxation exercises help this process significantly. Although you may not be able to completely eradicate all feelings of distress you will be able to reduce them enough to get started on the Anti-Candida/Anti-Allergy Program.

Just because you are locked into any of the aforementioned stressful situations don't give up hope that you will ever be able to start the Anti-Candida/Anti-Allergy Program.

COMMON STRESSES TO AVOID

While working on your attitude, breathing and mental relaxation exercises, avoid, wherever possible, the common stresses of modern life:

- Sunburn—even on small areas of the body, like forearms, hands and nose. Always wear a sunblock.
- Crash diets and skipping meals.
- Nutritionally deficient diets (hamburgers, frozen and tinned foods, dehydrated packaged foods, take-away, fast foods).
- Strict vegetarian (vegan) diets that exclude such important protein foods as fish, eggs and cheese.
- Dehydration—not drinking enough fluid, especially through the day.
- Shallow breathing—oxygen deficiency, carbon dioxide excess.
- Fasting—the total withholding of food from the body.
- Chills and colds.
- Chilling of the body due to: not wearing shoes in winter; rising in the morning without putting on slippers and dressing gown; sitting next to a heater while in a draught; working, sleeping, sitting or watching TV in a draught; surfing and swimming in winter without a wetsuit; playing sports in cold southerly winds; sleeping under a fan in summer (see chapter on asthma).
- Self-sabotaging attitudes. Habitually putting negative interpretations on what others say and do and on what happens to you in life. (See 'Self-sabotaging attitudes' later in this chapter.)
- Physical trauma, including surgical operations. (Get a second opinion if it's not a life-threatening emergency.)
- Over-work, lack of sleep and recreation, over-exercising.
- Pain—acute and chronic sports injuries, headache, neckache and backache from poor posture (mainly while sitting).
- Loneliness.
- Over-crowding.
- Excess noise.
- Poor posture. (See Chapter 16, 'Scientific explanations—Stress'.)

STRESS VERSUS DISTRESS

The facts are that stress is both good and bad for us. Many of life's enjoyable pleasures mobilise the stress hormones and it is the adrenalin in our blood that gives us the buzz we feel while experiencing these pleasures. A passionate kiss, orgasm, the thrill of a roller coaster ride, our team winning, a promotion, the achievement of a goal or the thrill of working towards a goal are all adrenal reactions that give us that familiar lift that makes life worth living. Such short-term bursts of stress are good for us, they create energy and enthusiasm and raise our resistance to disease. (See Chapter 16, 'Scientific explanations—Stress'.)

It is the prolonged stress of over-work, bad life situations, bad diet, dehydration, shallow breathing, negative attitudes and even too much of doing what we enjoy that does the damage. When going too hard at what we enjoy causes our body to become racked with pain and the symptoms of disease, we have stress with distress. At this point it's time to back off and accept that what once may have made us feel good is now making us feel bad. The stress hormones that in the short term gave us a buzz are now breaking down too much tissue and causing metabolic imbalances. It's now time for their levels to begin to drop. Rest and a change of attitude is now indicated.

Stress is a bit like drinking champagne. A little bit at a party makes you feel merry and light headed, too much makes you feel ill, depressed and heavy headed the next day. In this way the enjoyable things in life can distress us in the same way as the more easily recognised distresses previously mentioned.

RECOGNISING STRESS

The fact that we can stress ourselves out by doing too much of what we enjoy over too long a period of time makes recognising stress a problem for some people. Recognition of stress can be further complicated by certain physiological processes that take place in a stressed brain. When we're under significant stress the brain releases chemicals called beta endorphins. Beta endorphins belong to the opiate group of chemicals (the literal English translation of the Greek *endorphin* is the 'opium within') and are five times more potent than opium or heroin in producing euphoria and reducing pain. (The *Oxford Dictionary* defines *euphoria* as 'a feeling of well-being, especially one based on over-confidence and over-optimism.')

The high that long distance runners and other competitive athletes experience when they break through the pain barrier and receive their second wind is the result of endorphins. Many women have their first endorphin experience while giving birth.

Athletes and child-bearing women aside, the hard-charging, over-achiever type is the one most likely to experience a beta endorphin high and is therefore in danger of getting hooked on a stressful lifestyle. The painkilling and euphoria-producing effects of beta endorphins can so successfully mask the symptoms of stress that one is not aware one's adrenal glands are getting tired until one ceases the given activity and the levels of beta endorphin drop. It's at this point that the typical symptoms of adrenal fatigue manifest. Tiredness, irritability, drowsiness, loss of confidence and eventually depression are typical symptoms of adrenal fatigue. (See Chapter 16, 'Scientific explanations—Stress'.)

As a group, hard-chargers don't recognise these symptoms as a need to rest. Instead they reason that if working, exercising and socialising makes them feel good and slowing down makes them feel tired then the former is what their body needs. Non-hard-chargers reason that their bodies need rest until symptoms such as tiredness and depression go. Hard-chargers force themselves on until their adrenal glands fatigue to the point of incompetence and their bodies become racked with the symptoms of disease. Non-hard-chargers have learnt to pace themselves and enjoy good health. While hard-chargers are relying more and more on a chemical (beta endorphin) high for feelings of well-being, non-hard-chargers enjoy the natural high of normal good health. (A full description of the role and function of the adrenal glands is given in Chapter 16, 'Scientific explanations—Stress'.)

THE COMMON SYMPTOMS OF STRESS

Don't expect to have all these symptoms. Different people manifest different stress symptoms. However, the more stressed you are the more symptoms you will have. They are:

- Trouble getting off to sleep.
- Tendency to toss and turn and wake during the night.
- Waking up tired in the morning even after a good night's sleep.
- Feeling like lying in on waking.
- Grinding of teeth while asleep.
- Waking up with a sudden start just as you are beginning to doze off.
- Sweaty palms.
- Dry mouth.
- Feeling tired and drowsy to the point of nodding off in the middle of the day if you sit down to rest or read. At work this drowsiness can come on when you sit down at lunch or tea break. Truck drivers can experience it while waiting to be loaded.
- Feeling a reduction in the intensity of your allergy symptoms

while on the go—working, exercising and/or socialising—and a worsening of your allergy symptoms while resting.
- High cholesterol and triglycerides, especially when dietary intake of both is low.

If you seem to be forever eating on the go and experiencing a bloated abdomen as a result, you are almost certainly stressed. This is perhaps the most common of all symptoms and the one that most often brings hard-charging over-achievers to the doctor or naturopath in the first place. They have invariably read a book on food allergies or *Candida albicans* and they have recognised digestive tract symptoms. These people, after sticking strictly to the combined Anti-Candida/Anti-Allergy Program, are invariably no better by the end of the treatment program. They are still complaining that food is causing them to feel bloated and uncomfortable. This is because the high levels of adrenalin in their system are preventing the digestion of food. Instead it sits in their intestines and ferments giving rise to wind and distension of the abdomen.

Hard-charging, over-achiever types seldom experience dramatic improvements on any treatment regime—stress can mimic many of the symptoms of allergy and candida yeast infection. They seldom ever notice appreciable increases in energy as they burn up their new found energy as quickly as they get it by doing more, often without being aware of it. For them, stress is a very insidious thing and they are seldom aware of how much they are stressing themselves. A frequent remark I hear from hard-chargers is: 'No. I don't feel any more energetic since my last appointment, but I've got a lot more done in the last few weeks.'

HOW TO REDUCE STRESS
- Go on the Metabolism-Balancing Program. (Make sure you are drinking the required amount of fluid each day.)
- Reduce your work, exercise and socialising load.
- Get plenty of sleep and recreation.
- Do the deep breathing and mental relaxation exercises.
- Pamper yourself with regular warm baths and massages.
- Take time out to listen to music.
- Take time out to laugh. Read humorous books, watch comedies on TV or at the movies.
- Recent research has shown that watching nature documentaries on TV lowers stress hormone, cholesterol and triglyceride levels. Reading animal stories does the same thing. Many of my highly stressed patients have received great benefits from reading the *All Creatures Great and Small* series of books about the adventures of the Yorkshire vet, James Herriot, and the interest-

ing characters (both animal and human) he encounters on a daily basis. Read before bed for a restful sleep.
- Don't drive the car above the speed limit. Speeding will rev you up and keep you revved up for the rest of the day as you tend to move quickly at all other activities after speeding. It is when we speed that we discover the idiots on the road who get us uptight. When we slow down it's amazing how they disappear.
- Don't perch yourself on the edge of chairs. This tightens all your muscles from the lower back to the top of the neck. Sit back, use the backrest whether at home or work. (Follow the advice outlined under 'Poor posture' in Chapter 16, 'Scientific explanations—Stress'.)

DEEP BREATHING EXERCISES

The deep breathing exercises are a good prelude to the mental relaxation exercises as they have the capacity to significantly relax the muscles especially when combined with adequate fluid and vitamin/mineral intake. So effective are they that some people elect to use them alone as their vehicle for relaxation. Many hard-chargers who have a bloated abdomen and the symptoms of irritable bowel syndrome find that all these symptoms disappear after three to four weeks of the breathing exercises combined with a reduced workload, fewer commitments and the attendant rushing and speeding in cars.

This form of bloated abdomen and irritable bowel is caused by tight digestive tract muscles that cause food to get stuck in the intestines leading to fermentation, blockage and swelling. If three to four weeks of the deep breathing exercises don't significantly improve the condition then food allergy and/or *Candida albicans* infection is a safe diagnosis. Some people have all three factors contributing to their bloated abdomen or irritable bowel. In all cases treatment commences with the Metabolism-Balancing Program, adequate fluid intake and deep breathing. Otherwise the severity of any food allergies or candida infection will never be determined.

By relaxing the muscles, the deep breathing exercises also relax the brain. The muscles are connected to the brain by the sensory nerves. This makes it impossible to have relaxed muscles and a tense and agitated brain. (See Chapter 16, 'Scientific explanations—Stress—Oxygen and carbon dioxide'.) The deep breathing exercises relax the muscles by suffusing them with oxygen and removing from them carbon dioxide. Carbon dioxide is a major metabolic waste product of cellular respiration. Lying around in the muscles it acts as an irritant, causing them to contract, often to the point of spasm. Most importantly the breathing exercises lower the blood histamine levels, which reduces the number and intensity of one's allergies. Conversely, shallow, rapid breathing raises the histamine levels, aggravating allergies.

EXERCISE 1

This is a preliminary exercise for those who are habitual shallow breathers and have trouble getting the air down into the lower lobes. Lie on your back with your legs out straight in front of you. Place a light book on your abdomen. Empty your lungs by slowly sucking in your abdomen (Fig. 11.1). Now, breathe in deeply and slowly, concentrating on forcing the air down to your abdomen. As the diaphragm muscle descends with this deep inhalation, the abdomen will distend and the book will rise (Fig. 11.2). Concentrate on getting the book to rise up and down with each 'in' and 'out' breath. This may not come easily at first as you probably haven't used your diaphragm muscle properly since childhood. (Next time you get the opportunity observe the belly breathing action of a baby.) Keep persisting. Breathe slowly.

Practise each day for ten to fifteen minutes. If you are still having trouble try pursing the lips and breathing through your mouth (Fig. 11.3)—suck the air in slowly through pursed lips. Normally it is better not to breathe through your mouth but for the purpose of learning to use your diaphragm properly (the strong dome-shaped muscle that's attached to the lower ribs and separates the chest

Fig. 11.1: Exercise 1—the 'out' breath. The book drops (hold for 3 seconds).

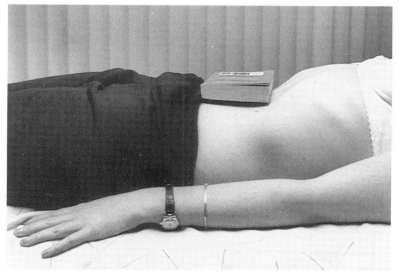

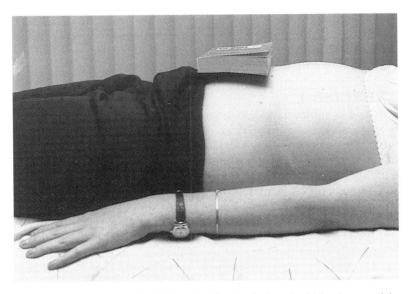

Fig. 11.2: Exercise 1—the 'in' breath. The book rises (hold for 3 seconds).
Fig. 11.3: Suck air slowly and deeply through pursed lips.

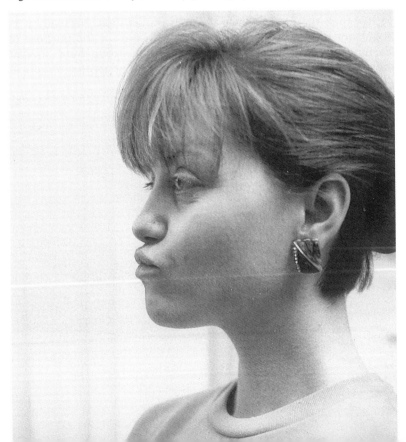

cavity from the abdominal cavity) it's important that you do so. Pursing the lips produces an obstacle to breathing that necessitates a vigorous sucking motion to get the air in. This vigorous sucking requires the use of the diaphragm. You can practise this pursed lips breathing at intervals through the day while driving or at work. Don't sit with a collapsed, forward hunched posture. This will make it difficult for the diaphragm to descend and will encourage shallow chest breathing (see the section under 'Poor posture' in Chapter 16, 'Scientific explanations—Stress').

You may notice that just as your belly breathing is progressing well, you will experience a sudden stalling as your chest muscles try to come into play and return you to your old shallow breathing habits. Don't be discouraged if this happens. We are creatures of habit and if we habitually breathe with our chest muscles it's perfectly natural that we involuntarily slip back into that habit while in the process of learning belly breathing. Besides, rib and chest expansion is normal during belly breathing but takes place only in the latter stages of the inhalation when the diaphragm is fully descended. If you experience a stalling in your breathing, concentrate even harder on pushing the book up with your abdomen. If you stall significantly and lose rhythm, relax and go back to the beginning—starting off with a new inhalation.

Chances are a lifetime of slumping in armchairs or at your desk, combined with shallow breathing, has left you with ribs that are tightly fixed to your spine and have lost their ability to articulate freely. If you are getting chest and back pains and/or repeatedly experience stalling in your breathing, it would pay to see your osteopath or chiropractor to have the ribs and thoracic/cervical vertebrae freed up. This will make all the difference.

EXERCISE 2—THE STANDING EXERCISE

Now that you have mastered the preliminary exercise it's time to commence the breathing exercises proper. There are many derivations of the standing, deep breathing exercises and all of them are good. If you have learnt Karate, Tai Chi or any of the martial arts, you may have one that feels good to you. By all means use it. If you have a favourite deep breathing yoga technique, practised from the sitting posture, then by all means use that.

If you are totally unacquainted with deep breathing techniques you may want to try my favourite. Taught to me by a Chinese Kung Fu master, it has the lyrical name of 'Scoop the Stream'. It is excellent for stretching the rib cage and expanding the lungs. Practised first thing in the morning, it is a good wake-up tonic. It raises the metabolic rate, giving you an immediate lift that makes you mentally alert and emotionally buoyant, yet calm.

1. Close your eyes or fix your gaze on a given object or point. Stand with your feet either together or 10–20 cm (4–8 in) apart (whichever is most comfortable for you), and arms hanging loosely at your sides. Relax your muscles (Fig. 11.4).

2. Breathe out until the lungs are empty then slowly and deeply inhale while at the same time raising the hands (palms down) until the fingertips touch above your head (Fig. 11.5 and Fig. 11.6). Now, turn the palms so that they are facing upwards (Fig. 11.7). Time it so that the fingers touch at the point of complete inhalation—when you are unable to take in any more air. Stretch upward and count to three silently. Now exhale slowly

Exercise 2—The standing exercise

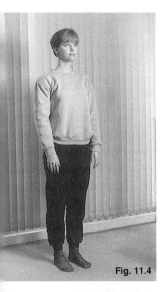
Fig. 11.4

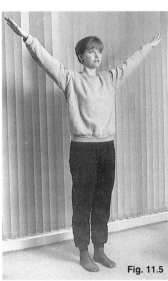
Fig. 11.5

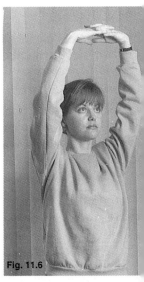
Fig. 11.6

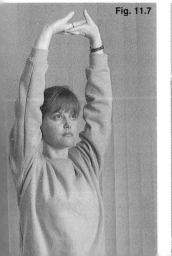
Fig. 11.7

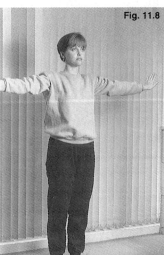
Fig. 11.8

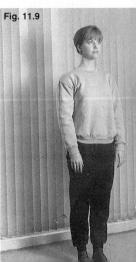
Fig. 11.9

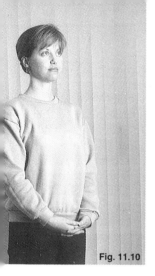
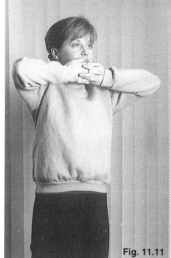
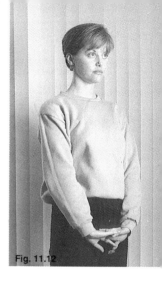

Fig. 11.10   Fig. 11.11   Fig. 11.12

Exercise 2—The standing exercise (cont.)

and steadily while slowly dropping your arms in the reverse motion to the previous action (Fig. 11.8). Have them reach the side of your legs at the point of complete exhalation (Fig. 11.9). To achieve complete exhalation contract your stomach muscles tightly so that the abdomen is concave at the point of total exhalation. Hold this position for the silent count of three. Count slowly.

3. Interlace the fingers with the palms up, forming a scoop (Fig. 11.10). As you slowly and deeply inhale, raise the scoop to the level of your lips with your bent arm in line with your shoulders and your elbows raised as high as possible (Fig. 11.11). Hold this position to the count of three.

4. Now turn the palms over and exhale slowly and steadily by tightening the abdomen muscles until the lungs are completely empty (Fig. 11.12). Slowly drop the overturned palms during exhalation.

5. At the point of ultimate exhalation your arms will be at complete extension. Press down as if pressing a spring and hold for a silent count of three. Return your hands to the side of your legs and start again. (Breathe and count slowly.)

Do these movements twelve times each. Take it easy, don't stand in a draught and make sure you are warm, yet loosely dressed (a tracksuit is good). Don't force yourself, you'll pull muscles otherwise. If you are out of condition and stiff it would pay to start off with six exercises only, building up to eight, to ten and then twelve when you feel you are ready. Concentrate on pressing the diaphragm down and letting the abdomen bulge out. Don't worry, this won't give you a pot. On the contrary, the tightening of the abdomen muscles on exhalation is excellent for removing a pot and slimming the figure.

To help you concentrate on your breathing you can count the breath 'in' and count it out again. To start with, breathe in to the count of six or eight, whatever is most comfortable. As you progress and your diaphragm descends further, and your rib cage expands further, you will need to expand the count to ten or twelve and even beyond. The further you extend the count, the more slowly you will be raising and lowering the arms. This is good, for the slower the exercise is, the more it will relax you.

Counting also gives you a yardstick to measure your progress. An increased count means your diaphragm is distending further and your rib cage is expanding further. Both actions increase the tone of the muscles needed to straighten your posture and improve your body shape. Breathe and count slowly.

WHEN AND WHERE TO BREATHE

The best time is first thing on rising after you've had your three, four or five 230 mL (8 oz) glasses of fresh water (warm or at room temperature). Make sure you are in a well-ventilated room. If it's not too cold open the window but close the door, this will prevent draughts.

If it's warm, you may do the exercises outside under a tree, or by a fountain, or on the beach. If you've slept in, do them before lunch in the park. Don't do them for at least three or four hours before bed. They give you energy which makes falling asleep difficult. Try and do the exercises every day but don't get upset if you can't. Even three or four times per week will do you good.

THE YOGIC WALK

Variety is the spice of life. If you want to vary your breathing exercise routine, you can do the yogic walk. The advantage here is that you can combine your breathing exercise with a gentle walk. Don't take the dog on a lead though, it will break your rhythm. The yogic walk can be done on the beach (hard sand only), through the park or on a country lane. Avoid traffic where possible as you don't want to be drawing in fumes. It can be done in the company of other yogic walkers. Like the standing and sitting breathing exercises, it's not to be done after a meal. Do the yogic walk on the flat or downhill only.

1. Empty the lungs by tightening the abdomen muscles. As you commence the walk, breathe in deeply to the count of your steps. As a beginner it may pay to breathe in to the first six to eight steps. Walk and breathe slowly.

2. When the diaphragm is fully descended and your rib cage full, hold your breath for the next three steps.
3. Breathe out, using the abdomen muscles for the next six to eight steps and when your abdomen is concave, hold your breath out for three steps.
4. Commence the inhalation again and continue for the duration of the walk. Results are disappointing if you walk too quickly.

Don't walk briskly—walk slowly and easily, letting your arms swing gently to the rhythm of your stride. As time goes by you will be easily breathing to ten, twelve, or more, steps. Don't raise the breath-holding time frame beyond three steps. The yogic walk has the advantage of gently moving the inhaled oxygen around the body, taking it to the peripheral tissues more quickly.

Walking encourages upright posture (jogging doesn't) by strengthening the back muscles. It draws oxygen into the major joints without straining them. It has all the advantages of vigorous exercise without placing strain on the adrenal glands. The adrenal glands can rest during a slow relaxing walk and take up lots of oxygen to prepare them for the rigours of the working day. Being a full weight-bearing exercise, walking is excellent for retaining calcium in the bones of the legs, pelvis and spine—preventing osteoporosis. Being a gentle exercise, it doesn't fill the muscles with lactic acid (the major waste product of muscle contraction). Lactic acid irritates the muscles causing spasms, aches, pains and stiffness. It is lactic acid build-up that causes the pain experienced after a hard game, heavy workout or long run. Lactic acid needs calcium to neutralise it and facilitate its removal from the muscles and elimination from the body. This puts demands on the body's calcium reserves and can cause calcium deficiencies which in turn can cause nervousness, irritability, lack of confidence and anxiety. Hard exercise is often a stress as most people engaging in it don't supplement their diet with adequate calcium. Hard-chargers produce the same amount of lactic acid by being overly busy. Carbon dioxide build-up is also a muscle irritant.

Yogic walking draws more oxygen into the body than jogging, yet doesn't raise the levels of carbon dioxide, lactic acid, adrenalin, cortisone and testosterone which cause metabolic imbalances (see Chapter 16, 'Scientific explanations—Stress—Oxygen and carbon dioxide').

BLOCKED AIRWAYS

Use whatever medication your doctor prescribes to keep asthma and infections at bay and your nasal passages clear. Obstructed airways interfere with oxygen uptake and carbon dioxide removal.

As you progress with the breathing exercises the increased oxygenation of the body will, along with the diets, raise your resistance to the point where the airways will clear naturally and the drugs can be discontinued. However, you have to get the oxygen in there first. Make sure you are on the Metabolism-Balancing Program and Formula Six supplements and if you have mucus in the nose, throat or chest, take two garlic and horseradish capsules (or tablets) with breakfast, lunch and the evening meal. These herbs are effective mucus clearers.

WATCH YOUR POSTURE

Poor posture will undo some of the good from your doing deep breathing exercises and will make it difficult to break the habit of shallow breathing. Slumping forward over desk and computer rounds the shoulders, which constricts the expansion of the rib cage. It also forces the lower ribs down into the abdomen cramping the action of the diaphragm. This gives rise to shallow breathing which predisposes to anxiety and panic (oxygen deficiency and carbon dioxide imbalance). Anxiety and panic gives rise to shallow, upper chest breathing.

Think back to the last time you were startled by someone or were frightened by something you saw on TV or at the movies. How did you breathe? Chances are high that you drew a sudden, upward breath in the top of the chest. I doubt very much that you drew a slow, relaxing, belly breath. It pays to keep away from anxiety-producing TV programs and life situations as much as possible while learning to breathe with the diaphragm.

Sit back after the evening meal in a relaxed posture and allow your belly to breathe unencumbered. Make use of your work chair's backrest as much as possible. Practise the posture techniques described in Chapter 16, 'Scientific explanations—Stress'.

MENTAL RELAXATION EXERCISES

'There are many paths to the top of the mountain but when we get there we all see the same moon.' (Old Japanese martial arts proverb)

There are lots of different forms of meditation, or mental relaxation exercises, and all of them work. If you have one that you are particularly fond of, by all means use it. If not, try this one. I have had great success with it.

For maximum results it pays to do the mental relaxation

exercises directly after the deep breathing exercises. The breathing exercises are relaxing exercises in their own right and prepare the body for meditation. Try and do the mental relaxation exercises twice per day. If that's not possible, do them once. I'd rather you have the extra sleep than see you getting up too early to fit them in. Some patients prefer to do the breathing exercises in the morning and the mental relaxation ones at night, before bed, or during the afternoon at work. As you become more proficient at them you'll be able to do them anywhere—on the train, waiting at the bus stop or in the dentist's chair (no kidding, I did it once, and had a tooth drilled without an injection—didn't feel a thing). Most people find it easy to fit the mental relaxation exercises in after the deep breathing on the weekend when they have more time.

THE EXERCISE
Duration ten to fifteen minutes.
Choose a *reasonably* comfortable chair. If it's too comfortable, your relaxation will come from physical comfort rather than the discipline of your mind. You need mental discipline if you are going to be able to relax anywhere at any time. As you become more skilled at this you will be able to do it in very uncomfortable positions. The yogis of the East deliberately contort themselves into painful lotus positions while meditating so they can develop deep mental relaxation as opposed to the superficial relaxation derived from reclining comfortably.

Only by learning deep mental relaxation can you calm yourself in difficult circumstances. Sit down, close your eyes or, if you prefer, fix your gaze on a distant point across the room and hold it for the duration of the exercise. Do this in an unhurried way, with pauses after each presentation, to give the idea time to register its effect in the brain. Say to yourself mentally: 'I feel relaxed—so relaxed. It's so good to feel so relaxed—my whole body feels relaxed—so heavy—so easy and so relaxed.'

When you begin to feel relaxed switch your attention to one area of the body and concentrate on relaxing it by visualising it and feeling it relax. It pays to start with the legs and work your way up through the body to the face. Mentally concentrate on one muscle group at a time, noting its presence and then feeling it let go. In the early stages this visualisation can be helped if you physically tense, hold and then relax the muscle in time to the mental commands: 'My right leg feels relaxed—I can feel the muscles let go—my leg is feeling heavy now—so heavy and relaxed—so easy—gentle—heavy and relaxed— no tension—just relaxed—I can feel my left leg now—it feels relaxed too—I can feel the muscles in it let go.'

So it goes on. The process is repeated as you shift your attention from one group of muscles to another and gradually work your way up through the legs, torso, arms, neck and, most importantly, the muscles of the face. There is a very close relationship between the muscles of the face and the mind. When the mind is relaxed it's mirrored in the muscles of the face. When the mind is agitated, the facial muscles tense and contort to reflect that agitation.

By the time you get up to the face you are already feeling pretty relaxed and you continue the exercise by feeling the relaxation in your face: 'Feeling so relaxed—feeling so relaxed in my face—I feel my forehead letting go—feel my jaw letting go—I feel easy all over—feel so relaxed—I feel my eye muscles letting go—I feel my teeth separate—feel easy in the face—feel easy all through my body—feel heavy in my body—feel easy in my face.'

It is at this point that you transpose the feeling of physical relaxation onto the mind: 'I feel so relaxed in my body—so relaxed in my face—I can feel the relaxation happening in my mind. My mind feels easy—calm—gentle—relaxed—just like my body—easy and relaxed.' If you have any significant metabolic distortions, such as fluid retention, or high cholesterol, now is the time to work on them: 'I feel my mind letting go—feel my body letting go—feel my tissues letting go—letting go of excess fluid—feel my kidneys letting go—letting go of excess fluid—it feels so good to be letting go—letting go of excess fluid.'

In the case of high cholesterol: 'I feel my stress levels dropping—feel the stress hormone levels dropping—dropping—dropping—so good to feel them dropping—I feel my cholesterol levels dropping—dropping with my stress levels—dropping—dropping—dropping—so good to feel them both dropping.'

If you have a skin problem: 'I feel my stress levels dropping—the stress hormone levels are dropping—dropping—dropping—dropping. The neurokinin levels are dropping too—dropping with the stress hormone—dropping—dropping—dropping—so good to feel the neurokinin dropping—skin is calming now—calm—easy—relaxed—quietening down—neurokinin is dropping—skin is calming—feels good—feels calm—easy—calm—gentle—relaxed.'

Don't feel cheated when you open your eyes and see your skin complaint is still there. It won't disappear in one session. It takes time. It's the cumulative effect of many sessions of mental relaxation that gives you control over your visceral functions. All you need for success is patience and persistence. IQ, education, personality type have nothing to do with it. Everyone has the ability to relax and control their stress hormone, cholesterol and neurokinin levels. Constant practice of the exercise produces longer tension and neurokinin free periods, and periods of cholesterol and metabolism balance.

HOW OFTEN?

Try and do the exercises every day if you can but don't upset yourself if you can't. Getting stressed out over missing a session or two defeats the purpose of doing them. Because life is unpredictable, circumstances that interfere with your routine will always arise. Don't worry about it. Some weeks you will be able to do the exercise every day, other weeks you will only fit them in three or so times. That's fine, so long as you keep patiently plugging away, the cumulative effects of your persistence will, in time, manifest. You won't slip back by missing a few sessions. The important thing is not to become fanatical. Fanaticism begets stress. Take your time, the inevitability of gradualness will reward you with the level of well-being you are seeking.

STRESS AND THE HARD-CHARGER

'Nothing can be more useful to a man than a determination not to be hurried.' (Henry David Thoreau)

Hard-chargers, as the name implies, are always on the go—busy, busy, busy. Some of them are impetuous; some of them have half a dozen projects going at once; many set high goals with unrealistic time frames for their achievement and all of them take on more than they can cope with. Because of this and because they are not quitters, they are always in a hurry. This lifestyle of perpetual rushing leads to bad habits.

Bad habit number one is frequent skipping of meals, particularly lunch which leads to a drop in energy and performance (hypoglycaemia) by mid-afternoon.

Bad habit number two is not drinking enough fluids through the day. This leads to dehydration and contributes to a drop in performance. Hard-chargers are too busy to drink, and by not drinking, don't have to make those time-wasting trips to the toilet, which they claim reduces their productivity. They practice thirst denial so often they no longer experience the subtle message of thirst, only the overt, serious ones. (See Chapter 10, 'The importance of water and oxygen'.)

Bad habit number three is shallow breathing. People who rush, automatically tense all the muscles in their body. Tense muscles don't expand through their full range of movement.This includes the muscles that facilitate breathing, giving rise to short, shallow breaths that don't take in much oxygen. A lack of oxygen causes muscles to tense and a vicious cycle is born. Lack of oxygen means the brain and nerves function below par giving rise to tiredness, irritability and anxiety. Hard-chargers tend to perch themselves on the end of chairs and hunch forward over desks, typewriters, computers. This posture further tenses the body and cramps the chest and diaphragm muscles, aggravating shallow breathing.

Because of these bad habits, the hard-charger is always performing below his or her full capacity. The great irony is that the maximising of one's potential, which is so important to so many hard-chargers, is seldom ever realised by them as they are in too much of a hurry to achieve it. Being of the non-quitter type, they continue to push themselves despite the fatigue and many other symptoms that dog them. The very practice of pushing themselves further lowers their energy and performance levels, giving rise to mistake making and the need to repeat work.

Hard-chargers are the classic Type A personalities described in life insurance company premium tables and popular psychology texts. They are forever tearing around like scalded cats. Type As in the workplace resent the Type B personalities who, being less ebulliently dynamic, are perceived as lazy under-achievers. At the end of the day, Type Bs are invariably more productive and make far fewer mistakes, a fact that is seldom ever admitted to by Type As.

I always remind my hard-charging patients of Aesop's fable about the hare and the tortoise and I always get them to tell me who won the race. Even with this technique, it's not easy to get through to the hard-chargers as they are all convinced they are coping and don't see their lifestyle and attitude as a problem. Their definition of coping is 'being on their feet and mobile'. They don't recognise that a body which is racked with chronic fatigue, aches, joint pains, allergies, skin rashes, bloated stomach, constipation, headaches or slow wound healing, is a body that is not coping. So long as they can force themselves out of bed in the morning, they think they are coping and all those symptoms they have, well, they are caused by something else and they will just have to drop in on the doctor or naturopath and pick up a pill or a diet to fix it.

Because we humans are such profound creatures of habit, it's quite easy to understand the hard-charger's point of view. They are so used to being stressed they see it as normal. This fact really hit home to me one night while watching a documentary on the Soviet gulags. One of the former inmates had returned to his particular Siberian gulag with a BBC cameraman and was recounting the horrors and privations of living in the abysmally subhuman conditions. I became quite distressed as more of this man's experiences were being revealed and then became amazed when he finished off by saying, 'Ah but we got used to it, humans can get used to anything.' That said it all for me; the penny finally dropped. It's no wonder hard-chargers argue that they are not stressed even when they are not responding to the Anti-Allergy Program they are so assiduously sticking to.

Hard-chargers fall into one of two camps, the adrenally competent and adrenally fatigued. The adrenally competent have all the symptoms of stress but have enough life left in their adrenal glands to be able to whip them along and keep themselves going. They are still able to produce enough beta endorphins to kill some of the pain and moderate the intensity of their symptoms. So long as they keep going they are OK. The moment they stop, they take a dive and start to feel lousy. Recognising that action is the only thing that makes them feel good they reason they should keep at it, so they get going again, not realising that it's an excess of that particular action that has them feeling the way they are.

The adrenally fatigued are those hard-chargers who have pushed too hard for too long. They can no longer produce enough adrenalin to force their tired bodies to perform. Chronic, unrelenting fatigue that reduces only a little when they push themselves is the main symptom. However, they seldom get to push themselves, for now they lack the enthusiasm to do so. The adrenally fatigued are easily recognised by the way they flop into the armchair in my office on their first visit and say, 'I don't really know why I'm here, I'm just a bit tired, that's all.' Having said that, they then proceed to verbalise a litany of symptoms.

RECOGNISING THE HARD-CHARGER

There are a number of categories of hard-chargers that I have come to recognise over the years. They are broad categorisations that don't take into account individual nuances. I've included them here to help you decide whether or not hard-charging is a problem for you. Because humans are such varied creatures they cannot be categorised rigidly. For this reason you may find you can fit into two categories, being, for instance, 60 per cent one and 40 per cent the other. If you can identify with any of these categories, but don't have any symptoms, take heed now. Ill health could be just around the corner if you don't slow down.

THE EARTH MOTHER

'One half the troubles of this life can be traced to saying yes too quick and not saying no soon enough.' (Josh Billings)
Kind, loving, caring, strong, patient, sometimes a bit self-effacing, she attracts leaners like a honeypot attracts bees. Seldom having a moment to herself as she always has visitors, most often girlfriends, who come to dump their problems on her, depart

175

feeling temporarily better while leaving her drained. Earth Mother gives good, commonsense advice to leaners and is continually frustrated by the leaner's tendency to keep repeating the same mistakes, despite her advice. Leaners phone at any time—meal time, TV-watching time and late at night—to dump. If she's not counselling, Earth Mother is baking cakes, cutting out patterns or sewing up dresses for leaners. Not surprisingly leaners are often possessive of Earth Mother. Earth Mother is often a houseproud, conscientious parent, who somehow has to fit in attention to house, children, husband/boyfriend, parents and in-laws. Parents, husband/boyfriend and in-laws are sometimes leaners too. Earth Mother's greatest stress is the guilt she feels when she's finally blamed for all that goes wrong in the leaner's life.

'Work out your own salvation. Do not depend on others.' (Buddha)
Earth Mother has to recognise that her health and the kids are suffering as a result of the time and energy she's putting into leaners. Furthermore, she is not really helping leaners by encouraging their dependency on her. Earth Mother has to acknowledge that sometimes the best kind of caring lies in encouraging others to stand on their own two feet and as much as she enjoys her role she has physical, mental and emotional limits.

The best course of action is to learn to say no. If you are an overstretched earth mother, get on the phone to everyone and explain to them that you need a rest and tell them why. If you explain that the demands everyone is placing on you has burnt you out, they will understand and back off. If you make up stories (because you don't want to hurt their feelings) they won't understand and resentment will develop on both sides. Tell them you'll phone when you are feeling better. If you don't feel up to phoning yourself get a parent, child, spouse or lover to do it for you.

Don't waste precious energy fuming and stewing over the fact that leaners have reduced you to the point of having the shakes, or binge eating in lieu of time to yourself, or feeling prostratingly fatigued. Leaners are not bad people. They are everyday people who have allowed the normal human desire for some support and emotional nourishment to get out of hand. They are not mind readers and that is why they don't know how you feel. Besides, you were always available and appeared to enjoy being so. This too is fine, and there is no reason to totally give up your supportive role when it's just as easy to define your limits of tolerance and notify yourself and others of them. Any leaner who refuses to acknowledge your need for rest is best extricated from your life. Fortunately, these types are few and far between.

It is important for home-based earth mothers to reserve some quiet moments through the day to indulge themselves. Reading, listening to music, doing something creative, before the afternoon rush of driving kids to and from activities, supervising homework and preparing the evening meal. Career-based earth mothers can try and organise some time off work to do the same.

Male earth mothers do exist, though in much smaller numbers than their female counterpart. Like female earth mothers, they too have to learn to let go of leaners as much as leaners have to learn to let go of them.

E-TYPES

'It is salutory to train oneself to be no more affected by censure than by praise.' (W. Somerset Maugham)

E-types are so called because they want to be no more affected by everything to everybody and burn themselves out trying to achieve this—you can't please all of the people all of the time. E-types are the archetypal approval seekers. They crave praise and fear detractors.

E-type women

E-types want to be the best mother, lover, wife, hostess, daughter, friend, tennis player, committee member. They burn up a lot of energy worrying about whether or not they are measuring up to their own and others' expectations. And they burn up a lot of anxiety energy over their perceived failure to do so. E-types burn out from running around doing things for others. They spend more time in the car and other people's homes than at home.

E-types tell themselves it's 'horrible', 'terrible', 'awful', if they fail to measure up or don't achieve at a given task. These gross over-exaggerations, in time, produce significant emotional disturbances—stress. What E-types have to recognise and accept is that we humans are all fallible, we all make mistakes and we all fail to achieve at given tasks from time to time. That is the way we humans are and it's OK. E-type career women strive in the belief that being the best will secure the approval of all others. Unfortunately, more often than not, others are jealous of E-type's ability and success and withhold the acknowledgement she craves.

For those women who have committed themselves to full-time careers the comments about the E-type man will be appropriate.

E-type men

'No one can make you feel inferior without your consent.' (Eleanor Roosevelt)

He is driven by the same guilts and insecurities as his female counterpart. E-type man tends to exercise his approval-seeking proclivities at work. The extrovert E-type male draws attention to himself by working hard and letting everybody know it. He moves quickly, acts dynamically and often boasts and whinges that no one works as hard as he. The introvert E-type gets stuck in and hopes he's noticed.

Typically all E-type males seek to gain approval by doing more and better than their fellows through 'application' and 'hard work', and to gain security by holding to a stable environment and a given system of excellent performance, even at a high cost of energy. This work and lifestyle pattern brings the E-type male some admiration but little of the love he craves. Instead, it brings him increasing responsibility, and greater and greater resentment for the pace he feels obliged to maintain.

This sustained resentment associated with repeated frustration, in time, gives rise to prostrating fatigue, providing fertile ground for the severe headaches so many E-types suffer from. The work and lifestyle pattern of the E-type male gives rise to the easily recognised personality traits of inflexibility, conscientiousness, meticulousness, perfectionism and resentment.

Suggested reading for E-types

Dr Wayne Dyer, *Your Erroneous Zones* and *Pulling Your Own Strings*.
Michael E. Bernard, *Staying Rational in an Irrational World*.
Albert Ellis and Robert Harper, *A New Guide to Rational Living*.
See 'Bibliography' for publication details.

THE ACHIEVER

'Success has ruined many a man.' (Benjamin Franklin)
Achievers are different to the E-types in that their desire for the approval of others is not as pronounced. They are more confident and self-centred. They seek to achieve partly for the status and kudos and certainly for the material rewards they desire and believe they deserve. They are very ambitious. In time, achievement for achievement's sake becomes a prime motivator. They thrive on challenge and in extreme cases believe their life has no meaning without it.

Achievers are always on the go. So busy are they, in fact, that they 'hardly have time to draw breath', an expression many of them use when describing a typical day in their lives. Such shallow breathing practices help to explain why so many of them are burnt out. They work hard and long hours. Being positive and highly motivated, many of them are into taking care of themselves, as they perceive 'taking care' to be. Many of them play some sort of sport, work out with weights, do aerobics, or jog or swim regularly.

The more extreme achievers get into heavy competition sport or take part in triathalons. Many of them stay away from junk food preferring wholemeal breads, sprouts, lentils, and other high-fibre natural foods.

The big problem is they never get time to rest. The irony is that high-fibre, natural foods are harder to digest than refined, fast foods and if they don't take time out to sit quietly they never absorb the nutrients from their food which, being high fibre, passes rapidly through and out of them. Insidious malnutrition is a big problem for achievers who are perplexed at feeling so tired when they are working so hard at keeping fit and eating properly (see Chapter 16, 'Scientific explanations—Food combining').

Extreme achievers take themselves, life and everything they do very seriously, often too seriously. They view life as a struggle for existence and remain stressed until they change this attitude. Some achievers pursue their chosen path in lieu of a relationship or because their present relationships are unfulfilling.

'Nature, time and patience are the three great physicians.'
(Proverb)

Achievers have to recognise that time out for quiet, restful moments in their day, plus eight hours' sleep, is imperative if they are to have it all. Reduction in work and exercise loads are also needed. Retaining the high goals they have set themselves is fine. Extending the time frames needed to achieve these goals is the answer. Apply the principle of the hare and the tortoise rigorously.

Achievers always argue that their exercise regimen is a release from stress and up to a point this is true. It is at least a diversion from work and it does at least get some oxygen into the blood and the blood moving. Unfortunately, high impact exercises also fill the muscles with lactic acid, which lowers the body's calcium reserves predisposing it to nervousness, headaches and irritability. The tension achievers incur through the course of a busy day has already put high levels of lactic acid in their muscles. To achieve true tension release from their busy schedule, achievers will benefit from taking up yoga, Tai Chi or yogic walking. The only good reason to go to a gym is for a sauna, swirl pool and massage. (See Chapter 10, 'The importance of water and oxygen' and Chapter 16, 'Scientific explanations—Oxygen and carbon dioxide'.)

Achievers burn out because they want results too quickly. If they can get the balance between work and rest right, they lead a fulfilling life and end up achieving more than they ever dreamed possible. High achieving is fine—over-achieving makes us ill.

THE DOERS

'A man is rich in proportion to the things he can afford to let alone.' (Henry David Thoreau)

Doers are positive, energetic people who are not as complicated as the E-types or achievers, though the more extreme ones exhibit some of the seriousness and competitiveness of the achievers. Doers simply have an urge to do and don't like sitting around wasting time. They would rather be doing something—anything. They have a lively appetite for novelty, exploration, challenge and adventure, which often drives them into situations which are fraught with difficulty, hardship and sometimes danger.

What drives doers? I've often wondered. Their urge to do is certainly associated with enjoying a challenge and could be genetic, their upbringing, astrological or a combination of all three. My records show that many of them are born under the sign of Aries.

'Nature is commanded by obeying her.' (Francis Bacon)

'Rest' is a four letter word to doers, E-types and achievers, yet it's one they have to get used to if they are to experience optimum health. Doers and achievers have to recognise that although the spirit may be eager and willing, the flesh is grounded by earthly limitations and requires rest. Those are the rules nature has set. Nature calls the tune here, not us. Those of us who humbly submit to nature's edicts reap the rewards of good health.

The word recreation means exactly that. Re-creation—a time to create. It is while we are taking time out to be still that nature repairs the worn-out brain, nerve and other tissues of the body. It's during this time that we replace the old, worn-out, white blood cells with new, young, dynamic ones (see Chapter 2, 'Allergies'). This re-creating of new cells can't be achieved while we are on the go and eight hours' sleep is not enough to do the job properly.

For those who argue they would rather be doing something 'constructive', bear in mind there is nothing more constructive than the rebuilding of the body during times of rest. Many achievers and doers like to kid themselves that a skiing holiday is a rest. It isn't.

THE FUN-LOVERS

'Fun is like life insurance; the older you get, the more it costs.' (Kin Hubbard)

Fun-lovers would not know what stress was if they tripped over it, and look in amazement when it's explained to them that they are doing too much. Fun-lovers embrace life with a great enthusiasm and are often impetuous. Being optimists they frequently bite off more than they can chew, long before they realise it. They burn out doing all those things they enjoy. Their personalities lack the intensity of the achievers and the urgency of the doers, though some doers exhibit some of the fun-lover traits.

Fun-lovers are into everything and often have lots of friends and a busy social life. They are not irresponsible. Most of them pursue interesting careers or at least hold down steady jobs. (In this context motherhood and domesticity are considered to be careers.) An over-abundance of enthusiasm is what drives them and they burn out trying to pursue all their interests and keep in touch with all their friends. Workaholic fun-lovers do exist. They differ from achiever and doer workaholics in that work to them is fun and they are just not aware of the hours they are putting in. Because of their lack of intensity they usually last longer than others before the effects of over-work set in.

Fun-lovers, like all hard-chargers, have to learn to pace themselves. They have to learn to get the balance right. Fun-lovers are like kids in a candy shop. Life to them is sweet, colourful and has so many different flavours they just can't wait to taste.

Most hard-chargers find it difficult to accept that their attitude and lifestyle is the root cause of their symptoms, as they invariably know someone with a similar lifestyle who is perfectly well. This may well be true and for a number of reasons:

- The other person doesn't have allergies or a candida yeast infection. The hard-chargers that seek me out have low-grade allergies which, prior to them becoming stressed, have never given them any symptoms. Since their cumulative stresses have built up over a period of time, their resistance has waned and the allergy symptoms have manifested.
- The other person hasn't been stressed for as long. The human body has remarkable powers of adaptation and can put up with stress for a long time before it's adaptive mechanisms break down. In a way this is not a good thing as it lulls us into a false sense of security. Because we are able to lead a stressful lifestyle for so long without any ill effects we naturally look for another cause when the symptoms of disease begin to manifest. If we are lucky enough to be born well nourished, with a genetically strong constitution, have no low-grade allergies or candida yeast infections and have had no pregnancies, terminations, or surgery, we can cope with high levels of stress and remain symptom free for a long time. However, symptoms in time do come and their cause is frequently misdiagnosed. Because we are so much in the habit of living a stressful lifestyle, we are actually comfortable with it

181

and feel uncomfortable at the thought of making changes to it. Such is the power of habit. Because it takes time to change habits we are patient and accept that it will take time for us to change. The best program to be on while reorganising our lifestyle is the Metabolism-Balancing Program. The deep breathing and mental relaxation exercises given in this chapter also help this process of change significantly.

LEARNING TO PACE ONESELF

'Choose what is best, habit will soon render it agreeable and easy.' (Pythagorus)

There are things in life that only we can do for ourselves and learning to pace ourselves is one of those. No one can do this for us because we all have such varying levels of tolerance to stress. It's up to us to discern our own tolerance levels and recognise our own early warning symptoms of overdoing it.

Perhaps the greatest hurdle to overcome is the guilt feelings that accompany resting and recreation. I have found that the best way to deal with these feelings is to take oneself aside, sit oneself down and give oneself a good talking to.

WHAT TO SAY TO YOURSELF

- 'There's nothing wrong with taking time out to rest. Rest is constructive. It's during times of rest that my tired cells and worn out tissues build themselves up and make necessary repairs. It's during rest that I make new, energetic white blood cells to replace the old tired ones.'
- 'Because my body can't do this while I'm busy and because eight hours' sleep isn't enough time to do it in, I have to take time out for recreation.'
- 'Recreation means exactly what it says, re-creation.'
- 'By recreating myself in this way I'll be more productive.'
- 'I'll do more in less time, with less mistakes.'
- 'This will more than offset the rest time I'm taking.'
- 'I'll enjoy sitting down after the evening meal with a good book/ to listen to music/to watch TV/to have a pleasant conversation.'
- 'I won't waste the evening by doing the ironing, putting on a load of washing, doing paperwork.'
- 'I'll hire someone else to do the washing and ironing or I'll organise the kids to do it.'
- 'I'll do the paperwork at work.'

By saying these things often enough for long enough it will start to filter through to your subconscious mind where all our habits are stored. At present, you have bad thinking habits.

ATTITUDE AND EXERCISE

'It is better to travel well than to arrive.' (Old Chinese proverb)
Many hard-chargers are committed to a life mode that has arriving as its prime objective. They are so busy rushing towards their goal they never get to enjoy the journey. Having achieved their goal they are usually unfulfilled, for being in a rush mode, when they arrive they feel disorientated and have to quickly find another goal to rush towards. They seldom, if ever, take time to savour the fruits of a given achievement. Many heart attack, cancer, arthritis, high blood pressure and diabetes victims live by this behaviour code and it's encouraging to see that more and more doctors are recognising this.

As a result, more and more physicians are using attitudinal healing as their main treatment modality. Attitudinal healing teaches enjoyment of the here and now and to not place more importance on a given achievement than on the process which made it possible. Such changes in attitude have the effect of relaxing us and removing the sensation that life is rushing past us. These attitude changes often necessitate an extension of the time frames needed to achieve our goals. They also encourage us to notice and enjoy more of the commonplace things in life that are so often taken for granted or go completely unnoticed.

The Eastern sages recognised that appropriate physical exercise was needed to help perpetuate attitudes of equanimity and appreciation of the banal. As a result such exercise regimes as Tai Chi and yoga came into existence. The slow rhythmic movements, combined with the deep, slow, rhythmic breathing of these disciplines, tone the muscles in a way that keeps them supple, young and strong. The sensory nerves that travel from the muscles to the brain carry calming nerve impulses that convey the relaxed state of the body to the mind which in turn enhances its relaxed state.

These exercise regimes compare favourably with the rip, tear and bust effect of jogging, aerobics, squash and weight training which, being more in time with a rush, do and bust lifestyle leaves the muscles full of lactic acid which makes them tight, shortened and overly toned (in spasm). Shallow breathing, stiff joints, headaches and awkward gait ensues. The uptight muscles send aberrant nerve impulses up the sensory nerves to the brain, imposing the agitated state of the body on the mind.

Such bodies and minds become rigid and lacking in stamina as evidenced by the frequent colds and 'flu hard-charging exercise buffs catch. A fit body is one that has a strong resistance to any type of disease and can survive a winter without as much as a sniffle. Unfortunately, the Western definition of a fit body is one that has bulging, hard muscles and can be pushed to inordinate lengths. The chronic pain that lingers after a sports injury has been incurred is an ongoing stress to the body which contributes to the lowering of its resistance and stamina.

WATER

'Right living is like the water, which of all things most yielding can overcome that which of all things is most hard.' (Old Tai Chi philosophy)

The Eastern sages were great observers of nature. They noticed that water, despite its softness, was so strong it could wear away the hardest rock, if it patiently and persistently dripped onto it for long enough. From this observation they formulated the 'Inevitability of Gradualness' principle, which they applied to everyday life. This principle holds that if we see our goals clearly, patiently and persistently, and despite all obstacles, work towards those goals, we will achieve them. They noticed that each drop of water that hit the rock momentarily disintegrated but quickly reformed to flow off the rock as a drop of water once more. Those who are successful and enjoy high levels of well-being have elected, like water, to bounce back after each hard knock. To regroup their forces, put that knock behind them and move on as a fully contained entity once more.

They noticed water's flexibility and that those who had a flexible body and mind were better equipped to cope with the vagaries, vicissitudes and hardships of life. Conversely, they noticed that those who have rigid, uncompromising attitudes are less tolerant and therefore more easily stressed by life's events. They noticed that water's flexibility enabled it, according to circumstantial dictates, to be as hard, cold and immovable as ice or as soft, warm and elusive as steam. Just as in life, there are times when a hard stand is appropriate and times when a diplomatic backing away is appropriate. That water readily returns to its neutral state when circumstantial catalysts are removed they equated with humans' capacity for forgiveness and urged that this capacity be regularly exercised as the main vehicle for keeping stress levels down.

Water, they noticed, is agreeable and impartial. It serves all species willingly and equally, it is not bigoted. Water is tolerant and adaptable. It readily adopts the shape of whatever container it is placed in. Water's ability and willingness to accept change is a quality we can exercise and develop, if our stress levels are to remain low and our levels of well-being high.

The Eastern sages also noted that, for the main part, the structure of a living species governed its functions. As humans are made up of 55–65 per cent water they reasoned that they would try, wherever possible, to emulate water's behaviour patterns. For this reason the movements of the exercise disciplines they devised were fluid and continuous rather than short, sharp, intermittent and jerky. These same fluid movements were incorporated into the self-defence regimes of the East, Tai Chi being one of the most effective.

'No rock so hard but that a little wave may beat admission in a thousand years.' (Alfred, Lord Tennyson)
The Eastern sages recommended watery behaviour and response patterns as the most effective way of dealing with conflict and confrontation. They recognised that human conflict was fuelled by intolerance, arrogance and aggression, which is represented by the element of fire. Water has the ability to extinguish fire and when used in sufficient quantities, always will. The aggressee can invariably disarm the aggressor by emulating water in his/her mental, emotional and physical response to aggression.

Bullies rely on a fiery retort from the bullied to work up their aggression and vindicate their attack. Equanimity and impassivity on the part of their victim comes as a surprise to them. It takes the steam out of their attack, putting them off balance and making them vulnerable to mental, emotional, verbal and physical control by the victim.

Nowhere is this principle of acquiescence and yielding more successfully employed than in the sticking hands technique of Tai Chi. Here the aggressor's strength is absorbed from and used against him by this flowing self-defence technique which exhausts and dominates him totally. Tai Chi's great forte lies in the fact that a calm mind is infinitely more successful at assessing and controlling a situation than an agitated and disturbed mind. A calm mind enables us to be more confident and watery in our behaviour than an opponent who is fiery in his. Two fires make a conflagration, fire and water make a nullification.

Traditionally (though less since World War II), Eastern humans have sought to learn from, and live in harmony with, nature and their environment. Conversely, European humans (though less of late) have sought to bend nature to suit themselves. This is not to say that our competitive, achievement-orientated society is wrong and we should all drop out to become yogis or Zen monks. Challenge and response is, and will always remain the catalyst for all growth and development.

The good news is, we are in a position to have it all, the material comforts, the good health and the peace of mind, if we adopt those attitudes that facilitate a day to day function that is more in line with our structure.

TAKING TIME OUT

It takes time to adopt new attitudes and for some people a change of attitude doesn't come easily. Action always speaks louder than words and action can greatly influence the way we think. For this reason, hard-chargers will find it of benefit to set aside specific time to do other things. Write this schedule down, post it on your mirror and rigorously adhere to it. The following checklist is one I suggest as the basis of such a schedule. It will bring balance to your life and in so doing will lower stress levels:

- Take time to work—it is the vehicle of success.
- Take time to rest—it is the foundation of health and vitality.
- Take time to think—it is the source of achievement.
- Take time to play—it is the secret of perpetual youth.
- Take time to read—it is the fount of wisdom.
- Take time to be friendly—it is the road to happiness.
- Take time to love and be loved—it is nourishment for the soul.
- Take time to share—it is too short a life to be selfish.
- Take time to laugh—it is the music of the heart.
- Take time to dream—it is the well of inspiration.

STRESS AND ATTITUDE

Feelings follow thoughts. The thoughts we choose to think determine the feelings we experience. We are all born with a free will. This enables us to choose the thought we wish to think.

So powerful is human thought it can over-ride the effect that external influences can have on us. Because of this, we have the power to remain minimally distressed through the greatest adversity, if we choose to. Our attitude has the greatest of all influences on our stress levels.

SELF-SABOTAGING ATTITUDES

These raise the stress levels. Avoid these:

1. 'Life, the world and others should provide me with everything I require to be happy, and if it and they don't, it's terrible and I can't stand it.'
2. 'One should be dependent on others. I must have someone strong to lean on.'
3. 'Things must go my way. It is terrible, awful and unbearable when they don't.'
4. 'People should treat me fairly at all times because I treat all others fairly. If they don't, they are damnable and should be severely punished.'

186

5. 'I must at all times be loved and approved of by all those who are significant in my life.'
6. 'I must be successful and achieve at all tasks. If I fail, I'm worthless and useless.'
7. 'All human unhappiness is caused by external events. Humans are victims of circumstance.'
8. 'I must feel anxious about perceived threats, be they real or imagined. I must ponder the possibility of their occurrence.'
9. 'It is easier to avoid than face self-responsibility and life difficulties.'
10. 'I should upset myself over the problems and disturbances of others.'

The words 'should', 'ought' and 'must' engender attitudes of inflexibility. They are demands that set us up for a life of frustration which, in time, leads to significant emotional disturbance. The world is impartial and does not respond to the demands of individuals. Substituting the words 'I prefer', 'it would be nice', 'I would like' (preferences), will do away with the emotional disturbance and the raised stress levels caused by 'should', 'ought' and 'must'.

SELF-ENHANCING ATTITUDES
These lower the stress levels. Adopt these:

1. 'My life is my responsibility. I will co-operate with others but won't demand continuous support from them.'
2. 'I will remain flexible in my views of others and will not make rigid rules for them or myself.'
3. 'No one is perfect. We all have the right to make mistakes. I will not condemn myself or others even when I intensely dislike my or their behaviour.'
4. 'I am adventurous enough to take risks that are not foolhardy and to do what I want even if there is a good chance I might fail.'
5. 'I am not the centre of the universe and although it would be nice if I was, I'm not. Therefore I will always be interested in others and will always act morally to protect their interests where possible.'
6. 'I am profoundly interested in myself yet I am willing to make sacrifices for those I care about—without becoming a martyr.'
7. 'My focus in life is not on being the centre of other's attention, but on those absorbing activities that I enjoy.'
8. 'I accept that I live in an impartial world that offers no guarantees for my well-being and that the uncertainty of life can upset my plans.'

187

Some bad luck is a mathematical probability for all of us during our passage through life. Fear of bad luck can significantly raise stress levels and is a waste of time—all the statistics prove that very little, if any, of what we fear ever befalls us. Fear, for the main part, is simply False Evidence Appearing Real.

In addition to imagining the worst, humans have a tendency to exaggerate the seriousness of any given life situation or predicament. This habit of 'awfulising' and 'catastrophising' can be overcome by vehemently disputing these thoughts as they arise. Looking for perfection in an imperfect world is a futile and stress-raising exercise that many fall victim to. Demanding ('should', 'ought', 'must') that we should find the perfect partner, have perfect sex, have the perfect friends, kids, house, car, job and that we should perform perfectly and always succeed, is expecting too much from life. It sets us up for bitterness, resentment and frustration, which can lead to anxiety and depression. The happiest couples are not those who are the most compatible, but rather those who are most tolerant of each other's differences.

Adopting the eight self-enhancing attitudes will not entirely do away with feelings of dissatisfaction—terrible and distressing things *can* happen in life. However, they will prevent feelings of dissatisfaction escalating into feelings of emotional disturbance; that is, they will keep stress down to non-health-affecting levels.

MAKING THE CHANGE

Like any change of habit, overcoming the tendency to think self-sabotaging thoughts requires time and effort. To achieve this task you need to:

1. Keep your energy levels up by eating well, getting adequate rest and taking in adequate fluid, oxygen, vitamins and minerals. It's easier to think positively when your energy is up.
2. Promptly dispute all self-sabotaging thoughts whenever they arise, attacking them instantly before they grow in size and intensity.
3. Each day, write down on a card one of the self-enhancing attitudes and take time to read and memorise it several times through the day. Carry them in your wallet. Cellotape them to your mirror.
4. Practise daily the mental relaxation exercises. It is far easier for new attitudes to filter down from the conscious mind to the subconscious when we're relaxed. Changing ones attitudes is less of a chore when we're relaxed. We tend to interpret people's words and actions more positively when we're relaxed and our reactions to them are more appropriate. Repetition is the key.

Keep repeating the self-enhancing attitude every day even if such an attitude feels unattainable. If you hear it often enough for long enough, you'll start to believe it. That's the way the subconscious works. Repetition is the powerful reprogrammer of the subconscious mind.

Remember: A willingness to accept change lowers stress levels. Those who enjoy high levels of well-being all have one thing in common—a willingness to risk change.

12.
Dangers of allergy drugs

'To live by medicine is to live horribly.'

Carl Linnaeus, 1707–78

In a recent survey, one-sixth of all hospital admissions were attributed to drug interaction or unintended reaction to drugs, many of them antihistamine or cortisone based.

ANTIHISTAMINES

These act in a similar way to tranquillisers, muscle relaxants, narcotics, painkillers and alcohol, suppressing brain and nerve function. For this reason antihistamines are a component of many commonly prescribed sleeping pills.

Suppressed brain and nerve function lower your performance physically and mentally, to a greater or lesser extent, depending on the doses of antihistamine taken. A combination of sedatives and antihistamines can cause tremors and mental confusion. If pain-killers are also taken, as they often are by arthritis sufferers, depression can ensue. Drugs that suppress brain and nerve function tend to intensify each other's effect and can lead to nutrient deficiencies by interfering with the body's ability to metabolise vitamins and minerals.

For instance, aspirin can cause vitamin C deficiency. This is bad news for arthritis sufferers—vitamin C is needed to repair the destroyed collagen of their affected joints. Indomethacin, another drug used to treat arthritis can cause psychiatric disturbances, epilepsy and Parkinson's disease by interfering with vitamin B, zinc and manganese metabolism. It also predisposes to infections and defects in the body's ability to coagulate blood. It impairs kidney function and, given time, can actually burn holes in the stomach wall, greatly interfering with digestion and absorption.

Dr Jean Mayer, Professor of Nutrition at Harvard University, believes a vast number of people suffer from iatrogenic (doctor-caused) malnutrition. My experience is that people on long-term Indomethacin most certainly do.

Although not particularly toxic in the short term, antihistamines can, even if no other drugs are taken, be toxic to the body over a period of time. It is because allergy sufferers take antihistamines for years on end that they end up joining the hospital admission list.

The following are the well-recognised side effects of commonly used antihistamines:

Atarax   Severe drowsiness may occur with the use of this drug. Patients should be warned against driving a car or operating dangerous machinery while taking it. Potentiates the action of sedatives and alcohol.

Benadryl   This medication may cause drowsiness. If affected do not drive a motor car, avoid alcohol. Potentiates the action of sedatives and alcohol.

Fabahistin   Same as above.

Polaramine   Same as above.

Phenergan   Drowsiness, dry mouth, dizziness, jitteriness, faintness, headache, nausea, allergic skin manifestations of rash and fluid retention, fatigue, disturbed co-ordination, tremor, irritability, blurred vision, palpitations, nervousness (and more).

Recent research in the United States has shown that long-term use of antihistamine nasal sprays can cause a permanently blocked nose—the very condition they are used to treat in the first place.

CORTISONE DRUGS

These are powerful anti-inflammatory hormones, produced naturally by the body during times of stress. Stress places the body on red-alert to potential physical danger and cortisone is released by the adrenal glands to reduce possible pain and inflammation from what the body sees as a potential threat.

The way in which long-distance runners tend not to feel sprained and inflamed ankle and knee joints until after the race is an example of how naturally released cortisone works. Similarly, footballers tend not to feel bruises until after the match. In both cases stress has abated after the sporting event and cortisone levels have returned to normal, no longer being high enough to act as a buffer against pain.

Nature never intended cortisone to stay in the blood any longer than the time of the stress, nor were we designed to endure prolonged stress. When high levels of cortisone are in the blood for too long, major imbalances in the metabolism develop. If un-checked, these metabolic imbalances become irreversible and the cells become addicted to or dependent on the cortisone.

The use of cortisone drugs for the treatment of allergies, particularly asthma, eczema and arthritis, will produce these major metabolic imbalances if used for too long.

CUSHING'S SYNDROME

This is the name given to the major metabolic imbalances caused by excess cortisone. The symptoms of Cushing's syndrome are:

1. The removal of fat from the arms and legs, which is deposited on the upper back and shoulders (buffalo hump), the torso and the abdomen.
2. The face develops a moon shape, due to the deposition of fat and the retention of fluid.
3. The skin becomes very thin due to the dissolution of the collagen and elastin. It bruises easily and tears, giving rise to stretch marks. Sores appear in the advanced stages.
4. The muscles become thin and weak, due to dissolved collagen.
5. The bones become thin and weak, due to a lack of calcium (osteoporosis).
6. Stomach ulcers develop.
7. Resistance to infections, allergies and cancer is significantly reduced.
8. The ageing process is significantly accelerated.

The sad thing about cortisone drugs is that they only treat the symptoms of allergy, not the cause. By the time you have developed the full-blown symptoms of Cushing's syndrome you still have your original allergies, only by this time they are usually worse. You are in a double lose situation as you have added a disease that is far more debilitating than your allergies.

192

CORTISONE CREAMS

These, if used too often for too long, will cause significant thinning and ageing of the skin (telangiectasia). When this happens bluish spider veins and purple-brown patches (purpura) begin to appear. It takes years on the Metabolism-Balancing Program to repair this damage.

CORTISONE PUFFERS

Although the cortisone in the commonly used asthma puffers can, in time, damage the lining of the windpipe and lung (telangiectasia again), it must be recognised that these puffers can save lives and should not be discarded without a doctor's advice.

The side effects of cortisone puffers are:

Becotide   The aerosol inhaler can produce candida yeast infections in the mouth and nose of those who use it for any length of time. This perpetuates the allergy and makes the patient more allergic.

Aldecin   Authorities admit there is no data on the long-term effects of Becotide and Aldecin inhalers on lung and gastric tissue. If you are currently using them and intend doing so for any length of time you are unwittingly volunteering to become a guinea pig for their database.

CORTISONE'S ROLE

In fairness to cortisone it does have a place in the overall treatment program of allergies. Cortisone creams are very effective at keeping skin rashes and eczema at bay while the programs are taking effect. Keeping the skin quiet during this time keeps stress levels down, the anxiety of looking at an affected skin being a major stress. Such anxiety reduces the efficacy of the programs. The short time that cortisone cream will be needed will not be long enough to damage the skin as the programs speed the rate of skin regeneration. Cortisone puffers allow a good night's sleep which is imperative for raising the body's resistance to colds, 'flu and asthma. Asthma responds quickly to the programs when body resistance is up. The programs lose some of their efficacy when sleep is broken by too many asthma attacks. The short amount of time cortisone puffers will be needed while on the program is not enough to produce significant candida colonies or tissue damage to the mouth, throat and upper windpipe.

CORTISONE WITHDRAWAL

This is a slow process. The time it takes depends on the amount you're on and the length of time you have been on it. Your doctor will probably reduce it by 1–2 mg only every two to four weeks. This gives the metabolism the chance to adjust and rebalance itself. My experience is that withdrawal from cortisone tablets is more successful if the patient is on the Metabolism-Balancing Program. If you are on cortisone and showing the early signs of Cushing's syndrome, don't panic. Follow the instructions listed in the recommended program. There is a 90 per cent chance you will get better.

If you allow yourself to be on the cortisone drugs (tablets taken orally) for too long you'll reach the point of no return. You won't be able to come off them.

FLUID TABLETS

In the short term fluid tablets (diuretics, water pills) remove excess fluid from the body. In the long term they cause fluid retention, the very thing they are supposed to treat.

Fluid tablets are often prescribed to sufferers of allergies, candida yeast infections and malnutrition to remove the puffiness from their fingers, ankles, eyes, face, legs and wrists or counteract the general weight gain that often accompanies these conditions.

Fluid tablets work by interfering with normal kidney function. They create metabolic imbalances in the tubule cells of the kidney. This inhibits the tubule cells' capacity to absorb water and nutrients as they pass through the tubules en route to the collecting ducts. As a result, water plus vitamins and minerals pass out of the body en masse, giving rise to insidious mal-nutrition.

After a while on fluid tablets, vitamin and mineral deficiencies begin to manifest as metabolic imbalances elsewhere in the body. Symptoms of these metabolic imbalances are many and varied. They can include: weakness, fatigue, light-headedness, dizziness, muscle cramps, thirst, flushing, prickly tingling of the skin (paraesthesia), blurred vision, rashes, low blood pressure on standing (postural hypotension), hypoglycaemia, aggravation of existing diabetes, increased blood uric acid levels, anaphylactic shock (usually in the severely malnourished), peripheral circu-latory failure (especially in the elderly), thrombocytopenia (low levels of blood platelets) and leucopenia (low levels of white blood cells).

Vitamin and mineral deficiencies are a significant stress to the body. When the body is under stress the adrenal glands work overtime and more adrenal hormones than normal are produced. Aldosterone is one such hormone. Its job is to regulate the body's fluid levels by stimulating the kidneys to retain sodium and water when the levels of these two are getting low. An excess of aldosterone means greater than normal quantities of sodium and water are retained. This is why people under stress have trouble losing weight while on a weightloss diet or put on weight without any change in their diet or eating habits.

Fluid tablets create a vicious cycle. By causing vitamin and mineral deficiencies they raise the body's stress and aldosterone levels which causes greater fluid retention and the need for more fluid tablets. The metabolic imbalances that this cycle of ever-increasing stress and quantity of fluid tablets cause are such that in time you become hooked on fluid tablets.

If you reach the stage of fluid tablet dependency you'll experience a significant weight gain the moment you stop taking them. Because it takes the aldosterone levels about fourteen to twenty-one days to come down the weight could last for that long. The Metabolism-Balancing Program plus the supplementary vitamins and minerals and rest reduce the stress and aldosterone levels within a week. Be patient, the weight will come down as the metabolism balances. Don't freak out and go back on the fluid tablets if your weight shoots up. Just wait it out and everything will be OK.

If you are already on fluid tablets for heart, lung or blood pressure problems, consult your doctor before doing anything.

If you are not on fluid tablets and your doctor wants to treat your allergy, candida, malnutrition or stress-based fluid retention problem with fluid tablets, refuse his or her offer and follow the treatment program outlined in this book with his or her supervision. Herbal, so called natural, diuretics create the same metabolic imbalances as the drug-based ones. Don't use them as they too treat only the symptoms of fluid retention and not the cause.

13.
The Metabolism-Balancing Program

'In every person, even in such as appear most reckless, there is an inherent desire to attain balance.'

J. Wasserman

It is best to start a get-well program with the Metabolism-Balancing Program. This program is nutritionally balanced and feeds the cells all the nutrients they need. In so doing, it balances the metabolism and increases the body's ability to perform on all levels. It also increases resistance to infection. When immune resistance is up, resistance to viruses, bacteria and candida overgrowth is up. By the same token sensitivity to allergens is down. A body built up on the Metabolism-Balancing Program shows up allergic to less things when tests are performed. The less things we show up allergic to the less restrictive the anti allergy program will be. This makes it: (a) easier to stick to; and (b) more nutritious.

This building up procedure contrasts sharply with the food challenge test procedure used by others, which so lowers the body's resistance it reacts to practically every food it's challenged with. Experience has taught me that building up the body prior to allergy testing gives a more accurate diagnostic picture of the patient and much better treatment results. And some people overcome their allergies on the build-up program alone.

Furthermore, because many of the symptoms of allergy, *C albicans* infection and stress are also the symptoms of vitar mineral deficiency, nutrient deficiencies must be eliminate allergy, candidiasis and stress can be accurately diagnosed.

On this program the cells burn more calories and produce more energy. Increased production of energy means excess fluid is pumped out of the cells, taken away by blood vessels and eliminated through the kidneys. Increased energy leads to increased activity—excess fat is used by muscle cells to provide fuel for this.

Because of this many people with slow metabolic rates experience a moderate weight loss when they first go on the Metabolism-Balancing Program. This is due mainly to the loss of excess fluid from the cells. The Metabolism-Balancing Program is too high in calories for weight loss to be from fat loss only. When the weight plateaus, it usually means that the metabolic rate has risen to normal. When your energy levels rise, you can be sure that your metabolic rate has also risen. The extent to which your energy levels have risen is the most accurate barometer of how much your metabolic rate and resistance to allergies and yeast infections has increased.

Many people remark that after six to eight weeks on the program their perceptions change and things others say and do that used to irritate and offend them, no longer do. Often people who complain of being in a crummy relationship at the beginning of the program, maintain the relationship is fine after six to eight weeks on it. This change in perception is inextricably bound up with an increase in energy levels. When our energy is up, our ability to cope is up. We are no longer over-sensitive and cease to over-react to threats which in reality existed only in our tired, over-sensitive minds.

The Metabolism-Balancing Program is excellent for getting our energy levels up, and our change in perception is mirrored in our white blood cells which also begin to perceive things more appropriately. They cease to perceive such innocuous substances as dust, pollen, mould or food as threats to the body and mitigate their over-zealous (allergic) reactions to these substances. They begin to correctly perceive viruses, bacteria and opportunistic yeast over-growths (candida) as the true threats to the body and do battle with them only. In this way, our resistance to these invaders increases on the Metabolism-Balancing Program, and our allergic reactions reduce. Less histamine is produced and, for this reason, many allergy symptoms reduce in intensity and some even disappear.

Don't make the mistake of overdoing it at work, sport or socialising when you feel your energy levels rise. If you burn up your new-found energy as quickly as you acquire it, your metabolic rate and resistance will drop right down again. Just as you save some of your earnings, so you should save some of your energy. You need to keep some in reserve if you want total health.

If you are the hard-charger type (see Chapter 11, 'Stress—Stress and the hard-charger') it's going to require a lot of discipline for you to be taking it easy when you feel so energetic. However hard this is, it must be done. Many hard-chargers erroneously believe that this program is a licence to go at full speed all the time. All diets, no matter how nutritious they are, have their limits and one can always push oneself to one's new-found energy limits. Those who misuse the Metabolism-Balancing Program in this way never get well. They only extend the time it takes for their health to break down.

The great forte of the Metabolism-Balancing Program is that it balances glucose metabolism. This in turn reduces hypoglycaemia (see Chapter 16, 'Scientific explanations—The metabolism'). Over-doing it causes hypoglycaemia and undermines the program's ability to contain it. Hypoglycaemia triggers allergies.

Sometimes an increase in appetite is experienced on the Metabolism-Balancing Program. If this happens, don't fight it. It's the result of the metabolism speeding up in a body that is deficient in protein, vitamins and minerals. Faster metabolisms require more nutrients. The more nutrients the metabolism receives, the sooner it will balance itself. If you put on weight on the Metabolism-Balancing Program, it will be from increased lean muscle density and tone, not fat accumulation, unless, of course, you are over-eating.

Within six to eight weeks on the Metabolism-Balancing Program the appetite will drop back to normal. When this has happened and your energy levels have significantly improved (which by now they would have), it's time to start the Anti-Candida Program and if necessary the combined Anti-Candida/Anti-Allergy Program.

Do not stop the Metabolism-Balancing Program and commence the combined Anti-Candida/Anti-Allergy Program if your appetite and weight initially increases. If you do, you will further strain and unbalance the metabolism. Wait until your appetite and weight have levelled out.

Never start the combined Anti-Candida/Anti-Allergy Program with an unbalanced metabolism.

If you are sticking to the amounts stipulated on the Metabolism-Balancing Program your weight will balance out with your metabolism. If you are over-indulging on this program, your weight will continue to rise. Make sure you don't eat or drink too much alcohol while on this program.

Don't despair if at first you feel nauseous or have stomach discomfort on this program. This indicates that the deep breathing exercises and your increased fluid intake are cleansing a toxic liver. Within a week or two your liver will be clean and the symptoms will abate. The liver is the great metabolic factory of the body and, while it's sluggish and full of gunk, it can't work at optimum capacity. An under-functioning liver means imbalances in the metabolism of the rest of the body and the brain. In particular, it means imbalances in glucose metabolism. The breathing exercises reduce the severity of allergy by lowering the overall level of histamine in the blood and are an important part of the Metabolism-Balancing Program.

Adequate rest, adequate fluid intake and adequate oxygen intake are integral components of this program. As many of the symptoms of allergy can be caused by a deficiency in rest, water and oxygen, such deficiencies must be eliminated if an accurate diagnosis of allergy is to be made. If you have followed the instructions in this program faithfully and have symptoms left after six to eight weeks on it, then candida/allergy is a safe diagnosis.

A word of warning about eating chicken: Listeria is a bacteria that has recently been found in the chicken population. Listeria can cause gut infections that mimic gut-mediated allergies. Symptoms include bloating, distension, pain and moderate to severe diarrhoea. Eating chicken has become 'Russian roulette', as any chicken can be infected, although free-range is safer. If you've been eating chicken and have any of the symptoms, don't automatically assume it's allergy.

THE METABOLISM-BALANCING PROGRAM

Immediately on rising, before you do anything else, drink from two to five 230 mL (8 oz) glasses of fresh spring, mineral or filtered tap water (warm water in winter). If these are not available you will have to have straight tap water either boiled for ten minutes (no lid on it) or left to stand overnight to evaporate the chlorine and settle the sediment. Have another glass about an hour later. The following is a guide to how much water to drink on rising:

Lean body weight
63 kg (10 st) and under	2 glasses
63–70 kg (10–11 st)	3 glasses
70–76 kg (11–12 st)	4 glasses
Over 76 kg (12 st)	5 glasses

Lean body weight should be calculated. This is your optimum weight before you started putting on weight. This is most important for kids.

You may, at first, find it hard to accommodate this much water first thing in the morning. Don't be put off by this. It only takes ten to fourteen days to get used to it. If your abdomen is bloating to the point of discomfort, add $^1/_4$–$^1/_2$ teaspoon of glucose powder to each glass of water. Glucose powder is obtainable from chemists, health stores and supermarkets. Glucose speeds the rate of absorption from the gut into the blood, reducing abdominal distension and the feeling of fullness. Switch to warm water if you are having trouble getting it all down; warm water has a relaxing effect on the stomach and gut muscles.

The early morning fluid is important for:

(a) flushing toxins from the liver;
(b) flushing the kidneys, especially of calcium oxalate, the major cause of kidney stones;
(c) cleansing the bowel: all the swallowing required to get the water down sets up peristalsis, the rhythmic contractions of the bowel muscles that move wastes along and out.

Try to fit fifteen minutes of deep breathing exercises in between the drinking of the water and the eating of breakfast. Don't eat for half an hour after the water.

Do not eat unleavened bread while on this program. Eat only those wholemeal breads that have been raised with yeast.

BREAKFAST

These breakfast options may be mixed and matched to keep breakfast interesting and varied. You can have two or more options at one meal if hunger or calorie expenditure dictates. You can mix the options in any way. You can borrow from any of the options to make up your own option. Make sure that any changes you make are conducive to sound digestion and appropriate food combining. (See Chapter 16, 'Scientific explanations—Food combining'.) The options pertaining to high cholesterol sufferers may also be used by those with normal cholesterol. The high cholesterol options normalise cholesterol levels, they don't reduce them to below normal. Try to vary your diet—it pays not to have the same option on two consecutive days.

OPTION 1

A fresh fruit salad (no canned fruits) with 60–180 g (2–6 oz) of raw nuts, sunflower and/or sesame seeds.

Weigh the nuts and seeds out and eat according to your size and how hungry you are. Purée the nuts and seeds in the blender for toddlers. Brown rice bubbles (the brown rice ones available at the health store) may be sprinkled over the salad in addition to the nuts and seed or instead of them—whichever you prefer. Puffed brown rice must be eaten if cholesterol levels are high. If they are very high add rice bran as well. Rice bran lowers cholesterol, just like oat bran. If constipation is a problem, add wheat/oat bran.

OPTION 2

Stewed fruits—any variety, as long as they are fresh. The same nuts, seeds and puffed brown rice mentioned in Option 1 may be added to the stewed fruit. Also a little milk (cold or warm) and honey or spices (see 'Recipes') may be added for flavour. Put nuts and seeds through the blender for toddlers. Puffed brown rice must be eaten if cholesterol levels are high. Add rice bran if the levels are very high. A dressing of cold pressed vegetable oil and lemon juice dressing may be used on the fruit salad or stewed fruit. Apricot kernel oil is good. Add wheat/oat bran if constipation is a problem.

OPTION 3

One to three eggs (depending on your size) cooked anyway you like with one to three slices of wholemeal bread (yeast-raised), toasted, with a thin spread of butter. You may have 30 g (1 oz) of bacon, salami, ham or a sausage occasionally.

Don't have Option 3 until, or unless, your cholesterol levels are normal—check with your doctor if you are unsure. If having your eggs scrambled, as an omelette or quiche, make sure you add the egg shells (crushed to a fine powder) to enhance the calcium content of the meal. If having sausages, have only those made on the premises by your butcher. These sausages have less MSG, metabisulphite, nitrates and other chemicals in them.

OPTION 4

Savoury mince (see 'Recipes' at the back of the book) on wholemeal toast (yeast-raised). Have a thin spread of butter if cholesterol levels are normal. If they are high, brush some olive oil on the toast (the way the Italians do). Eat according to your size and hunger. Don't overdo it.

OPTION 5

Wholemeal toast (yeast-raised) and 60–240 g (2–8 oz) of cooked fish (cooked any way—see 'Recipes') with parsley, onion and tomato.

Occasionally some canned fish such as tuna, salmon or sardines may be eaten. The wholemeal toast may be made from wheat, rye, oat, arrowroot, millet, buckwheat or soya flour—preferably stone ground. A thin spread of butter may be used—olive oil if the cholesterol levels are high. Don't fry the fish if the cholesterol levels are high—steam or lightly grill instead.

OPTION 6

A bowl of untoasted muesli or a bowl of puffed brown rice, either home-made or from the health store, with milk but no sugar in it.

Add oat bran to the muesli if the cholesterol levels are high. A little honey may be added for flavour. Eat according to size and hunger. Don't overdo it. Add wheat/oat bran if constipated.

OPTION 7

Wholegrain cereal or porridge made from oats, millet, buckwheat, cooked as kasha (see 'Recipes'), with some milk or cold pressed oil (olive, sunflower, sesame or apricot kernel) over the top.

Add oat bran if cholesterol levels are high. Honey may be added to flavour. No sugar. Eat according to size or hunger. Don't overdo it. Muesli tastes great cooked as a porridge—dried fruit and all. Add wheat/oat bran if constipated.

OPTION 8

$\frac{1}{4}$–$\frac{1}{2}$ cup of cooked brown rice (see 'Recipes') with olive oil over the top. This is for those with high cholesterol. If your cholesterol is normal you may add a little butter and a handful or two of cashew nuts to the cooked rice. Add wheat/oat bran if constipated.

OPTION 9

Steak and eggs: 120–240 g (4–8 oz) steak and one to three eggs with one to four slices of wholemeal toast (yeast-raised) with a thin spread of butter, though preferably olive oil, on it.

To be taken only if your cholesterol levels are normal and only if you have a day of strenuous physical activity ahead (for example, a surfing or windsurfing competition, mountain or rockclimbing, a long trek or a day spent concreting or loading trucks). Not to be had if you are sitting in an office or motor car all day, or visiting friends. Eat according to your hunger and size. Don't over-eat, or you won't be able to perform effectively.

OPTION 10

A toasted wholemeal cheese sandwich (on yeast-raised bread)— with onion, tomato or mushroom if desired.

OPTION 11

A glass of fresh fruit or vegetable juice (any variety) with 1 tablespoon of brewer's yeast powder, 1 teaspoon of dolomite powder and 1 dessertspoon of lecithin granules. Mix thoroughly and add a little honey to flavour.

This isn't everyone's cup of tea, even though the most nutritious of all the breakfast options. It is excellent for high cholesterol. Make sure you sip it slowly and mix it with the saliva in your mouth—it won't digest properly otherwise. Add wheat bran if constipated. Diabetics, pre-diabetics, hypoglycaemics and those who crave sweets should have this three times per week for the duration of this program, to balance the sugar levels.

OPTION 12

Three or four whole fresh fruits (any variety) and 60 g (2 oz) of nuts (any variety—or sunflower or sesame seeds).

About an hour after breakfast, or just before leaving the house for work, have a 230 mL glass of fresh juice (fruit or vegetable) or water with $^1/_4$–$^1/_2$ teaspoon of glucose powder if required.

MORNING TEA

You don't have to eat anything at morning tea if you don't want to. However, 230 mL (8 oz) of fluid is compulsory.

OPTION 1

A cup of herbal tea or ordinary tea or coffee. Milk may be taken if desired. The only sweetener to be used is honey, though it pays to try and go without a sweetener.

OPTION 2

A glass of mineral, soda, spring or filtered tap water. If none of these are available you will have to have boiled tap water. Add $^1/_4$–$^1/_2$ teaspoon of glucose powder if it's hard to get down, but try and do without the glucose if you can.

OPTION 3

A glass of fruit or vegetable juice. The canned ones are OK. Try to get one with minimal or no additives.

OPTION 4

If you are hungry, you may have a rice cake with a nut spread, or nut butter (any sort of nut), or one or two handfuls of nuts or seeds (any variety), or one or two pieces of fresh fruit (any variety). A sandwich for growing kids if they are hungry.

LUNCH

Not to be eaten any later than 1.30 p.m.
A little fruit juice or water (glucose if necessary) must be sipped before and during lunch.

If you've missed your morning deep breathing exercises then twenty minutes' yogic walking in the park before lunch is a good substitute—it will relax and energise you for the rest of the day.

The lunch options can be mixed and matched in the same way as the breakfast options.

OPTION 1

Good for those with high cholesterol, although suitable for anyone.
A garden salad using any variety of garden vegetables, lean meat (all the fat trimmed off), fish or poultry (peel the skin off). Have 120–240 g (4–8 oz) of meat fish or poultry.

Have also 120–240 g (4–8 oz) of a carbohydrate food, such as cooked potato, cooked brown rice, wholemeal pasta or whole-meal bread (not rice cakes), to keep the blood glucose levels normal.

You may have a dressing of cold pressed olive oil (only) with lemon juice or apple cider vinegar added. Any other herbs or spices that take your fancy may be added to the dressing. If you want to sweeten the salad dressing add crushed egg shells (crushed to a fine powder) to the vinegar. Egg shells are an excellent source of calcium in a calcium deficient world. Don't sweeten the dressing with sugar or honey.

OPTION 2

For those with normal cholesterol levels only.
The same salad as Option 1 with the addition of 30–60 g (1–2 oz) of cheese and occasionally some processed meats such as devon, luncheon sausage, ham, corned beef or salami.

No rice cakes. No more than 60–90 g (2–3 oz) of processed meat, no more than two or three times per week. Have only plain cheddar cheeses. The fancy ones (for example, blue vein and camembert) contain cancer-causing substances. Have Option 1's salad dressing—you can use any variety of cold pressed oil in preference to the olive oil.

OPTION 3

Three or four whole fresh fruits with 60–180 g (2–6 oz) of nuts and/or seeds and/or puffed brown rice (from the health store).

Or, a fresh fruit salad with the same amount of nuts, seeds or brown puffed rice (rice bubbles) on top.

Or, stewed fruit with nuts, seeds, brown rice, milk and honey. This option is the same as Options 1 and 2 from 'Breakfast'.

OPTION 4

Good for those with high cholesterol, although suitable for anyone.
A vegetable soup using any variety of garden vegetables thickened

with pearl barley, lentils and soya beans and one or two slices of wholemeal bread (no rice cakes) with a spread of olive oil. Make sure that soybeans are the main ingredient, they are excellent for normalising the cholesterol levels. Rice bran may be added as an additional thickener. It has an excellent cholesterol-normalising action as well. Any herbs and spices may be used.

OPTION 5
For those with normal cholesterol only.
The same soup as Option 4, with less soya beans and lentils and the addition of lean meat, fish or poultry (any variety) to it instead.

Any herb or spice that takes your fancy may be added. A thin spread of butter may be added to the wholemeal bread if your cholesterol levels are normal. (No rice cakes.)

OPTION 6
Wholemeal bread (no rice cakes) sandwiches (one to three depending on your size, hunger and activity levels) with a lean meat, fish or poultry filling, 30–90 g (1–3 oz) of each.

Other fillings such as tahini, peanut butter, almond, cashew or hazelnut paste may be used. You can have canned or smoked fish occasionally. Unprocessed, natural cheese may be included as a filling if the cholesterol levels are normal.

AFTERNOON TEA

Same as morning tea—again the fluid is compulsory. If going to night school, have a snack if you're having the main meal later in the evening. Don't have a big meal before bed.

EVENING (MAIN) MEAL

- You must have at least 120–240 g (4–8 oz) red meat (lean), three times per week.
- You must have at least 120–240 g (4–8 oz) seafood, twice per week.
- Poultry (skin and other fat peeled off) must be eaten twice per week. Egg and cheese dishes may be substituted for the poultry dishes.
- You may substitute one vegetarian meal a week.
- Egg and cheese may be used in any recipe.
- Green and coloured vegetables must be included with each meal, as must some form of carbohydrate (potato, brown rice, pasta, bread, sweet potato, yams, taro or pumpkin).

- The evening meal must contain salt—sea salt preferably, or iodised table salt if sea salt crystals are not available. A lack of salt in the diet will cause you to continue craving salted junk foods. Active kids have a lot of trouble giving up such things as crisps and Twisties if they are not getting salt in their main meal. It becomes impossible for those kids to stick to the Anti-Candida/Anti-Allergy Program later on. Active kids lose a lot of salt in their perspiration and in their urine if sunburnt. They need to replace this salt to keep their energy up.

- Any herbs or spices that take your fancy may be used.

- Sauces and gravies may be used if your cholesterol levels are normal. However, don't consume too much sauce or gravy or have very rich sauces too often.

- You may draw your recipes from any ethnic cuisine you like, be it Italian, French, Greek, Russian, English, German, or whatever. In fact it pays to eat a broad spectrum of ethnic cuisines. This way you are assured of eating as wide a variety of foods as possible. By not restricting yourself with the main meal of the day you won't suffer from that tied down and constrained feeling that so often accompanies diets. This feeling is a stress to many people and the Metabolism-Balancing Program is defeating its purpose if it's stressing you. Feel free to eat at restaurants—just make sure you follow the simple rules outlined in Chapter 16, 'Scientific explanations—Food combining', for optimum digestion and appropriate food combining.

- You may sip one or two glasses of wine or beer with the evening meal most nights. But not if you are a recovering alcoholic, member of AA, pregnant, breastfeeding, hypoglycaemic, have any sort of liver complaint, are diabetic or on any medication that conflicts with alcohol. Have at least three alcohol-free days per week.

- If you desire a dessert, have only a fresh fruit salad, or stewed fruit—yoghurt, dried fruit, carob powder and desiccated coconut can be added. Absolutely no chocolate or other cocoa derivatives should be consumed. The oxalic acid in cocoa blocks the absorption of minerals from the supplements and foods. It pays to have a small dessert and to wait thirty to sixty minutes after the main meal before eating it. Eating too much dessert, too soon, dilutes the digestive juices, interfering with the digestion of the main meal.

VITAMINS

Just before the evening (main) meal have 3 x Formula Six multivitamin and mineral tablets, that is, 1 tablet from each jar. Wash them down with sips from a 230 mL (8 oz) glass of juice (any variety) or water with 1 teaspoon of vitamin C powder in it (calcium or sodium ascorbate) and, twice per week only, 1 drop only of Lugol's iodine solution (from the chemist)—use an eyedropper. One-quarter to one-half a teaspoon of glucose may be added to the water. Sip a little more of the water to wash down the oil capsules after the meal. If you are a regular fish/seafood eater, then have the Lugol's once a week only. Tea, coffee or cocoa are not to be had one hour before and/or up to three hours after the vitamin and mineral supplements. Because hydrochloric acid is required to facilitate absorption of minerals, Formula Six must be taken at a time when there's maximum hydrochloric acid in the stomach, that is, just before a meal. (See Chapter 16, 'Scientific explanations—Food combining—Vitamins and minerals'.)

Because the Metabolism-Balancing Program is a broad spectrum food program and not a food restriction diet, the evening meal can be derived from any recipe book you like. The Metabolism-Balancing Program is designed to make you feel as relaxed as possible about being on a program and to impress upon your subconscious mind that 'being on a program' isn't so bad after all.

If you have high cholesterol levels there are some restrictions:

1. You are not to have rich or fatty sauces or gravies.
2. You are to go without poultry dishes and have two vegetarian meals per week in place of them. Make sure that soybeans and/or lentils are the principal foods in the vegetarian dishes.
3. No cheese or eggs until your cholesterol levels have normalised.
4. No deep fried foods, only light stir-fries using soya oil (or olive oil if you are not amine or salicylate sensitive).

OILS

After the main meal of the day have 2 x 1000 mg capsules of evening primrose oil (Nature's Own is a good brand) and 2 x 1000 mg capsules of marine lipid concentrate (MaxEPA). (See Chapter 16, 'Scientific explanations—Vitamins and minerals—Food combining'.) If you have high cholesterol make that 4 x 1000 mg capsules of marine lipid concentrate. Instead of taking the marine lipid capsules you can take cod liver oil from the bottle—1 dessertspoon per day, at any time of the day, except before the main meal. Have it in juice, on tuna or salmon, over cooked rice, in mashed potato or take it straight with a juice chaser. Blackmore's deodorised is the most palatable. This is for those who want to take a minimum of tablets/capsules.

Make sure that you have at least 1 teaspoon of some form of raw, cold pressed vegetable oil per day. Olive oil is the best as it's cholesterol free. Sunflower, safflower, linseed, sesame and apricot kernel oil may be used if you prefer them. Have this oil in addition to the oil you cook with. Either take it straight off the spoon or in salad dressing. Have it any time of the day except before the main meal, as too much oil blocks mineral absorption.

IRON

If you are very tired, have heavy or extended periods, have mid-cycle bleeding, have had a number of children or have had miscarriages or termination of pregnancy, you will more than likely need an iron boost. I recommend you go on a course of the FAB Co iron tablets available at the health store. (Not for men.)

Take one before breakfast, one before lunch and two with Formula Six just before the evening meal. Do this for four weeks, and if you haven't picked up in that time, do it for another four weeks. Then stop. Formula Six will do the rest.

FLEXIBILITY

The Metabolism-Balancing Program is flexible. Not only can you swap your options around, you can eat them at different times of the day, if you choose. You can have the evening (main) meal for lunch, if you like, and breakfast in the evening! It doesn't matter what order you eat your meal in, as long as you eat three meals per day, eat what's on the program and take the supplements before and after the main meal, whenever that is.

The Metabolism-Balancing Program is flexible enough to allow you 5 per cent junk food (see page 356 for junk food list). That's 5 per cent of the total weekly food intake, which means no more than five items of junk food per week. You may wish to take this in the the form of sweets at a dinner party once per week. Often it creeps in as sugar or white flour in sauces and gravies. Five per cent junk food will do you no harm if you are following the program seriously and taking your supplements.

Keep frozen foods to a minimum—have them only if fresh foods are not available. (See Chapter 16, 'Scientific explanations—Vitamins and minerals'.)

FLUID

You must consume at least 1 x 230 mL (8 oz) glasses of water or juice between the evening meal and going to bed.

You must consume daily the amounts of fluid for your weight shown in the following table. Your metabolism needs these amounts to stay balanced:

Lean body weight

10 st (63 kg) or under	9 glasses
11 st (70 kg)	10 glasses
12 st (76 kg)	11 glasses
13 st (83 kg)	12 glasses
14 st (89 kg)	13 glasses

And so on up to 15 glasses per day. Don't go over 15 glasses per day as most people over 16–17 st (102–108 kg) have an excess of fat tissue as opposed to muscle tissue. Fat, being a very inert tissue, doesn't require much fluid. If you are a lean athlete, footballer, weight lifter of 16 st (102 kg) or more, then drink as many glasses over 15 as you need.

These fluid tables are based on a sedentary lifestyle—after each significant physical work-out you must consume an extra 0.5–1 L of fluid. In summer, it would pay to add 1–2 teaspoons of Staminade to that litre of fluid. (Note: An hour's strenuous physical exercise can cause the loss of at least 1 L of fluid.)

Although the program sets down definite times for drinking, you may need to drink between these times to reach your optimum fluid intake. You can do this by having extra cups of tea or coffee while you are working.

Don't have more than five cups (and preferably only two or three) of tea or coffee combined per day and don't drink either of them for at least one hour before and three hours after taking your vitamins and other supplements. The acids in tea, coffee and cocoa interfere with digestion and absorption of vitamins and minerals. It's best to take a large bottle of water (with glucose if required) or juice with you to work, to sip at while working. (See Chapter 10, 'The importance of water and oxygen'.)

Note: Alcohol and the caffeine in tea, coffee and cocoa has a diuretic effect on the kidneys, causing water to be lost from the body. You must add an extra glass of water to your daily fluid consumption for every three glasses/cups of alcohol/caffeine-containing beverage you consume. These extra glasses are best consumed just before bed.

In summer, raise your sedentary fluid intake to 1 x 230 mL (8 oz) glass for every stone (6.5 kg) in lean body weight. That is, if you are 10 st (63 kg), then you need 10 glasses; 11 st (70 kg), 11 glasses, and so on.

Make sure you get all the fluid into your system through the day. To be drinking up your quota in the evening could mean too many trips to the toilet through the night. Broken sleep negates the energy-raising effect of the Metabolism Balancing Program. Sleep is the most potent of all medicines and is needed to overcome all illnesses including allergies.

ENTRÉES

Don't have soup, salad or pasta for entrée. Soup dilutes the digestive juices and salad/pasta absorbs them. (See Chapter 16, 'Scientific explanations—Food combining'.) Have only protein food entrées (oysters, mussels, meat, poultry, seafood). Eat entrées when dining out only, that way there is less chance you will put on weight.

ALCOHOL

Go easy on alcohol. Responsible drinking levels recommended by the National Health and Medical Research Council are as follows:

Safe:	Up to 4 standard drinks a day for men.
	Up to 2 standard drinks a day for women.
Hazardous:	4–6 standard drinks a day for men.
	2–4 standard drinks a day for women.
Harmful:	More than 6 standard drinks a day for men.
	More then 4 standard drinks a day for women.

Note: A standard drink = 1 middy of regular beer (285 mL), 1 glass of wine (120 mL), 1 glass of port or sherry (60 mL) or 1 nip of spirits (30 mL).

Don't think that saving up your daily safe levels of alcohol and having them all at once on a Friday or Saturday night is safe. It's not, and it will do your liver and brain significant harm. If you are on medication check with your doctor before drinking any alcohol.

The early warning signs of alcohol damage to the brain are:

1. Light sleep, shorter sleep duration, unrested after sleep, repressed dreaming, irritability, argumentativeness, denial.
2. Light tremors of the hand (most noticeable where fine motor performance is necessary, e.g. making model aeroplanes, plucking eyebrows or applying eye make-up).
3. Tendency to pessimism, depression and anxiety. Reduced foresight, judgement, creativity and memory. Difficulty in putting things back together—most noticeable when doing repairs on the car or around the house.

Take heart, the brain is resilient and will regenerate on the Metabolism-Balancing Program if over-drinking is stopped early enough. The body can recover from the occasional binge. It is regular alcohol abuse that does the damage. More than four drinks a day produces deficiencies in vitamins A, B3, B6 and C, minerals magnesium and zinc and the essential fatty acids. Remember, the female liver has less alcohol-burning enzymes (alcohol dehydrogenase) than the male liver and females have less muscle to burn alcohol.

DIETARY SUPPLEMENTS

The dietary supplements are an integral part of the programs in this book. Without them, the programs don't work properly and mediocre results are the best you can hope for. I have tried to balance body metabolisms with diet alone and have never succeeded. The supplements are not therapeutic agents in the manner that drug medications are, they are included to add to the overall nutrient content of the program. After twenty-two years of trial and error experimentation, I've learned which supplements give the best results and for this reason have included them in the book. In the case of Formula Six, the multi-vitamin and mineral tablets, I had to formulate them myself as there was nothing on the market that gave the results I was looking for.

In the first edition of this book I omitted to mention which brand of supplements to take and where to get them. This upset a few people because they didn't know what to buy or where to buy it and some were not getting the results from the programs the book had led them to expect.

Many people became stressed-out trying to hunt down what they hoped were the appropriate supplements. Many complained by phone and letter that they had wasted a lot of time searching for suitable supplements and still didn't have them. As a result of this a mail order service was born, as I felt obliged to procure the appropriate supplements and post them to those people.

The supplements described in this book should be available at your health store. However, experience has taught my readers, my patients and myself that some health store proprietors are not reliable at keeping stocks up and reordering when out of stock. If you are having trouble locating supplements, phone my clinic on:

(02) 981 2225,
(02) 982 7135

and we will procure and post them to you.

Do not start the programs without the supplements—their effects will be minimised and I don't want you to be disheartened, especially if you have been let down by other treatment regimes in the past. The programs are not complete without the supplements as even fresh foods are vitamin and mineral deficient these days. (See Chapter 16, 'Scientific explanations—Vitamins and minerals'.)

After you have completed the ninety-plus days on the Anti-Candida/Anti-Allergy Program, and are feeling well again, you must return to the Metabolism-Balancing Program and stay on it for the rest of your life.

If you want to be assured of optimum results I personally recommend you stay on all the supplements listed in this program, for all time. However, I realise that tablet taking annoys some people and the cost of long term supplementation is prohibitive to others. Both of these factors can be stresses, which undermine the good effects of the program. If you fall into either of these categories reduce the oils, vitamin C powder and Lugol's iodine by 50 per cent, but be prepared to raise them again if you feel your form dropping. Don't reduce the Formula Six. I wish there was an easier way than dietary supplementation to get and stay well, but unfortunately there is not.The age of dietary supplements is upon us, whether we like it or not.

Remember: The two most important nutrients are water and oxygen. If you are deficient in either, results from the program and supplements will be mediocre. Fluid levels can drop quickly (within an hour or so) and cause a corresponding drop in physical energy and mental alertness. Don't miss a drink. Consume the appropriate number of glasses every day. Consult the water consumption tables earlier in this chapter to make sure you are getting the right amount. These water tables are based on accurate scientific measurements of the fluid needs of body tissues (non-fat) and weight-to-water ratio. The amounts recommended are those needed to facilitate optimum metabolic function. See Chapter 10, 'The importance of water and oxygen', and Chapter 16, 'Scientific explanations—Water'.

Try and do the deep-breathing exercises every day.

Note: Because there is so much important data in this chapter that has to be remembered, I suggest you read it three or four times before getting started on the program.

14.
The Anti-
Candida Program

'One man's meat is another man's poison'

Hippocrates, 500 BC

D on't start this program until you have completed six to eight weeks on the Metabolism Balancing Program—you won't get good results if you don't first build your immunity up. Also, don't undertake the Anti-Candida Program while under a lot of stress or if you are breastfeeding. As you can't have fruit and milk, two sources of readily usable glucose will not be available to your body. Stress creates a greater than normal need for glucose and the blood glucose levels can drop when you are under stress if fruit and milk are not eaten.

The symptoms of stress are the same as the symptoms of candida yeast infection. For this reason, you may not feel that much better if you are stressed. You may begin to lose heart and feel the program isn't working, even though it is successfully killing the yeast. You may begin to feel tired and despondent on it, thus making it difficult to stick to. Take care of all your stresses before commencing this program and reduce them where possible. (See Chapter 11, 'Stress', and Chapter 16, 'Scientific explanations—Stress'.)

Smokers should not try to give up while on this program. Coping with the symptoms of yeast kill-off is difficult enough without adding the symptoms of nicotine withdrawal.

People with nightshade allergies are the exception to this rule. If you are allergic to any of the nightshade group of plants (tomato, chilli, cayenne, eggplant, green pepper, paprika, potato, red pepper, tobacco, belladonna) you must give up cigarettes. The nightshades are so closely related, being allergic to even one or two of them means that cigarettes will prevent the program from working.

Drugs, particularly marijuana, must also be given up, as they suppress the yeast-killing effect of the white blood cells.

There can be no standard anti-candida program that works for all of the people all of the time. This is because most candida sufferers also have allergies and are allergic to different things.

Because most people with a yeast infection are also allergic to yeasts, moulds and fungi, all yeasts, moulds and fungi have been withheld from the Anti-Candida Program.

One thing that all anti-candida programs do have in common is that they exclude sugar, honey, white flour and any food made from them. For the first four to six weeks, all fruits, milk and milk products are to be excluded from the program. Eggs are not dairy products and may be had on this program. The sugar in fruit, honey and milk feeds the *Candida albicans* yeast colony in the gut, causing it to grow larger. The Anti-Candida Program is an amended version of the Metabolism-Balancing Program. **Eat only what's on the program! If it's not written here, don't eat it!**

Children under four years of age are not to go on this program without supervision of a health professional.

You absolutely must eat the unleavened bread whether you like it or not. To not eat it means you will become short of the minerals chromium and selenium, and thus you will feel weak. If you are allergic to wheat, make the bread from millet flour, or rice flour, or buckwheat flour (see 'Recipes').

Don't go on this program if you are not prepared to eat the bread. One comforting thought is that even if at first you don't like it, you will develop a taste for it if you persist. Eat only those unleavened breads included in the shopping list.

All oat and rye products have been excluded from this program as experience has taught me that most allergic people have sensitivities to the common oat and to rye grass. These two are related to the cereal oats and cereal rye used in breads. Rice bran has been added to the recipes in lieu of oats as a cholesterol-lowering agent.

If you are a flight attendant on an international airline, you have to stay on fruit for the whole duration of the program. This may mean it will take longer to get well but this can't be helped. The long flights place too much strain on the body for it to go without the natural sugars found in fruit. If you are pregnant, you must also stay on fruit. Use crushed egg shells (crushed to a fine powder) in salad dressings, scrambled eggs, omelettes and in recipes. Egg shells are rich in calcium and preclude the need for milk.

Although I prefer my patients to go off fruit and milk concurrently for the first four to six weeks, you may go off them at any stage of the program and at separate times if you prefer—even the last four to six weeks if you like. Some people find that being on the fruit and milk at the beginning helps them to adjust to being on the program. They are used to being on it by the time they have to go off the fruit and milk. If you are allergic to milk or any particular fruits, you will go off them at the outset of the program. Don't have more than three to four pieces of fruit per day.

Sometimes a change of diet can cause constipation. If this happens to you on the Anti-Candida/Anti-Allergy Program take a mild herbal laxative (cascara sagrada is a good one) before bed and drink more water. As your bowels begin to return to normal, reduce the amount and frequency of the laxative until it's no longer required.

THE ANTI-CANDIDA PROGRAM

Don't start this program until you are getting adequate rest and sleep.

To make the program easier to stick to, each meal option has its own specific recipe—either in this chapter or in 'Recipes'. (You must use the low or negligible salicylate and amine options for at least the first four weeks.)

Cheese, dried fruit, grapes, bananas and melons must not be eaten. All other fruit must be excluded for four weeks. Milk must be excluded for six weeks. Pregnant women and international flight crew are to stay on fruit (but no melons, bananas or grapes).

Immediately on rising, before doing anything else, drink the appropriate number of glasses of clean water. Wait $1/2$–1 hour before eating breakfast. See the tables for appropriate water consumption laid down in the Metabolism-Balancing Program. Tap and soda water, although acceptable on the Metabolism-Balancing Program, are not acceptable on the Anti-Candida Program, unless they have been thoroughly filtered. Drink another glassful 1–$1^1/2$ hours after breakfast.

The adding of glucose to the water, which is acceptable on the Metabolism-Balancing Program, isn't acceptable on the Anti-Candida Program. This program's prime objective is to starve as many candida yeast plants as possible, and these plants can draw sustenance from glucose. By the time you start the Anti-Candida Program, your body will be used to the increased fluid intake which began on the Metabolism-Balancing Program, so the glucose won't be as necessary.

Drink only fresh spring water (home-delivered) or mineral water from a recognised spa. Commercially made mineral waters are derived from tap water. Try to get ten to fifteen minutes' deep breathing exercises done between the drinking of the water and breakfast. (See Chapter 11, 'Stress—Deep breathing exercises'.)

Many candida sufferers are chemically sensitive and find that the vaporised chlorine of a hot shower can aggravate their symptoms. Make sure the air extractor is on or the window is open, and run the hot shower for two to three minutes before getting in. This will clear the chlorine vapour that's released with the initial burst of hot water. Many people blame what they ate for breakfast for the symptoms caused by their morning shower.

While on this program it pays to shower before breakfast. While in the shower rinse the Nystatin powder around your mouth, swallowing it bit by bit. Use the early morning water to wash down the *Lactobacillus acidophilus* capsules and, if you are using them, the Nystatin and garlic capsules/tablets. If using Nystatin powder, use a little water to help dilute it and rinse it around your mouth before using the rest to wash it down. See instructions further on in this chapter.

BREAKFAST

As with the Metabolism-Balancing Program you can mix and match your breakfast options on this program. Read Chapter 13, 'The Metabolism-Balancing Program', for details on how to do this. Amend these options to keep high and moderate amine and salicylate foods out for the first four weeks.

OPTION 1

Untoasted wholemeal bread (one to three slices) (see 'Recipes') made from wheat, rice, soy, millet, buckwheat or arrowroot flour, depending on what allergies, if any, you have. Have a thin spread of butter (if you are not allergic to milk and have normal cholesterol levels) on your bread, though it is preferable to use cold pressed oil (olive oil is best unless you have a known salicylate sensitivity). Brush the oil on the bread.

Egg may be had on the bread if you are not allergic to it and your cholesterol levels are normal. Tahini, almond, cashew or hazelnut paste or butter may be used, but no peanut butter. Peanuts grow in the soil and have mould growing on them. Canned tuna, sardine or salmon (done in brine [salt and water] only—not oil) may also be eaten. Tomato and onion may be added for flavour. Candida Killer sandwich filling (see 'Recipes') may be used on the bread if desired. Consult the amine and salicylate lists at the back of the book. Have only cashew butter and soya oil for the first four weeks. After the first four weeks you may toast the bread.

OPTION 2

Any of the toppings from Option 1 on two to four brown rice cake/ wafers (the big round ones from the health store) instead of the unleavened bread or unleavened bread toast. Candida Killer

216

sandwich filling may be used on top if desired, but only after the first four weeks, when high amines and salicylates are allowed on the program.

OPTION 3

A bowl (as big as you like) of puffed brown rice (rice bubbles) from the health store with either freshly juiced carrot juice or soya milk over the top. This tastes great with nuts and seeds added. Be careful with soymilk though. The palatable ones tend to be thickened and sweetened with malt, maltose, maltodextrose and other sugar derivatives. Check with the manufacturer, and if it contains any ingredient that ends in -os, -ose, -one, ona or -ol it's sugared—don't have it. Wheat bran may be added. No carrot juice and only cashew nuts for the first four weeks.

OPTION 4

A bowl of cooked millet, buckwheat or brown rice (see 'Recipes') with butter melted over it (if you are not allergic to milk), though preferably cold pressed vegetable oil. Olive oil is best. Wheat bran may be added. Use soya oil until the inclusion of amines and salicylates is permitted.

OPTION 5

Raw nuts, such as almonds, cashews, brazil nuts, hazelnuts, walnuts, sunflower or sesame seeds (no peanuts—they have mould on them). Have as much as you feel you need without overdoing it. Don't have less than 60 g (2 oz). Cashews only for the first four weeks.

OPTION 6

A fresh fruit salad (no dried fruit and not from a fast food outlet), using any variety of fresh fruit except grapes, bananas and melons (all melons). You may have any of the nuts and seeds mentioned in Option 5 over the top—60 g (2 oz). Puffed brown rice bubbles may also be put over the top. A dressing of cold pressed oil and lemon juice may be used. Apricot kernel oil goes well with fruit salad, as do sunflower, sesame and saf-flower oils. Wheat bran may be added. Don't have fruit for lunch if you had it for breakfast. You may only have pears (peeled), golden delicious apples (peeled), paw paw, pomegranate and cashews for the first four weeks.

OPTION 7

Stewed fresh fruit (see 'Recipes'). Nuts, seeds and brown puffed rice may be added. No dried fruit. Wheat bran may be added.

Remember: Some time during this twelve week program you have to be off all fruit for four weeks and all milk for six weeks. It's preferable to go off them simultaneously, though not imperative. You may go off each one at separate times.

OPTION 8

Savoury mince (non-amine/salicylate version for first four weeks) on toast or bread or as a filling in a homemade pie or pancake or over noodles, brown rice or kasha (see 'Recipes'). No toast for first four weeks.

OPTION 9

Three or four whole fresh fruits and 60–90 g (2 –3 oz) of nuts and seeds, any variety according to any allergies that may exist. No melons, grapes or bananas. You can't have this option during your four weeks off fruit.

MORNING TEA

Drinking is compulsory at mid-morning, eating is not. No fruit juices, they are too concentrated in sugar. Keep high and moderate amines and salicylates out for the first four weeks.

OPTION 1

A 230 mL (8 oz) glass of vegetable juice, freshly juiced. You may have more than 230 mL if you like. Carrot juice is fine and mixed with celery it's even better. This is a good drink for kids.

OPTION 2

A cup of black, unsweetened tea or coffee—don't worry about the taste, you will be used to it in seven to ten days and won't be able to go back to sweet tea and coffee again. This is a good habit to get into as it helps you keep your weight down. A little lemon juice may be added to the tea. For the six weeks of the program that you are allowed milk you may add a little milk or cream to the tea and coffee. Otherwise a non-dairy coffee whitener may be used, though not if you are allergic to coconut. Non-dairy whitener is made from emulsified coconut oil as is the cream supplied with your coffee on airlines. Read all labels carefully. If any word on it ends in -os, -ose, -one, -ona or -ol it has sugar and is, therefore, prohibited.

Herb teas are permitted if you are not allergic to grasses or pollens. Have only those that are in a bag, not the powdered variety. Cereal coffees are malted and therefore not permissible.

OPTION 3

A glass of mineral water, office- or home-delivered spring water or filtered tap water. The water must be filtered as many candida sufferers are sensitive to chlorine and other chemicals in tap water. If a water purifier is not available then boil the water for ten minutes in a pot with the lid off to evaporate the chlorine. Boiling for more than ten minutes will solidify fluoride and that will place a strain on the kidneys. Pour the water into a half-filled bottle and shake it well. This will put oxygen back into the water and give it back its taste. Freshly squeezed lemon or lime juice may be added to the water.

OPTION 4

Only if you are hungry or feeling faint.
Brown rice cakes/wafers (the big round ones from the health store) with butter (if you do not have an allergy to milk) or with soya or olive oil brushed on them or one of the nut butters (cashew, almond, hazelnut, but not peanut). Tahini is OK but not the brands that are mixed with honey. Candida Killer sandwich filler/ dip may be used on top if desired.

Or, 60–120 g (2–4 oz) raw nuts and/or sunflower and sesame seeds.

OPTION 5

A sandwich for growing kids if they are hungry. Stay away from the nut butters that have sugar added. Read all labels carefully. *Remember:* -os, -ose, -one, -ona and -ol.

LUNCH

Lunch is not to be eaten any later than 1.30 p.m. If it is, you run the risk of hypoglycaemia and will blame the resulting tiredness, lethargy, mood swings, poor concentration, weakness, light-headedness on the program, suspecting you are allergic to a food,

A 230 mL (8 oz) glass of water or vegetable juice must be sipped with lunch. Glucose cannot be added to the water on the Anti-Candida Program.

If you missed your morning deep breathing exercises then twenty minutes' yogic walking in the park before lunch is a good substitute and will relax and energise you for the rest of the day.

As with the breakfast menu, the lunch options may be mixed and matched, swapped or changed with other meals. Again keep high and moderate amine and salicylate foods out for the first four weeks—study the lists.

OPTION 1

A home-made garden salad (not from fast food outlet) comprising any variety of garden vegetables that you are not sensitive to. Include 120–240 g (4–8 oz) of lean unprocessed meat (all fat trimmed), seafood or poultry (skin and all fat trimmed off). Eggs may also be had if you are not allergic to them and your cholesterol levels are normal. Nuts and/or sunflower and sesame seeds may be added to give the salad variety and flavour. 90–150 g (3–5 oz) of a carbohydrate food such as boiled, baked or mashed (with oil) potato must be eaten. Cooked brown rice, wholemeal pasta and wholemeal unleavened bread (see 'Recipes') are other acceptable alternatives. No rice cakes.

Home-made chips (French fries) may also be eaten—not if you have high cholesterol though, and not the commercially prepared chips or the little round potato balls served at restaurants and take-away outlets, or bought frozen from the supermarket. These contain chemicals that many people are allergic to. Carbohydrate foods must be eaten at lunch to prevent the blood glucose levels dropping by mid-afternoon (hypoglycaemia). You can have a dressing of cold pressed vegetable oil with lemon juice (no vinegar) and garlic if you like. Add any of the permissible herbs and spices to the dressing. (See the amine and salicylate lists in 'Food tables'.) Candida Killer dip may be eaten on the side or over the salad (see 'Recipes') after four weeks.

OPTION 2

Good for lowering cholesterol levels, although suitable for anyone.

A thick bean and lentil stew (see 'Recipes'). Add lecithin granules if your cholesterol is high. One to three slices of wholemeal unleavened bread (see 'Recipes') may be eaten with it (not rice cakes). Have the bread dry or with a thin spread of butter if you are not allergic to milk and your cholesterol levels are normal. Preferably, brush olive oil on the bread.

You may still have this dish if your cholesterol levels are normal as it only lowers *high* cholesterol levels, it doesn't lower normal cholesterol levels. A rice bran muffin (see 'Recipes') may be eaten in place of the bread if your cholesterol levels are high.

OPTION 3

A thick vegetable soup. Include any variety of garden vegetables that you are not sensitive to. Lean meat, fish or poultry may be included in the soup (see 'Recipes'), as may any of the permissible herbs and spices. One to three slices of unleavened wholemeal bread (not rice cakes), with butter (though preferably oil) on it, may be eaten.

Toast the bread (after first four weeks) if you like. If your cholesterol levels are high, a rice bran muffin (see 'Recipes') may be eaten instead of bread, and rice bran may be added to thicken the soup. The soup may still be eaten if your cholesterol levels are normal as it won't lower them below normal.

OPTION 4

Sandwiches—two slices of bread per sandwich, as thick as you like. Unleavened wholemeal bread (not rice cakes) or muffins (see 'Recipes') may be used for sandwiches. The fillings may include salad with lean meat, fish or poultry. Canned fish (done in brine [salt and water] only) may also be used.

Egg filling is permissible if you are not allergic to egg and your cholesterol levels are normal. Cashew, almond and hazelnut pastes (and butters) and tahini are good fillings. No peanut butter though. You may have a thin spread of butter (if you are not allergic to milk and cholesterol levels are normal), though oil is preferable.

Candida Killer sandwich filling may be used if desired. Savoury Mince (see 'Recipes') may also be used. Have one to three sandwiches, depending on your size, hunger and activity levels.

OPTION 5

Not for hypoglycaemics.
60–120 g (2–4 oz) of raw nuts and/or sunflower and sesame seeds. Two to three fresh fruits (but no melons, grapes or bananas) may be eaten with the nuts and seeds for eight weeks of the twelve week program. *For four weeks you are to have the nuts and seeds only.*

Have nuts and fruits in accordance with any allergies that you may have. Keep high and moderate amine and salicylate foods out for the first four weeks.

Note: You cannot have this option if you had fruit salad for breakfast.

AFTERNOON TEA

Same as morning tea. A 230 mL (8 oz) glass or cup of fluid (water, vegetable juice, black coffee or black tea) is compulsory at mid-afternoon. Drink one or two more between now and dinner. If you are going to night school, have something before you go, either the evening meal early or a snack and then the evening meal later. But don't have a big meal just before going to bed.

EVENING (MAIN) MEAL

Because the Anti-Candida Program is strict and restrictive, the individual meal options will be clearly stated. Unlike the Metabolism-Balancing Program which is flexible, the Anti-Candida Program must be followed to the absolute letter—no deviations.

- You must have red meat three times per week as the main meal of the day.
- You must have fish twice per week as the main meal.
- You must have poultry or soya beans on the remaining two nights.

VITAMINS

Start the meal by sipping on a 230 mL (8 oz) glass of freshly juiced vegetable juice (from the low and negligible amine and salicylate lists for first four weeks), or mineral, spring or filtered tap water with 1 teaspoon of vitamin C powder (calcium or sodium ascorbate—any brand) in it and, twice a week, 1 drop only of Lugol's iodine solution (from the chemist); use an eyedropper for accuracy. Use as little as possible of the fluid to get the before and after meal supplements down. Finish the remainder off later in the evening.

Just before eating, swallow 3 × Formula Six multi-vitamin and mineral tablets, that is, 1 tablet from each jar. Because hydrochloric acid is needed to facilitate absorption of minerals, Formula Six must be taken when there is maximum hydrochloric acid in the stomach, that is, just before a meal (see Chapter 16, 'Scientific explanations––Food combining—Vitamins and minerals'). Keep high and moderate amine and salicylate foods out for the first four weeks.

OPTION 1

120–270 g (4–9 oz), depending on your size, hunger and activity load, of grilled steak, or veal, pan fried in oil; 60–120 g (2–4 oz) of steamed, boiled, mashed or dry-baked potato; potato chips (French fries) or roast potato may be eaten as long as they are done in olive oil or other cold pressed vegetable oil; and 60–120 g (2–4 oz) steamed or lightly stir-fried green, yellow, orange or red vegetables.

Cooked brown rice, millet, buckwheat or pasta noodles (see 'Recipes') may be eaten in place of potato. If gravy is desired have only the one from the 'Recipes' section.

Salt the meal with unadulterated sea salt crystals (Malden or Russell's are OK; Celtic salt is best). No table salt unless the label guarantees it to be free of chemical additives such as free flow agents or anti-moisture agents.

Don't use any butter, margarine or animal fat for cooking.

A side salad (not from a fast food outlet) may be eaten in addition to the vegetables. Candida Killer dip/dressing may be eaten with the side salad (see 'Recipes') after the first four weeks.

OPTION 2

120–270 g (4–9 oz) grilled or steamed fish (see 'Recipes')—any sort of fish, the oilier the better. Potato or brown rice and vegetables prepared as for Option 1. If allergic to potato have brown rice, millet, buckwheat or pasta noodles instead.

OPTION 3

Fish, lightly fried in cold pressed vegetable oil. It may also be cooked in bread crumbs as long as wholemeal bread crumbs are used (see 'Recipes'). The same vegetables as Option 1.

OPTION 4

A roast of beef, lamb, pork, venison or rabbit—cooked in its own fat or in cold pressed vegetable oil (preferably olive oil). Roast potato and other roast vegetables are to be included. The only gravies to be eaten are those recommended in the 'Recipes' section. If allergic to potato have cooked brown rice, millet, buckwheat or pasta noodles instead. See 'Recipes'.

OPTION 5

Roast chicken, duck, turkey, goose, quail or guinea-fowl—prepared in the same way and with the same vegetables as Option 4.

OPTION 6

A meat, fish or chicken casserole made in strict accordance with the recipes in the 'Recipes' section.

OPTION 7

Good for lowering cholesterol, although suitable for anyone.
A bean and lentil stew made in strict accordance with the recipe in the 'Recipes' section.

OPTION 8

Spaghetti bolognese made strictly according to the recipe in the 'Recipes' section.

OPTION 9

Lasagna made strictly according to the recipe in the 'Recipes'.

OPTION 10

Spaghetti marinara made strictly according to the recipe in the 'Recipes' section.

BEVERAGES

You should drink fresh spring water (those delivered to the home and office are good) or mineral water from a spa—not commercially made. Deep Spring and Taurina are good spa waters. No more than five cups (combined) per day of tea and coffee (no whitener of any sort, no sweetener of any sort). Diet Coke or diet lemonade may be used as a treat for adults and kids—no more than two to three times per week. Raw lemon or lime juice may be squeezed into water to give variety of taste. No alcohol.

No fruit juices on this program—they are too concentrated in natural sugars and many have mould growing in them.

No tea or coffee for one hour before taking the supplements or for three hours after. The acids in tea and coffee block the absorption of the minerals. No cocoa or hot chocolate.

DESSERT

Raw fruit, fresh fruit salad (only from the low and negligible amine and salicylate list for the first four weeks) or stewed fruit are the only permissible desserts (see 'Recipes') and they can be had for eight of the twelve weeks of the program. No dried fruit, yoghurt or sweetener of any sort (including honey) is to be added to the dessert. Have the dessert thirty to sixty minutes after the main meal. This time span is important if the water in the fruit is not to dilute the digestive juices and interfere with the digestion of the main meal.

Only one fruit salad per day is to be eaten on this program. If you have one for breakfast or lunch, you must go without dessert at dinner.

OILS

After the main meal of the day have 2 × 1000 mg capsules of evening primrose oil (Nature's Own is a good brand) and 2 × 1000 mg capsules of marine lipid concentrate (MaxEPA). If you have high cholesterol, have 4 × 1000 mg capsules of MaxEPA. (See Chapter 16, 'Scientific explanations—Vitamins and minerals'.) Have a herbal laxative before bed if constipation is a problem.

For those who don't like taking capsules and tablets, instead of the marine lipid concentrate you can take 1 dessertspoon of cod liver oil from the bottle, at any time of the day, except just before the main meal—too much oil reduces mineral absorption. Have it in vegetable juice, on tuna or salmon, on cooked brown rice, in mashed potato or take it straight with a vegetable juice chaser. Blackmore's Deodorised Cod Liver Oil is the most palatable.

Make sure you have at least 1 teaspoon of some form of raw, cold pressed vegetable oil per day. Soya oil is best as it's salicylate-free. Have this oil in addition to the oil you cook with. Either take it straight off the spoon or in a salad dressing. Have it at any time of the day except just before the main meal. If having it over the salad make sure you consume a full teaspoon's worth. It might pay to pour at least 1 dessertspoon of oil over the salad to ensure this.

NYSTATIN POWDER

Ask your doctor to prescribe Nystatin for you (see Chapter 5, 'How to cure your allergies—Approaching the doctor'). Twenty to thirty minutes before breakfast, and before going to bed, have ½ teaspoon of Nystatin powder. Dump it on your tongue, mix it with your saliva and rinse it around your mouth, swallowing it slowly, bit by bit, over a one to two minute period. Some people find they need to sip a little water to help this process along. Do not mix it with food as it reduces vitamin absorption.

OTHER CANDIDA KILLERS

Although Nystatin is the best candida-killing agent it isn't easy to get hold of in powder form. If you cannot get it, use 4 Nystatin tablets for each ½ teaspoon of the powder. If you cannot get the Nystatin tablets, garlic is best. Take 2 × 600 mg odourless garlic capsules (from the health store) immediately on rising, just before lunch, and just before bed. Eat as much raw garlic as possible.

candida treatment.) Eat as much raw garlic as possible.

Odourless garlic must be taken for the full twelve weeks of the program even if you have elected to use Nystatin as the principal source of treatment. Chew some garlic every day for the first seven days then two to three times per week after that. Although the odour is disagreeable to some people fresh garlic has to be chewed to kill those candida plants growing in the mouth, throat and on the tongue. Keep going with it even if you feel a bit nauseous or experience heartburn. These are the symptoms of candida kill-off, not garlic sensitivity. Nystatin powder is best because it kills the mouth- and throat-borne candida without affecting the breath. You don't have to use garlic if you are using Nystatin.

Use only Mycostatin brand of Nystatin powder. Nilstat powder is easier to get than Mycostatin powder. Unfortunately, some people react adversely to it. If your abdomen is still bloating after ten to fourteen days on Nilstat, you are allergic to it. Take 2 × *Lactobacillus acidophilus* capsules at the same time you take the Nystatin. Take only the Bio-Organics Megadophilus brand of *Lactobacillus acidophilus*, which is not adulterated with milk, malt, sugar or preservatives. I find that all the other brands are likely to cause allergic reactions—especially in the gut. Take lactobacillus as directed by this book not by the label on the jar.

Nystatin tablets are available from the chemist on a doctor's prescription. Wash them under a warm tap to remove the outer, coloured coating. Don't have the Nystatin capsules as they contain milk and allergenic preservatives.

BEFORE BED
Take the Nystatin powder and the *Lactobacillus acidophilus* capsules. If not using Nystatin, take the garlic capsules.

THE KILL-OFF
Don't be dismayed if at first you feel worse. Your symptoms may well flare up at this time. This is the result of the Nystatin or garlic and Caprinex killing off the yeast, not the result of an allergy to Nystatin. As a result of the yeast drying, extra acetaldehyde and bits of dead yeast are released into the blood. The waste products are carried right through the body to the kidneys for elimination.

As these waste products pass through the system they can make you feel ill. The symptoms vary from mild to severe depending on the size of the yeast colony and can last for two to seven days. All you can do is drink lots of fluid between meals to dilute the toxins, stay on the regime and rest. Painkillers won't work, just bear with it. Sometimes extra Nystatin or garlic helps to shorten the kill-off period. Use cortisone creams if eczema flares up and keep asthma medication handy. Some people find that going back to antihistamines helps mitigate the kill-off symptoms. Use cortisone puffers if asthma is bad.

Don't be alarmed if your urine is dark and odorous and your bowel motions greeny yellow in colour. This is the result of your bowel, blood and liver cleansing themselves. It indicates a significant candida infection and a toxic liver and that your body is responding positively to the program. This is a good sign.

INHALING NYSTATIN
If your sinus, hayfever, stuffy nose or post-nasal drip isn't responding, you might have a candida colony in your nose. Just before taking the Nystatin powder, shake the bottle vigorously,

unscrew the lid and inhale the smoke. This will help kill candida in the nose. Don't do this if you suffer from asthma unless your doctor gives you permission. Have your asthma medication handy just in case inhaling the powder triggers an attack. This is less likely to happen if you inhale gently.

PREGNANCY

Nystatin is listed by the health authorities as completely safe for pregnant women, as it's not absorbed. However, if pregnant, check with your doctor before taking Nystatin. Get him or her to assess your particular situation. I have never had any problems with pregnant patients taking Nystatin—but you can never be too sure and it pays to err on the side of caution.

HUNGER AND WEIGHT LOSS

If you are over-weight and don't over-eat you will find you will lose some weight on the Anti-Candida Program. Your weight loss will be accompanied by increased energy, greater mental activity, clear skin and good muscle tone. You won't feel hungry. You will feel and look better than before.

If you are losing weight and are hungry, lethargic, depressed and experiencing 'the fades' each afternoon, you are making one or more of the following mistakes:

1. You are filling up on fruits and not including enough nuts and seeds or brown rice bubbles on the fruit salads.
2. You are filling up on vegetables and not having enough meat, seafood or poultry at the main meal of the day.
3. You are skipping meat, seafood and poultry altogether and having vegetables only as the main meal.
4. You are not having a carbohydrate food (potato, bread, pasta, rice, etc.) or a protein food (meat, seafood, poultry, egg) at the midday meal. That is, you are having salad (rabbit food) only.
5. You are not drinking enough fluid. No one aged 12 or over should have less than 9×230 mL (8 oz) glasses of fluid per day (see water tables in Chapter 13, 'The Metabolism-Balancing Program') and most people need more. Most of the dry, wrinkled skins, constipation and gaunt, drawn, expressions that sometimes develop on the Anti-Candida Program are due to dehydration. (See Chapter 10, 'The importance of water and oxygen'.)
6. You haven't properly addressed the stresses in your life and are doing too much and resting too little. Check to see if you are getting eight hours' sleep. You need at least eight hours' sleep per night for the candida program to work properly.

A WORD OF CAUTION

Anti-candida and anti-allergy programs are by their very nature food restrictive. The restriction on the number of foods eaten means that over a period of time nutrient deficiencies could develop. This is unfortunate but there's not much that can be done about it.

To make sure nutrient deficiencies don't develop:

- Take the supplements every day without fail.
- Stick to the program so that you only have to be on it for three months, after which you can start reintroducing the foods you were allergic to. Three months' total abstinence is usually enough to overcome a sensitivity to a food and/or to kill off a candida yeast infection.

Nutrient deficiencies are most likely to occur if you are allergic to such staples as wheat, fish, rice, oats, egg, baker's yeast, milk, corn or beef.

If you are allergic to wheat and have to go off bread you should eat liver (calf's or lamb's) at least once and preferably twice a week. Liver contains the minerals selenium and chromium you were receiving from the yeast and wheat. Selenium and chromium help insulin regulate the blood glucose levels. A deficiency in them can cause hypoglycaemia (see Chapter 16, 'Scientific explanation—Vitamins and minerals—Cholesterol'). A long term deficiency can predispose to diabetes. Have only lamb's liver if you are allergic to amines (see amine and salicylate charts in 'Food tables').

On no account should you break the program for the time you are on it (three months minimum). Skipping meals is breaking the program. Eating only *some* of the advised foods is breaking the program. Eating rice cakes instead of bread for lunch is breaking the program. Having fruit twice a day is breaking the program. The program offers a number of options so you can rotate foods and prevent over-exposure to any one of them. Eating less than three meals a day is breaking the program. Skipping lunch is a cardinal sin. Don't skip meals, the program won't work if you do.

Note: The Anti-Allergy Program is the Anti-Candida Program minus those foods to which you are allergic.

THE LIST OF DO'S

1. Do study carefully the 'Food tables' at the back of the book pertaining to yeasts, amines and salicylates, moulds and ferments (don't eat unleavened breads from your baker—bakers use yeast plus sour dough), malt, monosodium

glutamate (MSG) and milk (for the appropriate six weeks). Do this before starting the program to make absolutely sure you do not eat any of these foods.

2. Do eat liver at least once, preferably twice, per week (see 'Recipes'). The nutrients in liver can make the difference between average and excellent results. Lamb's liver is best. Chickens are force fed with chemical pellets, so don't eat chicken liver.

3. Do wash all fruits and nuts in warm water and soap to remove mould (unshelled nuts don't need to be washed). Don't leave them in the water too long. Just in and out for a quick brisk wash then dry them quickly before they go soggy. Rinse off all the soap. Sunflower seeds are grown locally and therefore are fresher than nuts. Only wash them if they smell a bit mouldy.

4. Do chew wholemeal, unleavened bread thoroughly, taking the time to mix it well with saliva. Unleavened bread requires more chewing than ordinary bread as it's harder to digest.

5. Do cut your freshly baked, unleavened bread up into slices. Wrap them individually in greaseproof paper and keep them in the freezer. Leave them out overnight to thaw. This way they won't grow mould.

6. Do rinse and wipe clean the blade of any cutting utensil before cutting any food you are going to eat. Black, brown and greeny blue coloured film on the crust of bread or on the surface of vegetables is mould. Wash off before cutting through fruit or vegetables, you will drive the mould in otherwise.

7. Do seek out all mould in the house and remove it. Cracked pipes that leak into brick, concrete and carpet underlay are insidious mould producers. If the house is the slightest bit musty after one to two days of being shut up, there is hidden mould—find it.

8. Do wear a mask if cooking a food you are allergic to as the smell of it can trigger your symptoms. This is applicable to those who are cooking for others who are not on their program.

9. Do drink mineral water with a drop of freshly squeezed lemon or lime juice in it when out socially. If they are available have a Diet Coke or diet lemonade as well. Dry roasted cashews, hazelnuts, almonds and macadamia nuts (the latter three have salicylates) may also be had as a treat or at parties. As a treat at home you may have popcorn (see 'Recipes'). Be careful about salted nuts. If the manufacturers can't guarantee they haven't used adulterated salt don't touch them.

10. Do test all nuts by biting and tasting them before eating them. If nuts are getting old they turn rancid and lose their sweet fresh taste. Rancid nuts can cause enough of an adverse

reaction as to mimic your allergy and candida symptoms. Many patients in the past have erroneously believed they are allergic to nuts because they have eaten rancid nuts. Fresh nuts are more nutritious. However, roasted nuts can be eaten once per week as a treat. No need to wash roasted nuts.

11. Do chew nuts properly. All nuts must be reduced to a purée before they leave your mouth. Bits of nut have sharp edges that can irritate the bowel lining to the point of causing diarrhoea. Many patients have erroneously believed they were allergic to nuts because they had diarrhoea that showed bits of (unchewed) nut.

12. If dining out at friends' houses, do send over a photocopy of the 'Recipes' in the back of this book, so they can feed you in accordance with your food restrictions. If it's a drinks party, get them to make popcorn and the Candida Killer dip with plain Kettle Chips (provided you are past the first four weeks) for you. You can drink diet lemonade or Diet Coke at the party. My experience is that friends are only too willing to help.

13. If you are pregnant do stay on fruit for the duration of the program. This will slow your rate of healing down but that can't be helped. Stay off milk for the mandatory six weeks of the program and for the whole program if you are proven allergic to it or belong to any of the Asian, African or Mediterranean ethnic groups. Crushed egg shells plus Formula Six and sardines or salmon three to four times per week will give you all the extra calcium you need.

14. Do take a herbal laxative if at first you are a little constipated. Any type is OK and won't affect your allergies, as laxatives are not absorbed.

15. Do substitute soymilk for cow's milk as long as the soymilk doesn't contain malt and other additives. Have only the soymilk shown on the shopping list.

16. On completing the Anti-Candida/Anti-Allergy Program, and successfully containing all your symptoms, do return to the Metabolism-Balancing Program, plus Formula Six, for the rest of your life. Go back onto the Anti-Candida Program once a year for four weeks to give yourself a clean out.

LIST OF DON'TS

1. Don't attempt this program if you are not guaranteed ninety uninterrupted days. Breaking it will enable Nystatin and garlic resistant candida colonies to grow back. Birthdays, weddings, house guests, business trips, holidays, moving house and home renovations disrupt your routine, causing an unplanned breaking of the diet. Plan these out of your ninety days. This program works best the first time around.

2. Don't overdo it. Rest is needed for any treatment regime to work, be it antibiotics for pneumonia or a strep throat, acupuncture for headaches or diet for candida infection. Nothing works without adequate rest.

3. Don't buy fruit or garden salads ready made from take-away outlets. Invariably they have been sprinkled with MSG or metabisulphite to prevent discolouration and loss of flavour. Often these salads have been made early that morning or even the night before. Be very careful in restaurants for the same reason. Quiz the waiter/waitress.

4. Don't eat Chinese or Italian food unless the restaurant owner guarantees it's free of MSG and metabisulphite.

5. Don't eat sauces and gravies in restaurants—the risk is just too great. Eat only the sauces and gravies recommended in this book (see 'Recipes'). Pre-cooked meals, such as roasts, are usually sprinkled with MSG and metabisulphite—be careful.

6. Don't eat chips (French fries) or potato balls in restaurants. They have been delivered in large plastic bags with toxic chemicals to prevent them sticking together and discolouring. Eat only whole or halved fresh potato. Home-made chips are OK, cooked in an oil you are not allergic to.

7. Don't drink any alcohol whatsoever,

8. Don't take the contraceptive pill for the duration of the program. The program won't work if you do. Oestrogen replacement therapy for those at the menopause is OK. Progesterone is the hormone that encourages candida.

9. Don't use toothpaste. They all contain sugar. Use a mixture of bicarbonate of soda and sea salt crystals. Don't use your old toothbrush. Buy a new one and hang it up so that it drips dry. Wet toothbrushes grow mould.

10. Don't do anything to increase the chances of catching a cold or 'flu while on this program. Antibiotics will send you back to square one. Study the section on 'Colds and 'flu' in Chapter 6 to prevent this. Study the section on 'Asthma' as well.

11. Don't buy cut meat from the deli—it will have MSG and/or metabisulphite or nitrates on it.

12. Don't buy frozen, pre-cooked meals, especially Chinese or Italian. They contain MSG and/or metabisulphite. Buy all meats fresh from the butcher and all fruits and vegetables fresh from the greengrocer or supermarket.

13. Don't take gelatin capsules if you are allergic to beef. Slit them or pull them apart and empty their contents onto a spoon.

14. Don't eat leftovers. Leftovers grow mould very quickly, even when left in the fridge. Eat only those foods that are cooked or prepared that day. The exception to this rule is frozen food.

Leftovers may be put in several small plastic containers (soup, casserole, etc.) and taken out one serve at a time to eat. Cuts off the roast may be wrapped in greaseproof paper and taken out to thaw one serve at a time.

15. Don't buy unleavened breads from the local baker. Invariably, these breads are made with yeast or from sour dough. See shopping list for the only permissible breads.

16. Don't have any tofu or miso—these are fermented foods. Have homous if you like. Add it to any lunch/main meal option.

17. Don't go on this program until your baby is weaned from your breast (10–12 months)—(a) because of the reduced spectrum of nutrients, and (b) because the kill-off could turn the baby off also. (See Chapter 15, 'Questions and answers'.)

ANTI-CANDIDA/ANTI-ALLERGY PROGRAM SHOPPING LIST

Because the Anti-Candida/Anti-Allergy Program is so particular, you must be careful about what you buy. The wrong brand can make the difference between success and failure. Twenty-two years spent taking care of allergy sufferers has taught me what brands are safe. I have listed these brands so that you may get optimum results from this program. Some of the material is the result of my research and some of it the result of trial and error experimentation by my patients. I would like to now thank those former patients on behalf of myself and all those who are going to benefit from their efforts.

FROM THE HEALTH STORE

EVENING PRIMROSE OIL: Nature's Own brand only, 1000 mg capsules.

MARINE LIPID CONCENTRATE: Nature's Own MaxEPA, 1000 mg capsules.

COMPLETE MULTI-VITAMIN AND MINERAL FORMULA: Formula Six brand only, available from better health food stores or by mail order (see phone numbers at end of this chapter).

VITAMIN C POWDER: Any brand, either sodium or calcium ascorbate.

IRON TABLETS: FAB Co brand only. For women only, for four to eight weeks only, if required. Wash coating off the tablets.

COD LIVER OIL: Blackmore's deodorised brand is good but any brand will do. For those who don't want to take MaxEPA capsules.

ODOUR-CONTROLLED GARLIC: Kyolic Garlic—won't repeat on you as garlic normally does.

LACTOBACILLUS ACIDOPHILUS CAPSULES: Bio-Organics brand only—marketed as Megadophilus.

Other candida killers: Kyolic garlic capsules.

Herbal laxative: Cascara Sagrada—Nature's Sunshine brand is mild and won't give you gripe pains. Take only if required.

FROM THE CHEMIST

Lugol's iodine solution (plus eye dropper): No doctor's script is necessary. The chemist will mix this up in the dispensary. Keep Lugol's iodine away from children, it's toxic in large doses.

Nystatin powder: Mycostatin is the first choice. Nilstat is the second choice. Doctors script is needed.

Nystatin tablets: Doctor's script is needed. Wash coloured coating off tablets before use. Don't use Nystatin *capsules*—they contain milk products.

Dust mite covers, sprays and nose masks: Allersearch brand only.

FROM THE SUPERMARKET OR HEALTH STORE

Wholemeal pasta (wheat), a number of varieties: Eden

Wholemeal pasta and a wide range of wheat-free, gluten-free pastas: Freedom Foods—Orgran.

Wholemeal spaghetti (organic): Pureharvest.

Wheat noodles (egg-free): Demeter.

Corn spaghetti (wheat-free): Westbrae Natural.

Corn noodles (gluten/wheat/egg-free): Country Harvest.

Wheat flour (stone-ground): Russell's or any other stone-ground brand.

Rice bran (extruded): Russell's.

Brown rice baking mix: Abundant Earth brand·only—especially for wheat and gluten sensitive people. The bread recipe on the back of the packet may be used by those who are wheat and gluten allergic though not milk, egg or soya bean allergic. The amount of milk and honey in the recipe won't affect the candid-killing effect of the program if only one loaf per week is consumed. Going without the sustenance of bread will do more damage than the milk and honey (to those who are not milk allergic).

Popped brown rice: Abundant Earth.

Popped corn: Abundant Earth.

Popping corn: Russell's.

Tomato paste: Leggo's brand only.

Potato flour: Selected Foods brand.

Salt: Celtic Ocean Salt.

Soymilk: Soya King Soya Drink (no malt) by Tixana Pty Ltd.

Soya powder (to make milk): Herbal Valley Natural Soya Bean Powder.

RICE MILK: Rice Dream by Imagine Foods; Aussie Dream by Pureharvest.

SOYA FLOUR, BARLEY FLOUR AND BUCKWHEAT FLOUR: Russell's.

POTATO CRISPS: Plain Kettle Chips (contain salicylate—not in first four weeks of Anti-Candida Program).

MINERAL WATERS, STILL (NITRATE FREE): Koala Spring, Crystal Spring, Mt Franklin Still, Russell's.

MINERAL WATERS, CARBONATED/SPARKLING: Taurina Spa.

BREADS FOR THE METABOLISM-BALANCING PROGRAM: There is no brand restriction on the Metabolism-Balancing Program. Pritikin, Demeter and any other wholemeal bread (not wholegrain), raised with yeast, are all suitable.

BREADS FOR THE ANTI-CANDIDA PROGRAM: Any of the self-made unleavened breads mentioned in 'Recipes'; Pure Life sprouted wheat unleavened bread; or PAVS Allergy Bakery yeast free wheat.

BREADS FOR PEOPLE WHO ARE WHEAT SENSITIVE: Peter and Vicky's bakery 100 per cent unleavened rice bread.

There are many more varieties of bread; some contain yeast or sourdough. You must read the labels carefully.

CHEMICAL FREE SPRING WATER: Neverfail Spring Water, home delivered. Telephone (02) 9481 9888.

CHEMICAL FREE SOAPS, SHAMPOOS, CONDITIONERS AND DEODORANTS: As tastes are so individual it is best that you choose your own from the health store.

MOST IMPORTANT

Don't tell anyone in a health store you are on the Anti-Candida Program. Some health store attendants fancy themselves as physicians and offer conflicting advice on treatment or try to sell products they believe to be superior to those recommended in this book. Inevitably you will react adversely to what they sell you. This will leave you confused and disheartened. If a health store doesn't have the brand you are looking for, decline all substitutes and go to another store. It's not worth taking supplements you are going to react allergically to. To get results from the programs, you must have the recommended brands. This is the only way you can be sure of not reacting allergically to a given food.

MAIL ORDER

If you are having trouble procuring any of the recommended items on the shopping list phone my clinic on:

(02) 9981 2225 or
(02) 9982 7135

and we will post them to you as part of our mail order service.

IMPORTANT

As with the Metabolism-Balancing Program you may need to take a bottle of water to work and sip from it steadily through the day as you work. This is to reach your optimum fluid intake levels.

FORMULA SIX

Now that you are well you must keep taking Formula Six for the rest of your life. The vitality of your white blood cells will fall otherwise and candida plants will slowly grow back on the gut wall. There are not enough vitamins and minerals in our foods (even fresh fruits and vegetables) to maintain optimum candida-killing power of our white blood cells. See Chapter 16, 'Scientific explanations—Vitamins and minerals'.

I have tried to get people well without supplementary vitamins and minerals only to find that fresh food alone is not enough to achieve a cure.

Note: As there is so much important data in this chapter to be remembered, I suggest you read it three or four times before getting started and several times more through the course.

15.
Questions and answers

'Know Thyself.'
'Nothing in Excess.'

Carved by the ancient Greeks on the portals in front of the
temple of the oracle at Delphi

FASTING

Q. You're down on fasting but I feel better when I fast?
A. There are two reasons why you would feel better when you fast:

1. The withholding of all foods from the body is an effective way of
removing the symptoms of food allergy. This is the reason many
chronic fatigue syndrome sufferers experience a significant
burst of energy while fasting. Unfortunately this 'drift net'
approach to treating allergies has its drawbacks as vitamin and
mineral deficiencies quickly develop on fasts. Recent reports in
the newspapers have described how parents have fasted their
babies to rid them of allergic asthma and eczema and that
although the symptoms disappeared while off food, the babies
became so malnourished they died in their sleep. By following
the treatment program in this book you will get rid of your
allergies safely, you won't develop nutrient deficiencies and you
will feel as good as you did on your fast. Fasting doesn't cure
allergies it only removes the symptoms for the period that you
are on the fast. When you start eating again, the symptoms
return.
2. Non-allergic people can also experience a short-term physical
and mental boost from a short fast. The total withholding of food
from the body is a stress (see Chapter 16, 'Scientific explanations—Stress'). Stress causes the release of the hormone

adrenalin and adrenalin sends extra blood and oxygen to the brain, eyes and muscles. This makes us feel mentally alert and physically stronger. This process has been used for thousands of years to increase mental agility, inspiration and readiness for action. Einstein claimed that some of his flashes of brilliance were the result of 'frugal fare' and Shakespeare captured the essence of the fasting principle in describing the demise of Julius Caesar: 'Have about me men that are fat. Yon Casca has a lean and hungry look. He thinks too much.'

However, just because great men have used and advocated fasting, that doesn't make it a desirable practice. Granted, twelve and twenty-four hour fasts won't do much harm if they are not practised regularly and you are not pregnant, diabetic, hypoglycaemic or on medication. In my experience though, most people take the view that if a little bit makes you feel good, more will make you feel better, and this doesn't hold for fasting. These people begin practising longer fasts more frequently. By the time they consult me they are suffering from vitamin and mineral deficiencies and look and feel terrible.

The deep breathing exercises in Chapter 11 will put more oxygen in your brain and muscles than the adrenal surge of a fast. You'll feel brighter and stronger permanently, rather than have your mental acuity go up and down with your adrenalin levels.

Remember: the effects of fasting are cumulative and if you're not taking a complete multi-vitamin and mineral supplement you will, in time, develop deficiencies. I don't recommend you try fasting, the probability of things going wrong is too great.

VEGETARIANISM

Q. Why do you recommend so much animal protein in your program. I'm a vegetarian and find that meat tends to sit heavily in my stomach?

A. Animal protein (red meat, veal, fish, eggs, cheese) contains all the essential amino acids and many of the essential minerals in easily absorbable form. Soya beans and lentils also contain these essential amino acids but it's harder for the body to digest and absorb them as they also contain chemicals called trypsin inhibitors, haemagglutinins and phytates. The trypsin inhibitors reduce the action of the protein-splitting enzyme trypsin, the haemagglutinins line the wall of the intestine and slow down protein absorption and the phytates reduce mineral (zinc especially) absorption. These chemicals can have their actions negated if the legumes are sprouted, fermented or cooked slowly over a prolonged time. (Bear in mind, however, that fermented foods are prohibited on the Anti-Candida Program.) Most busy city people don't have time to sprout or ferment beans and lentils.

Many of the vegetarians I've treated who have been on Stage 7 macrobiotic diets have been zinc deficient. It is zinc deficiency that is responsible for the feelings of light-headed detachment they so frequently experience. These symptoms disappear when supplementary zinc is taken. Unfortunately, many vegetarians believe this light-headed detachment to be the beginnings of esoteric ascension and so continue their very restrictive diets.

Legumes and grains are low in zinc (meat is rich in zinc) and devoid of vitamin B12. Vitamin B12 is found in animal products only and those on strict, vegetarian diets (vegans) are in danger of developing deficiencies in these two essential nutrients. Lacto-vegetarians (those who include milk and cheese in their diet) are less likely to be B12 and zinc deficient. Lacto-ovo-vegetarians (those who eat eggs as well as dairy products) can enjoy superb health if they complement their diet with a complete multi-vitamin and mineral formula, brewer's yeast, kelp and spirulina. Lacto- and lacto-ovo-vegetarians should not have their eggs and dairy foods at the same meal as grains, soya beans, lentils and other legumes. The phytates in the legumes block the absorption of the minerals from the eggs and dairy products. Sprouting and fermenting legumes and grains neutralises the phytates. Cheese and egg sandwiches are fine if wholemeal leavened (yeast-fermented) bread is used.

Many vegetarians don't salt their food and are usually salt deficient. Salt and minerals zinc, calcium, magnesium and manganese are needed to make hydrochloric acid in the stomach. Hydrochloric acid is needed to digest protein. Animal protein will sit heavily in the stomach if there's a hydrochloric acid deficiency. An animal protein deficient diet helps to produce a hydrochloric acid deficiency. To break this vicious circle take a hydrochloric acid tablet just before eating animal protein. I find Digestivezyme by Bioglan gives the best results.

Hydrochloric acid is needed for us to absorb iron. Iron is more plentiful in red meat and more easily absorbed from it than from vegetables or grains. Iron deficiency anaemia is common among female vegetarians. Thirty per cent of the population lack the enzymes necessary to convert vegetable protein into animal protein inside the human body and there's no way of knowing if you're in that category until you turn vegetarian.

Q. Won't eating meat make me aggressive?
A. There is no scientific data to support this claim. Eskimos are predominantly meat eaters. They are a friendly people and wars

among them are rare. Hindus, who are vegetarians, are not any more peaceful than the Eskimos. It is true that wolves, lions, tigers are meat eating and aggressive and that rabbits, cows and horses are vegetarians (herbivores) and easily domesticated. No, you probably would not leave a lion to mind a baby. But would you leave a rabbit to mind a lettuce?

Q. If meat is so good for you, how come all the statistics show that vegetarians are healthier than most meat eaters?
A. The statistics are misleading. Most of the vegetarians cited in these studies were from certain religious sects who, in addition to not eating meat, didn't smoke, drink alcohol, take drugs or keep late hours. There is no doubt that such abstinence contributed to their good health. The meat eaters, conversely, were lumped together in one category. Alcoholics, smokers, drug addicts, down and outers, over-indulgers and fast food addicts were all lumped together as meat eaters, the inference being that meat eating was the reason for their poor health. Had the comparison been drawn between vegetarians and those meat eaters who didn't smoke, drink or take drugs, didn't stay out late at night or eat fast food and who took regular exercise and got plenty of rest, the statistics would have told a different story. In my experience meat eaters of this ilk are stronger and healthier than the average vegetarian.

Vegetarianism is fine if (1) you have the time to prepare the food properly, to make sure that meals have a balance of all the essential amino acids; (2) you live in a warm climate; and (3) you are not under stress. Yogis and people living in ashrams survive happily on a vegetarian diet. Those working forty-plus hours per week, in temperate zone winters, who have all the stresses and time constraints of big city life, don't fare as well.

Most of the vegetarians I have treated have diligently prepared their balanced meals for the first one or two years, after which time constraints seem to get the better of them and they start cutting corners. Because it can take a number of years for vitamin B12 deficiencies to develop it is hard for them to accept that an established lifestyle is the cause of their problem.

From the allergy standpoint, the lack of variety in vegetarian diets can lead to problems in those who are genetically predisposed to allergy. To get the essential sulfur amino acids, vegetarians have to eat cheese and eggs every day. This can lead to over-exposure to these foods. By eating meat, fish and poultry, the sulfur amino acids and minerals are obtained from a wider source and there is less chance of developing food allergies.

The Anti-Candida/Anti-Allergy Program can present a significant problem to vegetarians. Cheese is not permitted on the Anti-

Candida Program and eggs are a common allergen. If you're on the Anti-Candida Program and are allergic to eggs you have to include fish in your program. You'll become malnourished if you don't.

Q. You recommend the eating of liver, but isn't liver full of toxins?
A. North American and European liver is. The toxic content of Australian liver is miniscule by comparison with overseas liver and is far outweighed by nutrient content (see 'Recipes' for preparation guidelines). North American and European pastures are contaminated by acid rain and acid snow. Australia, with its small population, small industrial base, and its vast grazing areas and small rainfall, doesn't have this problem. Furthermore, the open range is not aerially top dressed. Australian pastures are clean.

Northern hemisphere stock is barn/stall fed on growth hormones and grain fodder. The grains have been sprayed with herbicides and insecticides. Hormone and spray residuals end up in the liver and fat of the meat. Grain-fed stock produce marbled meat, meaning the fat is evenly disseminated through the meat making it soft and easy to chew. Range-fed beef is lean on the inside with the fat on the perimeter of the cut. Nature sends the liver toxins to the fat tissue for storage. Being a very inert tissue, the toxins can do less harm to the body while sitting in the fat. Eaters of range-fed meat can trim the fat, and what little toxins there are in it, off. Range-fed livers are clean in comparison to stall-fed. Everything you read about the toxins in meat and liver is true for the northern hemisphere, barn-fed animals. The book you read it in was probably written in the northern hemisphere.

However, Australian poultry is force fed, so I wouldn't recommend you eat chicken, duck or turkey liver. Americans and Europeans claim range-fed Australian beef is too tough. This is the price we pay for cleaner meat, and is that so bad? All that chewing tones up the facial muscles so they can resist the pull of gravity and keep us looking younger for longer. You need liver on the Anti-Candida Program to get minerals you were previously getting from the yeast in bread. Lamb's liver is best but no more than twice per week as it's very rich. Calf's liver may be eaten by those without an amine sensitivity.

DIETING

Q. I don't want to go on a diet, I'm thin enough.
A. Not all diets are weight-loss diets. The programs in this book are health-promoting programs. By optimising your health they automatically optimise your body weight and shape. If you are overweight, they bring your body weight down to normal, if you are

under-weight, they will build your body weight up. If you are already at optimum weight, they leave you there, that is, providing you follow them properly.

Q. I've been dieting for some time. The Metabolism-Balancing Program includes more food than I've been having. I'll freak if I put on weight.
A. If you need less food than is on these programs to hold yourself at your optimum weight, you are malnourished. Malnutrition produces metabolic imbalances which, in turn, cause fluid retention which manifests as weight increase. Fluid retention worsens over time if the metabolism isn't balanced. While the metabolism is balancing itself, your weight will fluctuate up and down a bit. This is normal so don't be concerned. When the metabolism has fully balanced, your weight will normalise, this should take only three to six weeks. Don't get on the scales during this time.

We are what we think. If you focus on over-weight and get emotional (depressed) about it, over-weight is what you will get. If you put the scales away and focus on getting healthy and get emotional (excited) about it, optimum health is what you will get. Optimum body weight and shape is a spin-off of optimum health. To help ease your worries about putting on weight with these programs, don't eat any nuts, limit your bread intake to two slices per day (eaten in the middle of the day) and don't eat deep fried foods. Include nuts when your weight has normalised. If your weight doesn't normalise on the Metabolism-Balancing Program you are retaining fluid because of candida and/or allergies. The weight will normalise when they're treated.

Q. I haven't lost the weight I expected to on the Anti-Candida Program. Why haven't I lost weight?
A. Reduce the size of your meals by 40 per cent. Over-size meals is the main reason body weight doesn't normalise on these programs. Cut out nuts and deep fried foods until your weight normalises.

Q. If Formula Six is a concentrated food will I put on weight if I take them regularly? Do they contain many calories?
A. The calorie content of Formula Six is minuscule. It helps you lose weight by helping to raise your metabolic rate. It will never put weight on.

DRINKS

Q. How much fruit juice can I have daily and are the commercial brands OK if the label states 'No Added Sugar'?

A. Have as much fruit juice as you like—within reason—on the Metabolism-Balancing Program and none if you are on the Anti-Candida Program. Fruit juice carries mould and is too concentrated in natural sugars for the Anti-Candida Program. The commercial brands are OK if you are not allergic to anything in them.

Q. Can I have tea or coffee when I first get up?
A. Yes. After you have had your water.

Q. Should I avoid tea and coffee?
A. Not completely. Only one hour before taking your supplements and three hours after. The acids in tea and coffee block absorption of the minerals. No more than four or five cups of tea or coffee (total) per day. Sometimes mould can grow on tea and coffee if it's been in storage for too long. If you are not responding to the Anti-Candida Program as you feel you should, go off tea and coffee and observe your response.

Q. What can I drink after dinner?
A. Fruit juice or water if you are on the Metabolism-Balancing Program. Vegetable juice and water only if you are on the Anti-Candida Program. A squeeze of lemon juice may be added to give the water taste. (No lemon if you are amine and salicylate sensitive.)

Q. Is rainwater OK?
A. Yes, if you catch it in a clean pan in the garden. Don't catch it off the roof. Chemical fall-out from industry and agriculture collects on rooves and runs off in the rainwater.

Q. Are all the commercial mineral waters the same?
A. No, they are not. Some are made from tap water, others are from European Alpine streams (=contaminated by acid snow), and others from European springs. Unfortunately, the European subterranean water table has been polluted by seepage from toxic chemical dumps and is high in nitrates from nitrogen fertiliser run-off. The Australian water table is vast, and for the main part, pristine. Very rarely does it contain any nitrates at all. Drink only those mineral waters from recognised Australian spas. Look for the name of the spa or spring on the label. The recommended ones are included in the shopping list in Chapter 14. Nitrates are not only potent allergens, they can cause cancer and will reduce the amount of oxygen carried by the blood. Babies under three months can turn blue from nitrate-containing water. See 'Food tables—Sensitising chemicals in foods' at the back of the book.

Q. What type of water filter should I buy? Do I need one?
A. Tap water is so full of chlorine and other chemicals it frequently causes allergic reactions. The only tap filters that work are the expensive ones (they cost around $500, with regular replacement cartridges at about $100). You would be better off getting home-delivered, fresh spring water. I've found it gives the best results.

OILS

Q. Which of the cold pressed vegetable oils is best? Why do we need them?
A. They are all good. Choose an oil that you are not allergic to (see amine and salicylate lists in the 'Food tables' at the back of the book). Read Chapter 16, 'Scientific explanations—Vitamins and minerals', for a full explanation of why we need oils.

Q. Will I put on weight if I have the oil?
A. Not if you take only the quantities recommended in the programs.

Q. Which is the most stable oil for cooking?
A. Olive oil. But it contains amines and salicylates. Use one of the others if you suspect you are amine or salicylate sensitive.

Q. Is cod liver oil safe to give to children?
A. Most certainly, if you can get them to take it. If not, give them the MaxEPA marine lipid capsules. Not for toddlers though, they may choke on tablets or capsules.

Q. Which is better, butter or margarine?
A. Butter. Margarine has preservatives, colourings and often milk sugar and milk protein. Butter is pure fat.

VITAMINS AND MINERALS

Q. Why take Formula Six before a meal?
A. So they make contact with the digestive juices that are waiting in the stomach for the food to arrive. This ensures maximum absorption of the vitamins and minerals in Formula Six. Have them just before your first mouthful of food.

Q. I don't like taking tablets—why can't I spread them out through the day?
A. For vitamins and minerals to work optimally they must be taken all together, at the same time, with food. You will not get the potentially good results from the programs if you space the tablets over the day. Try and get them down with half a glass of water or juice using the other half to get the oil capsules down after the meal.

Q. Is Formula Six free from sugar, yeast, amines, salicylates, and artificial colourings?
A. Yes. The yellow colour of the urine is the natural residue of vitamin B1. It's normal for your urine to turn yellow at this time. There's no need to go off the tablets because this happens.

Q. Don't we excrete most of the vitamin/mineral supplements in our urine?
A. No. See Chapter 16, 'Scientific explanations—Vitamins and minerals'.

Q. Why is Formula Six divided into three tablets?
A. To put the quantity of vitamins and minerals in Formula Six into one tablet would make it too big to swallow.

Q. The kids won't swallow tablets.
A. Pulverise the tablets by dropping them into a blender with the blades going. When reduced to a fine powder, stop the blades and pour in a warm drink of 50 per cent home-made juice and 50 per cent hot water with ½–1 teaspoon of honey or glucose powder. Blend drink and powder together for twenty seconds. Keep stirring it between sips to keep the heavy minerals from settling to the bottom of the glass. Orange and lemon juice are best for disguising the taste of the vitamins.

This is no problem for those on the Metabolism-Balancing Program. If they still won't take tablets by the time they start the Anti-Candida Program, the vitamins will have to be continued in the drink with honey or glucose powder. However, they will have to remain on the Anti-Candida Program for four months instead of the usual three as the juice and honey/glucose will slow down the rate at which the candida yeast can be contained.

Q. Is it safe to take Formula Six while pregnant?
A. Most certainly. In fact, it's advantageous. A recent report from one of the American universities stated that taking vitamin/mineral supplements during pregnancy significantly reduced the chance of physical and mental birth defects in babies and improved the baby's IQ. Facial shape abnormalities are common in babies born to vitamin/mineral deficient mothers.

NYSTATIN

Q. Will Nystatin and garlic kill Lactobacillus acidophilus?
A. No. Nystatin kills only yeast organisms and garlic is not a broad spectrum killer of bacteria. It only kills unfriendly bacteria. Lactobacillus is a friendly bacterium.

ANTI-CANDIDA PROGRAM

Q. Yoghurt contains Lactobacillus acidophilus, *shouldn't I be taking it?*
A. No, not on the Anti-Candida Program. Yoghurt is fermented milk and aggravates yeast allergies. It also contains milk sugar. That is why the capsules of pure *Lactobacillus acidophilus* are taken instead.

Q. If the kill-off symptoms only last one week, why must I stay on the program for three months?
A. The symptoms of kill-off are your body's reaction to the new experience of having *Candida albicans* killed. After a week or so your body gets used to it and doesn't react adversely to the process for the remainder of the program. Kill-off doesn't mean that all the yeasts are killed off in a week. It takes at least three months to kill them off.

Q. I am tired of my candida/allergy symptoms, I want to go on the Anti-Candida/Anti-Allergy Program now.
A. You will only get mediocre results if you skip the six to eight weeks on the Metabolism-Balancing Program first. I suggest you read the preamble in Chapter 13, 'The Metabolism-Balancing Program'.

Q. I react to dust, pollen and mould. How can a program help me?
A. By raising your overall resistance to all allergens. By removing the food correlates of inhalant allergens you desensitise yourself to those allergens. This is explained in greater detail in Chapter 2, 'Allergies', and Chapter 5, 'How to cure your allergies'.

Q. Are avocados and tomatoes fruits? Should I avoid them during the fruit free period of the Anti-Candida Program?
A. Yes, they are fruits. However, because they contain very little sugar, they are permitted during the full twelve weeks of the program, unless you are amine and/or salicylate sensitive.

Q. I'm only eating rice cakes because I'm allergic to yeast. Does this mean I can avoid the unleavened bread in the Anti-Candida Program?
A. No. You must eat the unleavened breads listed in the recipe section. You will become run down if you don't. Rice cakes aren't substantial enough.

Q. Should I avoid sprouts, especially alfalfa, because they grow mould easily?
A. I suggest you do if you don't have the time to wash the mould

Q. Are sweet potato, pumpkin and carrot juice too sweet for the Anti-Candida Program?
A. No. Despite their sweetness they are vegetables not fruits and their carbohydrates are the complex sort that don't feed candida.

Q. Why can't I eat wholegrain bread?
A. Wholegrain bread is white bread with bits of whole grains in it. Whole grains are indigestible and pass straight through the body. Wholegrain bread is not nutritious. It feeds candida and shouldn't be confused with wholemeal bread. Wholemeal is whole grain ground up into a flour that is digestible. Whole grains are akin to birdseed and humans don't have the digestive mechanisms that birds have.

Q. I've been told I'm gluten sensitive, should I avoid all grain foods?
A. No. Avoid only those gluten foods listed under 'Gluten' in the 'Food tables' at the back of the book.

Q. Why is it I can have fresh but not dried fruit?
A. Dried fruit is treated with chemicals—metabisulphite being the major one—and also grows mould. It is also concentrated in natural sugars as is fruit juice. For this reason, fruit juices and dried fruit are not allowed on the Anti-Candida Program.

Q. Why can't I have frozen vegetables, aren't they as nutritious as fresh vegetables?
A. No, they aren't. See Chapter 16, 'Scientific explanations—Vitamins and minerals'. One cannot avoid frozen vegetables completely but try to keep them to a minimum.

Q. Why can't I continue eating my breakfast cereals. All the ads claim they are healthy foods?
A. The breakfast cereals in question have had most of the vitamins and minerals removed in the manufacturing process. Because four or five vitamins and minerals have been put back, these cereals are touted as 'fortified' and, therefore, healthy. They are still very vitamin and mineral deficient and have been adulterated with sugar, malt, artificial flavourings, preservatives and colourings. Because of this, many people react allergically to them. They also feed *Candida albicans*.

Q. Are commercially prepared herbs and spices suitable?
A. Yes, provided they are not the mixed varieties. Use only the one-herb-per-jar variety. Stay away from those with a number of ingredients. These tend to have chemical additives.

Q. Is arrowroot flour classed as white or wholemeal flour?
A. Arrowroot is similar to potato flour which puts it halfway between white and wholemeal flour. Use it as an inclusion in recipes only, not as the principal ingredient.

Q. I find it difficult to relax during meals as I'm always jumping up and down getting things for the kids.
A. This is a problem when you have small children. All you can do is try to remain as calm as possible for the duration of the meal and make sure you relax well after the meal when they are in bed.

FISH

Q. I don't eat fish as I've heard it's polluted by the water?
A. Only fish caught from the shallow waterways around major cities and industrial areas are polluted. All the others are fine. Before buying, ask where the fish were caught. There's no species that is considered completely clean as a group, as those that can be caught in clean waters can also be found close to cities.

CHOLESTEROL

Q. I don't eat eggs because I don't want a cholesterol problem.
A. The humble egg has been much maligned by the cholesterol issue. Eggs are very nutritious as only healthy hens can lay eggs, and although they contain cholesterol, they also contain lecithin, vitamins B1, B2, B3, B5, B6 and B12 as well as the minerals calcium, magnesium, sulfur, selenium, zinc and phosphorus. These nutrients keep egg cholesterol soluble in the blood and prevent it sticking to the artery wall.

The cholesterol the body makes from junk food is the big problem. Junk food/fast food doesn't have the vitamin and mineral content needed to keep cholesterol soluble and off the artery walls. When eaten in association with junk food, eggs get the blame for rising cholesterol levels and cholesterol build-up on artery walls. Junk food/fast food never rates a mention. The facts are that two eggs per day raise the blood cholesterol levels by only 2 mg per cent (not enough to contribute to atherosclerosis) in non-smokers, and by 27 mg per cent in smokers. (Smokers inhale the toxic heavy metal cadmium from the smoke of their cigarettes. Cadmium negates the cholesterol-lowering and -dissolving effect of zinc, selenium, and calcium. This can also happen to passive smokers.) Non-smokers on the programs in this book will not see their cholesterol levels rise from eating eggs.

Eggs are close to being a complete food. They are one of the few foods that food manufacturers haven't adulterated. Their high sulfur content builds strong joints, nails, hair, skin and brain cells. Eggs are good for arthritis and slow the ageing process.

Try to have eggs at least two or three times per week. However, if your cholesterol levels are high, you should wait until they have normalised. That way you won't have well-meaning family and friends badgering you and spoiling your egg meal. Vegetarians will enjoy good health if they include eggs in their program.

A teaspoon of vitamin C powder in a glass of juice or water, taken daily, is excellent for normalising cholesterol levels and keeping them normal. Remember only 30 per cent of the cholesterol in our blood comes directly from the food we eat. The rest is manufactured from the liver, mostly from fats and oils. However, any food eaten over and above the body's calorie requirement can be converted to cholesterol. Junk food/fast food is very high in calories.

Q. I'm a breastfeeding mother, what program should I be on?
A. The only program to be on while you are breastfeeding is the Metabolism-Balancing Program. This will keep the nutrient content of your milk high. The Anti-Candida/Anti-Allergy Programs are too food restrictive for breastfeeding mothers. Breastfeeding, and the broken sleep that goes with it, is too stressful for these programs. However, if you have *severe* reactions to certain foods, stay off them. (1) It could turn your baby off your milk, and (2) the stress of such a reaction could affect milk production.

Recently the British medical journal, *Lancet,* reported that babies breastfed beyond seven months had stronger immune systems than formula-fed babies. The crux of allergy prevention and treatment is strong immunity. Wean the baby at ten to twelve months, then start the Anti-Candida/Anti-Allergy Program.

Mothers of African, Asian or Mediterranean extraction should stay off cow's milk while breastfeeding. Use crushed egg shells for calcium (see 'Recipes' for details on preparing these).

The Anti-Candida/Anti-Allergy Program is OK during pregnancy.

16.
Scientific explanations

'It is highly dishonourable for a reasonable soul to live in so divinely built a mansion as the body she resides in, altogether unacquainted with the exquisite structure of it.'

Robert Boyle, 1627–91

CHOLESTEROL AND SALT

Cholesterol is an essential substance. We can't live without it. It is a constituent of every cell in the body, particularly the cell membrane. It is needed to make the bile acids (needed for fat digestion) and the steroid hormones, which comprise the sex hormones and the stress hormones of testosterone, adrenalin and cortisone (technical name cortisol). Around 70 per cent of all the body's cholesterol is made in the liver and every cell of the body has enzymes that enable it to make its own cholesterol should the levels begin to fall. Only 30 per cent of the body's cholesterol is obtained from the diet and changes in the diet can bring about moderate falls in cholesterol levels.

There is significant evidence to link high blood cholesterol levels to blood vessel wall deterioration and heart attacks, though heart attacks occur in those with normal cholesterol levels as well.

To date, dietary restriction and drug therapy have been major vehicles of blood cholesterol lowering. However, there is more to it than that. Any textbook of pathology states that blood cholesterol levels rise (1) when there is a deficiency in thyroid hormones in the blood, (2) when the body is under stress and (3) when late onset diabetes is present.

The highest concentrations of cholesterol in the body are to be found in the adrenal glands. Habitually stressed people use vast quantities of stress hormones. (See Chapter 11, 'Stress', and section on stress in this chapter.) The liver has to keep making the cholesterol to satisfy this demand. The high cholesterol reading in stressed people is the measure of cholesterol travelling from the liver to the adrenal glands to make stress hormones.

Stress further aggravates blood cholesterol levels because cortisone breaks down tissue to be burned for energy. The breakdown of body cells releases their cholesterol content into the blood. This is how crash diets and fasting help raise the cholesterol levels. Prolonged stress puts inordinate demands on the thyroid gland as it labours to keep the body's energy level up. In time it tires and produces less thyroid hormones and the cholesterol levels go still higher. (See any good physiology or pathology text for details of thyroid hormone influence on cholesterol.)

To try and keep the energy levels of an over-stressed body up, the adrenal glands produce more adrenalin, which requires still more cholesterol. The body is now running on false energy. Instead of relying on normal cell respiration for its energy supplies, it's relying on the stimulation of adrenalin. Many hard-charging, over-achiever types (see Chapter 11, 'Stress') rely on this 'adrenal buzz' to get them through every day. They get so used to living on it they consider it normal and cannot understand why they have high cholesterol levels. In extreme cases their cholesterol levels resist dietary measures to lower them which can lead to ever stricter diets to achieve the desired results. If the diets become too restrictive they become a stress in themselves and a vicious downward spiral is born. Seriously restrictive diets are short of the mineral chromium which leads to late onset diabetes and still higher cholesterol levels. Stress-based high cholesterol levels often give way to diabetes-based high cholesterol as the hard-charger reaches mid-life and beyond.

The Metabolism-Balancing Program is designed to maximise body energy levels by providing ample nutrition to all the cells including those of the thyroid gland. Co-related with sensible work loads, exercise loads and socialising loads the body maintains high energy levels and the cholesterol levels normalise. The deep breathing exercises help keep us calm and relaxed as well as vital. This helps prevent anxiety which is also a cholesterol raiser. The mental relaxation exercises are excellent for 'talking down' cholesterol levels and have worked wonders with many of my patients. The more you practise the exercises, the more proficient you'll become at lowering, and keeping low, your cholesterol levels.

Because high cholesterol is essentially a metabolic problem the answer is easy. Balance the metabolism and you balance the cholesterol levels. By following the Metabolism-Balancing Program and doing the breathing and relaxation exercises your cholesterol levels will normalise without recourse to the drastic diets and toxic drugs so often used. Many people become so miserable on these drastic diets they go off them with a vengeance and binge eat on all the high fat foods (cakes, chocolates, desserts) which only sees their cholesterol levels rise again. Drastic diets don't work for people in the early stages of late onset diabetes. Diabetes can be fully corrected by the Metabolism-Balancing Program only. When the diabetes is corrected the cholesterol levels automatically balance out.

SALT

Like cholesterol, salt (sodium chloride) is an essential substance. Sodium is intimately involved in the transfer of energy within every cell of the body. A deficiency in it sees a drop in energy levels and cramping of muscles—all muscles—including the heart and blood vessel wall muscles. Too much of a good thing can be bad for us and salt, the great preserver of food, is consumed in too high a quantity by those who eat preserved foods. Canned, frozen and packaged foods from the supermarket are highly salted. Processed meats, pickled foods, TV dinners and pre-cooked foods that require only heating up are all highly salted. If you are living on them you are in danger of hardening your arteries and contributing to heart attacks. If you keep these foods to 5 per cent, or less, of total food intake (see the Metabolism-Balancing Program) you will be OK.

The unfortunate thing about the information on excess salt's bad effect on the body is that only the health-orientated people read it and this information was meant for the sedentary, junk food, over-indulgers. The health buffs who weren't living on junk foods, weren't overdoing it on salt, went for over-kill by cutting it out of their diet completely. Because too little salt can do as much damage as too much, these people begin to see an inexorable decline in their vitality. This decline is aggravated by the fact that health-orientated people tend to be more active and thus evaporate more salt and water from their bodies than sedentary over-indulgers.

It is common these days for doctors and naturopaths to be treating people for the symptoms of salt deficiency. If you are eating only 5 per cent junk foods and 95 per cent fresh, natural foods, you need to salt your food each day—$^1/_4$ teaspoon a day is fine for most adults of average size. If you are physically active raise it to $^1/_2$ teaspoon. If you are physically active and big have $^3/_4$ teaspoon each day. If you have spent a day in the sun and have a bad headache have a whole teaspoon in a large glass of water—

251

drink it all. Take 1 teaspoon in a large glass of water if suffering from diarrhoea. Take one every day until the diarrhoea is over. Stress (particularly sunburn) causes salt to be lost in the urine. Salt is needed to make adrenalin (one of the major stress hormones) and to make the digestive juices (hydrochloric acid) of the stomach. A deficiency in salt means a deficiency in digestion and absorption and therefore in protein, vitamins and minerals. Because sodium is so easily disposed of by the body it doesn't hurt to take a bit more than is needed.

I've found that a lot of the hard-charger, health buff types I treat don't salt their food and are suffering from bloated stomachs as a result of this. What little salt they are getting from the fresh fruits and vegetables is going to sustain their heavily exercised muscles. There is no salt left over to make hydrochloric acid. By the time they come to see me they are deficient in minerals. Minerals need hydrochloric acid for their absorption. Food sits for long periods of time in their stomach and they are always tired. All because they didn't salt their food.

DIABETES

Late onset diabetes is one of the most common symptoms of a significant imbalance in the body's metabolism and is caused by a deficiency in the mineral chromium. Late onset diabetes develops slowly over the years and is recognised as a glucose resistance to the hormone insulin. Insulin's job is to latch onto glucose in the bloodstream, take it to the cell and push it through the cell wall into the cell where it's burned to produce energy. Chromium's job is to bring glucose and insulin together and ensure a secure bond between them. If there is a deficiency in chromium, glucose and insulin float through the blood ignoring each other. Because the cells are now missing out on their major energy source they have to fall back on their second choice energy source, fat.

The blood fat and cholesterol levels rise as these reserves are mobilised for energy production. High fat and cholesterol levels born of this metabolic imbalance don't respond well to strict anti-cholesterol diets that are designed to treat cholesterol born of over-indulgence in saturated fat foods (all processed meats, fried foods, hamburgers, chips, TV dinners, packaged foods, butter). This is because such foods as beef and liver that are considered too high in cholesterol to eat are rich in chromium. Whole wheat also contains chromium. White flour has all its chromium removed in the milling process.

The only other significant source of chromium is brewer's yeast and there was a time when beer provided plenty of it. Unfortunately these days very few brands of beer are brewed from yeast (they're now chemically brewed) and a good source of chromium has been lost. Very few people will take brewer's yeast in its natural form. Is it any wonder that late onset diabetes and high cholesterol are on the rise? Chromium deficiency is on the increase as more and more manufactured foods are replacing natural foods at the dinner table. Imbalances in glucose metabolism are on the increase and account for under-functioning, sluggish livers, lack of mental acuity and intractable over-weight problems as well as late onset diabetes and high cholesterol levels.

Not only dietary deficiencies are involved in overall chromium deficiency. Each pregnancy can cause white blood cell chromium to drop by 50 per cent. (No wonder so many mothers develop allergies after childbirth; see Chapter 2, 'Allergies'.) The glucose drips that accompany surgical operations cause chromium levels to drop to one-third of normal and if the patient has a post-operative viral infection the end results can be disastrous if chromium supplements are not taken.

Diabetes, like heart attacks, offers very few early warning signs. Most people don't know they've got it till they've got it. Intractably high cholesterol levels are seldom recognised as an early diagnostic sign. The gradual loss of tolerance to alcohol from mid-life on is a classic sign of chromium deficiency and impending diabetes.

The removal from the diet of such cholesterol-containing foods as beef and liver doesn't help reduce cholesterol in those with late onset diabetes or the beginnings of it. In fact it aggravates the condition. These foods are rich in chromium and actually help to lower the cholesterol levels in those whose high cholesterol is linked to chromium deficiency diabetes. I've found that those patients of mine whose cholesterol levels are still above normal despite sticking to the standard cholesterol-lowering diet are invariably chromium deficient. It's amazing how many high cholesterol sufferers fall into this category and how quickly they respond to chromium (plus all the other vitamins and minerals) supplementation. High cholesterol, for most people, is the result of imbalances in the metabolism. Balancing the metabolism with the Metabolism-Balancing Program is the best way to treat it.

Evidence to support the importance of balancing the metabolism with adequate vitamin and mineral intake can be found in the dietary habits of different groups. Eskimos eat a diet high in saturated fats yet rarely have atherosclerosis. Liver is prized among these people, and with good reason, as it contains just about every vitamin and mineral known. It is rich in chromium and all the support vitamins and minerals needed for chromium to be effective. Vegetarians who eat a diet low in saturated fats often develop atherosclerosis. This is not surprising as most vegetarians do not supplement their diet with brewer's yeast or sugar beet molasses. Both these foods are rich in chromium and the principal support nutrients of iron, selenium, manganese, vitamin B12 and folic acid needed by chromium to complete its metabolic chores. Guinness stout (made in Ireland) is a good source of sugar beet molasses and brewer's yeast. Australian stout is made from cane molasses which isn't as nutritious. Don't overdo it though. If too much stout (alcohol) is consumed the liver will be damaged and the metabolism unbalanced once more. (See the alcohol tables in Chapter 13, 'The Metabolism-Balancing Program'.)

It's no coincidence that Grandma took molasses during and after pregnancy and that she mulled stout and gave it to those with infections and those recovering from surgery. The mulling process involves the plunging of a hot poker into the stout to burn off its alcohol content. Her winter/spring remedy of molasses and sulfur powder was a great tonic as well as a cleanser.

FOOD AND MOOD

The exact biochemical pathways that mediate the effect of food on brain cells are still a subject of controversy among scientists. However, scientists generally agree on the following:

1. Allergies can target the brain cells as readily as they can target the skin, nose, joint and bronchial cells of the body.

   The histamine released into a brain cell during an allergic reaction can significantly disrupt the function of that cell. Some authorities maintain the swelling (localised fluid retention) that accompanies allergic reactions puts undue physical pressure on the cell, slowing down its release of waste products while at the same time reducing the flow of oxygen, water and nutrients into it. Others maintain that the histamine revs up the metabolism of the cell to the point where it fatigues very quickly and that symptoms of brain allergy are symptoms of brain fatigue.

   All seem to agree that the brain cells are the most sophisticated of all the body's cells. They are not unlike the engine of a high performance motor car, very delicate and finely tuned. The more complicated and sophisticated a motor car engine, the more likely it is to break down. In other words, the more parts there are to it, the more there is to go wrong with it—high performance motor cars are more temperamental. If moisture gets into them on a rainy day and they stall at the lights it usually takes a mechanic in a workshop to get them fully operational again. A spray of WD40 will often get a standard car going but not the sophisticated one. In like manner, allergies tend to upset the delicate and finely tuned brain cells more profoundly than they do the less sophisticated body cells.

Because allergies can target different parts of the brain in different people we can get a variance in symptoms. Some people become emotionally disturbed yet remain fully functional intellectually. Some remain emotionally balanced and content yet intellectually impaired. Some become both emotionally and intellectually affected.

2. Vitamin and mineral supplementation improves and increases the body's ability to make neurotransmitters. Neurotransmitters are the chemicals that form a bridge between individual brain cells. Over this bridge pass the nerve impulses that are the communication medium of the brain cells. It is the travelling around from brain cell to brain cell of these nerve impulses that allows a group of brain cells to co-ordinate their functions to produce thoughts, feelings, memories, decisions, etc. These neurotransmitters are made from proteins, fats, vitamins, minerals and nucleic acids. One neurotransmitter called acetylcholine is made almost entirely from the B vitamin called choline. Nucleic acids are found abundantly in fish which gives some credence to the old wive's tale that fish is brain food.

On this point it's interesting to note that in 1929 a survey was done to ascertain why there was a disproportionately high number of Scottish graduates from English universities. The survey concluded that the only major difference between the Scots and English was that the Scots ate more fish and more porridge. This is not as far fetched as it may seem. The cold water fish of Scotland are rich in marine oils that keep cholesterol down as well as the nucleic acids and vitamins and minerals needed to build neurotransmitters. The oats the Scots used for porridge in 1929 were unprocessed. Being rich in oat bran, porridge helped keep the cholesterol down and the blood vessel walls clean, allowing good passage of oxygen and nutrients into the brain cells. Oats are among the most nutritious of all the herbs, being rich in a broad spectrum of vitamins and minerals. Oats are herbal calmatives (not to be confused with the full-blown, sedative effect of other herbs) and help produce a state of mind that is conducive to study and learning. European and Nordic cultures have for thousands of years used oat straw tea and various tinctures of oat as nerve tonics and anti-depressants.

FOOD COMBINING

It's not so much the food we eat that determines our health, it's the food we manage to digest and absorb that counts. If food is not successfully absorbed from the digestive tract into the body proper it passes out of the body with the bowel movements of the following day.

Stress is the great inhibitor of digestion and absorption. Adrenalin (see Chapter 11, 'Stress', and the section on 'Stress' in this chapter) shuts down the digestive tract by directing the blood away from it to the muscles, brain and eyes to prepare us for action. Food in the pipe at this time just sits there doing nothing save causing the abdomen to bloat and distend. (The digestive system is simply an 8.5 m (28 ft) pipe stretching from mouth to anus.)

Insidious malnutrition afflicts those who are too busy, committed, or anxious to sit down to eat and to relax after eating to let the food digest. The great irony here is that nutritious foods like wholemeal bread, nuts, seeds, fresh fruits and vegetables, with their high fibre and complex carbohydrate content, are harder to digest and absorb than the refined foods of white bread, tinned fruits, TV dinners, pies or potato crisps, that have a slower passage through the pipe and are more likely to yield their limited nutrients to absorption.

The fact that whole, natural foods require adequate rest and relaxation for their digestion is often missed by the hard-charging, health buff type who works forty to fifty hours per week, jogs three nights, plays competition sports such as squash or touch football and is always eating alfalfa sprouts, wheat grass, wholemeal bread, nuts and seeds on the go and yet feels tired all the time. (See Chapter 11, 'Stress—Stress and the hard-charger'.)

These types always seem to have a brother-in-law who 'is a bit of an under-achiever', doesn't exercise, eats pies for lunch in the pub, is a bit over-weight, but seems energetic enough and never catches the amount of colds and 'flu that the hard-charging health buff catches. In short, he annoys the hard-charging health buff who cannot understand why this brother-in-law seems to have a higher resistance to infection and a greater *joie de vivre* than the hard-charging health buff, who is so fit and has such regular bowels. The regular bowel movements are, unfortunately, where most of the hard-charger's food intake ends up.

Often the hard-charger tries to rectify the situation by coming in late from a busy day and cooking a balanced nutritious meal. Being that it's late and there is a busy day ahead, the hard-charger goes to bed with a full stomach, a practice that interferes with digestion as during sleep all body processes slow dramatically, including those of digestion and absorption. The hard-charger wakes next morning and cannot face breakfast as part of last night's meal is still lying undigested in the stomach.

Young, New World civilisations have a lot to learn from the historically successful and well-established Old World civilisations. The Italians, for instance, have some of the sanest and most health-promoting eating habits of all. They have their main meal in the middle of the day and they take the afternoon off to relax, enjoy and digest it. Before their leisurely midday meal they often sip such appetisers as Campari and Vermouth to enhance the flow of their digestive juices in readiness for the food. With the main meal they eat bitter salads that help to maintain the acidity of their stomachs. Optimum stomach acidity is needed to ensure digestion of protein and absorption of minerals. They get maximum nutritional benefit from their food which gives them energy when they need it most, during the waking hours. Could this be one of the reasons Italy has contributed so much to the world of art, music, architecture, education and scientific thought?

Cultures that are predominantly Anglo Saxon–Celtic tend to have their main meal at the end of the day. Although this is not as wise as the Italian practice, it's OK if the evening meal isn't too big or eaten too late and if the rest of the evening is spent relaxing. However, watching drama and violence on TV does not constitute relaxation, for this gets the adrenalin levels up again and reduces digestion and absorption. Using the after-dinner hours to do the ironing, put on a load of washing, sit over a desk doing paper work, phone customers, colleagues or employees to discuss work is not relaxing and will help to reduce your digestion. If you are one of these workaholic, hard-charging types, are guilty of these practices and habitually drive your car above the speed limit, you will find you will probably have a distended abdomen through the week that flattens out on the weekend—if you slow down. Many people think this see-sawing pot tummy is the result of candida or over-eating and so go on a strict, often crash diet to get rid of it. Such restrictive diets add to their already high stress levels and cause malnutrition.

CORRECT FOOD COMBINING

Correct food combining ensures optimum digestion and absorption. However, it's not necessary to be as strict as some exponents of food combining claim. To live on a daily fare that sees one eating protein only at one meal and carbohydrate only at another, with fruits and vegetables separated at opposite ends of the day would be incredibly boring for most people. Such boredom can so stress the body as to raise the adrenalin levels which then interfere with digestion and absorption. Food and the eating of it is one of the greatest sensual experiences nature has bestowed on us. The more it's enjoyed the better it is digested—ask any Italian. For eating to be a sensual experience the meal must have flavour and aroma. Flavour and aroma are best achieved by combining two or more foods in a given dish. It is the aroma and anticipation of a meal that helps to get our digestive juices flowing and it's the flavour of the meal that perpetuates that flow. The secret of optimum digestion and absorption is optimum digestive juice flow. Certain food-combining practices aid and abet the digestive juices.

The practice of drinking large quantities of water or eating a fruit or garden salad or a large bowl of soup before the main meal dilutes the hydrochloric acid secreted from the stomach walls for the digestion of protein foods (meat, poultry, seafood, eggs and cheese). These foods contain minerals (zinc, manganese, iron) and minerals need a good supply of hydrochloric acid if they are to be absorbed. Protein can't be broken up without hydrochloric acid. Small amounts of water taken before and sipped during a meal is fine. Pineapples and paw paws contain protein-splitting enzymes and may be had in small quantities just before or with a protein meal as may bitter salads which help promote hydrochloric acid secretion. It's the little exceptions to the rule like these that make strict, uncompromising food combining invalid.

It's best to eat at least half of the meat, seafood, poultry, egg, cheese (protein) component of the meal before starting on the carbohydrate (potato, rice, pasta, yam taro, sweet potato, pumpkin). The bottom part of the stomach is where the hydrochloric acid is secreted and because this acid only works on protein it pays to get a good measure of protein food down there first. When the bottom part of the stomach (pylorus) is full of protein it closes off and the rest of the food is stored in the top part (fundus) until the bottom half has emptied its semi-digested contents into the small intestine.

It works out well for the second part of the meal to be the carbohydrate foods as most of their digestive enzymes are found in the mouth. While waiting in the closed-off top section of the stomach their digestion, which began in the mouth, continues unhindered by the acid in the lower portion of the stomach. Hydrochloric acid stops the digestion of carbohydrate foods, which don't resume their digestion until they pass through the lower part of the stomach into the small intestine. Too much carbohydrate soaks up the hydrochloric acid (like a sponge does water), reducing the acid's contact with the protein food. Furthermore, the alkaline carbohydrates tend to neutralise the acid. However, if the bulk of the protein has passed to the small intestine by the time the carbohydrate foods are released into the lower stomach, their passage through it into the small intestine will be quick as small amounts of protein food in it tends not to hold its passage up.

In the small intestine protein and carbohydrate food can be digested simultaneously and if small quantities of protein foods are carried through with the carbohydrates they don't strain the small intestine's capacity to digest them, even if they haven't first been broken up by hydrochloric acid. Most importantly the bulk of the minerals in the protein food have already been absorbed in the strong acid medium that existed before the carbohydrates reached the lower stomach.

Ideally, all the protein foods should be consumed before starting on the carbohydrates, green and coloured vegetables and sauces. However, some people find that this practice detracts from the enjoyment of the meal. So, as long as half the protein food is consumed first there will be enough minerals absorbed to sustain the average healthy person, though I suggest the seriously run-down eat all of their protein first until such time as they have built themselves up.

Remember, everything that leaves the mouth should be in a fluid state. The digestive juices are designed to mix with fluid food, they do not work as effectively on chunks of this and that. Don't bolt your food. Take your time and chew it properly. Don't sit hunched forward for the duration of the meal. Draw your chair in closer and periodically lean back against the back rest while you chew. This way you won't compress your digestive organs and reduce their function. The main reason for sitting back and relaxing after the main meal of the day is to prevent the compaction of the digestive organs.

Formula Six has been designed to aid digestion and promote optimum absorption. It contains the vitamins and minerals needed to help achieve this, and for this reason must be taken with a little water just before the main meal of the day. This way you can be sure hydrochloric acid is waiting in the lower part of the stomach to receive your protein food and that there will be optimum absorption of the minerals in Formula Six. Many people are hydrochloric acid deficient due to a lifetime of vitamin and mineral deficiencies and for this reason don't receive optimum benefit from the food they eat. Hydrochloric acid deficiency is most prevalent in the over forties.

Most people, by instinct and commonsense, combine foods appropriately. For example, most meals that are essentially protein in nature are served with only a small portion of potato, rice or other carbohydrate, and vegetables and salad. (The Italian scallopine dishes are an example of this.) Dishes that are essentially carbohydrate by nature usually have a small portion of meat on top. (The Italian spaghetti dishes are good examples of this.) Conversely, most people instinctively know that eating large dollops of carbohydrate (for example, mashed potatoes) with a large portion of meat, seafood or poultry doesn't sit well, takes longer to digest and gives rise to that typical sign of incomplete digestion, wind, at both ends. Often, steak dishes have pineapple included and many salads contain pineapple and paw paw (papaya), which aid in the digestion of proteins.

Those with an appreciation of food and refined eating habits usually wait an hour or so after the main meal before eating sweets. This gives the top half of the stomach time to empty into the bottom half leaving it free to take the sweets without mixing them up with the carbohydrates and vegetables. The sweets are held in the top half of the stomach until the bottom half has emptied the carbohydrates into the small intestine.

Too much water with meals will dilute the digestive juices in both stomach and small intestine as water is fairly slowly absorbed and can only be absorbed from the lower portions of the small intestine. Sugar and alcohol, however, are efficient transporters of water through both stomach and upper small intestine wall. This is why wine or fruit juice can be sipped during a meal without making us feel bloated, whereas a comparable amount of water leaves us feeling heavy and uncomfortable.

I have found that the principles and practice of adequate rest and relaxation, plus the eating and food-combining habits advocated in this section, have done wonders for improving the nutritional state of those I have treated.

WHAT ABOUT SANDWICHES?

If you are eating a meat, seafood, poultry, egg or cheese sandwich you have no choice but to eat protein and carbohydrate together. This is not the end of the world. Granted, it's not the ideal way to eat, but it's better than going without food. If you eat it slowly, masticate it thoroughly and don't stuff yourself the sandwich will be reasonably well digested in the small intestine. Although it won't yield as many nutrients as it would if you ate the protein content first and the carbohydrate bread later, it will still give you enough sustenance to get by on. Don't be fanatical about food combining. The stress of fanaticism will undo the good of the food combining. So long as the main meal of the day is being properly combined you will get enough nutrients into your body to sustain optimum health.

THE METABOLISM

The metabolism can be broadly described as the sum total of all the chemical reactions which take place inside all the cells of the body. Perhaps the most important metabolic processes are those which turn the food we eat into energy or into body chemicals such as hormones, enzymes and antibodies. These chemicals are made from protein, fat, carbohydrate, vitamins, minerals and trace elements. If a deficiency exists in any one of these nutrients certain chemicals cannot be made and this will adversely affect the function of the other chemicals, thus producing an imbalance in the metabolism.

Most metabolic imbalances are associated with over-weight which in turn is frequently the result of eating the wrong type of food. Take white bread for example. It is both fattening and capable of causing serious disturbances in the metabolism. It is fattening for two reasons:

1. Because white bread is refined it is quickly digested and therefore rapidly absorbed into the blood as molecules of glucose which arrive in the bloodstream in such large quantities that the blood sugar levels immediately shoot up. To normalise the blood sugar levels the pancreas releases the hormone insulin which removes the glucose from the blood by converting it to fat. Years of eating white flour and sugar can so sensitise the pancreas that it over-reacts and releases too much insulin. This causes the glucose levels to drop too low, causing the metabolic imbalance known as functional hypoglycaemia. This usually happens to those who are vitamin and mineral deficient and/or under stress.
2. Because white bread is refined it lacks the vitamins and minerals required for normal carbohydrate metabolism and, because it cannot be metabolised properly and used by the body as a carbohydrate energy source, most of it must be converted to and stored in the body as fat. Thus, the body has increased in weight but its carbohydrate needs have not been fully satisfied. This usually manifests a desire to eat more carbohydrate and all too often white bread is again the choice.

To be correctly metabolised, any carbohydrate food needs to contain vitamins B3 (niacin), B1 (thiamine), B2 (riboflavin), B6 (pyridoxine), B5 (pantothenic acid) and the minerals phosphorus and magnesium. During the milling process of whole grain flour to its white refined state the magnesium, phosphorus, pyridoxine and pantothenic acid are removed and not replaced. If this white flour (refined carbohydrate) is to be metabolised at all the body must steal these four nutrients from other glands and tissues, thus creating imbalances in the metabolism. It steals phosphorus from bone, thereby impairing its growth and ability to repair and magnesium from heart muscle, predisposing it to spasm and, in time, arrest. Pantothenic acid (B5) is stolen from the nerves and brain, rendering us liable to lowered energy levels and increased irritability, and pyridoxine (B6) is stolen from the white blood cells, particularly the T-lymphocytes (which attack viruses, yeasts, bacteria and cancer cells) causing them to become very weak and lethargic.

Sugar, be it white, brown or raw, requires the same vitamins and minerals to be metabolised and is thus responsible for creating the same metabolic havoc. How much of our processed foods contain white flour and white sugar? Most of it. Even frozen turkeys contain added sugar! Any manufactured food with a word in the list of ingredients on the label ending in -ol, -ole, -one, -os or -ose has sugar in it. You'll be amazed how many do.

It is the complex interaction between all the vitamins and minerals which maintains a balanced metabolism and a healthy body. Foods picked fresh from the garden have a far greater chance of containing all the necessary nutrients. The foods on the Metabolism-Balancing Program, especially when supplemented by a complete vitamin and mineral formula, ensure that our bodies receive the required nutrients. No vitamin or mineral can work on its own and must be aided and complimented by all the others. For a single vitamin or mineral to be effective it must arrive in the system with all the other vitamins and minerals and at the same time. That's why you take your vitamin and mineral formula just before the main meal of the day. Unrefined foods ensure a balanced metabolism and are also the foods which are least (if at all) fattening.

THE WHITE BLOOD CELLS

By robbing our T-lymphocytes of vitamin B6 (pyridoxine) white flour and sugar predispose us to cancer, colds, 'flu, candida yeast infections and allergies, while at the same time causing us to pile on the weight. For the T-lymphocytes to have the vitality to fight viruses, cancer, candida yeast and prevent allergies they need a daily supply of vitamins C, B12 and B6, folic acid, choline and zinc as all of these vitamins and minerals interact chemically to help produce the energy supply for the cells. If just one of these nutrients is missing the necessary chemical reaction will not take place and the cells become fatigued, less numerous and have a shorter life span. These six nutrients are the principals of T-lymphocyte metabolism. However, they still need the support of the full spectrum of vitamins and minerals for optimum T-lymphocyte function.

THE THYROID GLAND

While white flour and sugar are responsible for the theft of vitamin B6 from the T-lymphocytes they also cause a deficiency in the thyroid hormone. Thyroxine, the hormone produced by the thyroid gland, regulates the speed at which the cells burn glucose for energy. A thyroxine deficiency means that the cells burn glucose less efficiently and therefore lack energy. Because most of the body cells rely on thyroxine, a lack of thyroxine causes a slowing of the metabolic rate and a slow metabolic rate means that less of the food we eat is burned for energy and more of it is stored as fat.

The T-lymphocytes also rely on thyroxine to burn glucose for energy, therefore a thyroxine deficiency causes the T-lymphocytes to lack vitality and diminishes their capacity to kill cancer cells and resist allergies. To produce thyroxine the thyroid gland needs adequate supplies of vitamin A, B6, C, B12 and E as well as the minerals iodine, zinc, manganese and copper. The complex inter-action between all of these nutrients enables the thyroid gland to manufacture thyroxine and if one of these nutrients is absent no thyroxine is produced. A vitamin B6 deficiency, caused by eating too much white bread and products containing white sugar, can in time, single-handedly cause an under-active thyroid gland.

DIETING INDUCES METABOLIC IMBALANCES

White flour and sugar are the most fattening foods and it is a sad fact that most people who are over-weight eat far too much of these foods. If they are not taking vitamin and mineral supplements they will incur severe nutrient deficiencies as well.

Most weight-reducing diets are vitamin and mineral deficient which further aggravates the metabolic imbalance created by these deficiencies. High protein diets lead to deficiencies in vita-mins B6 and B3 as large quantities of these vitamins are needed to metabolise protein. As we have already seen, a vitamin B6 deficiency interferes with thyroid gland and T-lymphocyte metabo-lism. A vitamin B3 and B6 deficiency aggravates carbohydrate metabolism.

Some of the high fibre diets advertised are high in tinned peas, beans and corn. The chemical preservatives used in the prepara-tion of these foods can build up in the liver over time and disrupt its function. As the liver is the great metabolic factory of the body, any disruption in its function can lead to disruption in the metabolism of the body as a whole.

ALLERGIES

Allergies can severely disrupt the metabolism by causing a daily loss of the mineral zinc and vitamin B6 through the urine and thus deficiencies of both of these are created. Zinc is necessary to the pancreas for the manufacture of the hormone insulin and an insulin deficiency means that not enough glucose reaches the cells (including the thyroid gland and T-lymphocyte cells) to provide necessary energy and vitality. A severe insulin deficiency leads to diabetes at which point resistance to cancer and infection is extremely low and cholesterol levels rise. The foods that contain zinc also contain chromium. Chromium is needed for insulin to work. A deficiency in insulin and chromium means diabetes. Diabetes is one of the serious metabolic diseases.

THE PEAR-SHAPED FIGURE

Histamine is a chemical needed to transmit nerve impulses from one nerve to another. A deficiency means that the metabolism slows and fat accumulates around the hips and thighs. Most cells manufacture histamine by way of a complex interaction between vitamins B12, B3, P (rutin) and folic acid and if there is a deficiency in any of these, histamine cannot be produced. If there is a deficiency in B12 and folic acid the T-lymphocytes function below par—yet another example of the way metabolic imbalance can be responsible for a weight problem, a predisposition to cancer, colds, 'flu and allergies.

CRASH DIETS

Crash diets, fasts and mono fad diets are so dangerous they deserve special attention. Many cases of arthritis, diabetes, allergies and cancer I have treated include a history of crash dieting. As well as creating severe vitamin and mineral deficiencies and the attendant metabolic imbalances which follow, these diets release large quantities of toxic chemicals, particularly DDT, into the bloodstream. Nature in her wisdom stores the DDT we ingest from fruits and vegetables and the chemicals from refined, processed foods in the fat of our bodies where they can do the least harm to our bodies.

Fasts and crash diets cause sudden fat and lean tissue loss which, in turn, suddenly liberates DDT and the other chemicals into the blood in large quantities. Because there is a dearth of vitamins and minerals in the blood of the crash dieter the toxic chemicals are not neutralised and can therefore irritate the delicate tissues of the kidneys, urinary tract, brain, liver and, of course, the white blood cells. The latter giving rise to allergies in those genetically predisposed.

DRUG MEDICATION

Drugs can also be responsible for metabolic imbalances by creating vitamin and mineral deficiencies. Fluid tablets cause potassium to be lost from the body in urine. Antacids prevent the absorption of vitamins A and B complex. Antibiotics cause vitamin K, iron, calcium and magnesium deficiencies. The contraceptive pill gobbles up vitamins B12, B6, C, folic acid and the mineral zinc. As we already know the effects of deficiencies in these nutrients are detrimental to our bodies. Without adequate vitamin and mineral supplementation the pill can contribute significantly to metabolic weight gain, via fluid retention.

The bad news is that white bread, white flour, sugar, or any foods which contain these items, create metabolic imbalances and weight gain. The good news is that they need not do so. If you select 95 per cent of your foods from the Metabolism-Balancing Program and only 5 per cent from refined forms, while remaining on a complete vitamin and mineral formula, the effects of the junk food will be negligible. All foreign chemicals, be they drugs or food flavourings, preservatives, colourings or chemical pollutants of air and water, will try to interfere with the normally occurring chemical reactions in cells. Whenever they succeed in getting involved in these chemical reactions they alter their outcome and so disrupt the metabolism.

The Metabolism-Balancing Program has a minimum of foreign chemicals in it. The supplementary vitamins and minerals that form an integral part of the program help prevent foreign chemical intervention by latching onto (chelating) and neutralising these chemicals before they get involved.

These days we need enough vitamins and minerals left after the cells, needs have been fulfilled to protect us against foreign chemical invasion. For example, extra zinc neutralises the cadmium released from motor vehicle tyres driven along the road; vitamin C neutralises the pesticide DDT and calcium neutralises the lead from car exhaust fumes.

MIND AND THE METABOLISM

The thoughts we choose to think give rise to the feelings we experience both emotionally and physically. For example, the feeling of butterflies in the stomach experienced before delivering a speech is the result of extra adrenalin triggered by anxious thoughts. Extra adrenalin changes the chemistry of the blood by causing the levels of glucose and free fatty acids to rise.

Prolonged stress also causes cortisone and testosterone to be released by the adrenal glands. Cortisone breaks down muscle cells into amino acids releasing cholesterol into the blood. Testosterone affects the metabolism by negating the effect of oestrogen. This can give rise to the growth of body and facial hair in women. Many women experience a thickening of their body hair or growth of a light moustache when under prolonged stress.

It has been demonstrated that tears of happiness are chemically different to tears of sadness. The bile secreted by the liver to help digest fats is normally green in colour yet when we're depressed it turns black. The word *melancholy* means literally 'black bile'.

Feelings of anger, rage and hostility can cause the release of the chemical neurokinin from the end of the sensory nerves into the skin, blood vessels and sub-skin tissues, so disrupting the metabolism in the area of release as to cause significant inflammation. (See the section on skin complaints in Chapter 6.) The ruddiness of face seen in those who're angry and the blush of those who are embarrassed are examples of neurokinin's ability to change the metabolism of the skin.

The deep breathing and mental relaxation exercises included in the chapter on stress help the programs to balance the body's metabolism.

DEEP BREATHING AND THE METABOLISM

The deep breathing exercises described in the chapter on stress are particularly important for maintaining a balanced metabolism.

Prolonged or excessively shallow breathing causes a build-up of carbon dioxide in the blood. Too much carbon dioxide causes the significant chemical imbalance of the blood called acidosis. Acidosis has far-reaching effects on the metabolism of the body.

As carbon dioxide retention in the blood progresses the degree of metabolic imbalance increases and the symptoms of acidosis become more numerous. The early symptoms are a quickening of the pulse, stomach upsets, heart burn, gas, panic and anxiety attacks, moist warm hands, muscle cramps in neck, shoulder and back, constricted pupils and elevated blood pressure. Severe carbon dioxide retention leads to drowsiness, dizziness, fatigue, confusion, tingling and numbness in arms, legs and hands, and tremors. Hallucination, fainting and coma are the severest symptoms of all. Some people experience sleep disturbances.

Although the blood has special buffer substances to neutralise the carbonic acid (retained carbon dioxide in the blood) and the kidneys are also able to neutralise it, the body still relies heavily on the lungs to blow most of it off. This can only be done if we breathe deeply as most of the carbon dioxide sits in the lower lobes of the lungs.

Drugs, especially morphine, Valium and the barbiturates, will also cause carbon dioxide retention. Deep breathing is imperative for those who are being treated with these drugs.

Those whose shallow breathing is the result of stress also have a build-up of lactic acid in the blood. An excess of lactic acid robs the body of its calcium reserves as calcium is needed to neutralise lactic acid. A deficiency in calcium contributes to anxiety. The deep breathing exercises help to reduce the levels of lactic acid as well and are even more successful at this if the mental relaxation exercises are also practised.

Deep breathing helps to maintain a steady, elevated, metabolic rate which helps keep the body weight normal. (See Chapter 16, 'Scientific explanations—Oxygen and carbon dioxide', for a full description of how and why this happens. See also Chapter 10, 'The importance of water and oxygen'. Chapter 11, 'Stress', contains a full description of the deep breathing exercises.)

GLUCOSE METABOLISM AND HYPOGLYCAEMIA

Hypoglycaemia means that the levels of glucose in the blood have dropped so low that cells of the body and brain are being starved of this vital energy-producing food. Tiredness, depression, mood swings, confusion, poor concentration, low frustration tolerance, temper tantrums, the shakes, poor memory, disorganisation and all of the other symptoms of allergy listed under 'Mental and behavioural' in Chapter 2, 'Allergies', are also caused by hypoglycaemia.

Hypoglycaemia is not, as many think, a disease in itself. It is a 'symptom' of many different disease conditions. For instance, hypoglycaemia can be caused by:

- stress;
- too much white flour and sugar in the diet;
- skipping meals;
- allergies;
- a malfunctioning liver;
- vitamin and mineral deficiency;
- an under-active thyroid.

Just as allergies can cause the blood glucose levels to drop, a drop in blood glucose levels caused by other factors can trigger allergies. Low-grade, non-symptom-producing allergies can be exacerbated into full-blown, symptom-producing allergies when hypoglycaemia is caused by any of the above factors.

By providing three balanced meals a day and supplementary vitamins and minerals, the Metabolism-Balancing Program removes all the other causes of hypoglycaemia. Chromium helps insulin to get the glucose into the cells. Vitamins B3, B1, B6, B12 and C help the thyroid hormone speed up its conversion to energy. Mineral iodine, vitamins B12, folic acid, B6, B5, E, A and B1 help the thyroid gland to make thyroid hormone and iron facilitates the carriage of oxygen that makes all the other processes possible. This balanced inflow of glucose into the cells, and its subsequent conversion to energy keeps all the cells (especially the white blood cells), tissues and organs of the body functioning in a balanced way.

The brain manifests this state of balance by remaining calm, yet mentally alive and on the ball. The white blood cells manifest it by not over-reacting and causing allergic reactions when non-life-threatening substances, such as dust, pollen, grasses, moulds or foods enter the body. The liver manifests it by not allowing too much glucose to be released into the blood during times of stress and the pancreas manifests it by not over-reacting to glucose's presence in the blood. (It's the secretion of insulin by the pancreas that causes the blood glucose levels to drop precipitously.)

In this way the Metabolism-Balancing Program removes the causes of functional hypoglycaemia and in so doing removes one of the major triggers of allergic reactions.

This leaves allergy as the only other cause of hypoglycaemia and glucose imbalance. As explained in Chapter 2, 'Allergies', an allergic reaction can take place in any tissue or organ of the body. If allergies inflame the thyroid gland they can disrupt glucose metabolism by making the gland over- or under-function—the latter causing hypoglycaemia and over-weight. If allergies attack the liver, pancreas or adrenal glands their metabolisms can become so distorted that hypoglycaemia develops immediately. Allergic hypoglycaemia is a whacky, unpredictable thing that can be here today and gone tomorrow, whether treated by drug medication or not. This is because allergies are migratory by nature and can move randomly from one tissue to another.

For this reason many people erroneously believe that they've 'outgrown' their allergies, not realising that the new set of seemingly unrelated symptoms that have sprung up elsewhere in their body is caused by the same allergy.

The random, unpredictable nature of allergies means that 'allergic hypoglycaemia' can be turned on and off to no set pattern, leaving the sufferer as confused as the physician. This is particularly so if the thyroid gland is the target organ, as the drugs taken for the affected thyroid can cause adverse reactions when the gland suddenly rights itself.

It is only with sound nutrition, sensible eating habits, appropriate exercise, adequate oxygen, water and rest, and by containing allergies, yeast, bacterial and viral infections, that the metabolism can ever be fully balanced.

OXYGEN AND CARBON DIOXIDE

Oxygen (O_2) is the most important nutrient of all and must be constantly supplied to the cells. A few minutes of oxygen deprivation causes death. Oxygen makes up 20 per cent of the air we breathe, the rest being made up of an inert gas called nitrogen. Oxygen is inhaled into our lungs with each 'in' breath and diffuses across the thin wall (alveoli) of the lungs to be picked up by the blood passing through the blood vessels (capillaries) that surround the lungs. It is then transported to every cell in the body where it helps to ignite the flame of life. Cellular respiration (combustion) can only take place in the presence of oxygen. Cells cannot produce heat and energy in a vacuum, just as a motor car engine cannot ignite petrol to produce the energy to drive its wheels without oxygen. Similarly, fires won't burn in a vacuum. (Humans are slow burning fires!)

Oxygen is a gas and like all gases it diffuses down a pressure gradient from levels of high concentration (high pressure) to levels of low concentration (low pressure). To optimally oxygenate our blood we must create high concentrations of oxygen in our lungs. By breathing in deeply and filling our lungs to full capacity, we create significant air pressure in them. A significant quantity of oxygen is then forced under pressure into the blood and rapidly transported to all the cells of the body. Shallow breathing only partially fills the lungs creating a weaker air pressure in them. Not only is less oxygen taken in but less of it is forced into the blood. The deep breathing exercises described in the chapter on stress require the holding of the breath for three seconds. This gives extra time for oxygen to diffuse under pressure from the lungs to the blood.

Most of the oxygen is carried by the red blood cells though some is absorbed and carried by the water content of the blood. To get full benefit from deep breathing, red blood cell and water content of the blood must be at maximum levels. A diet rich in iron and all the other vitamins and minerals must be adhered to and adequate fluid consumed.

Shallow breathing is epidemic in modern affluent societies. Lethargy, low resistance, low frustration tolerance, mental confusion, allergies and infections are just some of the spin-off effects of widespread oxygen deficiency. Not surprisingly a number of 'blood oxygenation' treatment programs have evolved and have become very popular.

Some doctors are administering the ozone treatment, whereby the blood is drawn out of the veins, 0.5 L at a time, treated with ozone and replaced.[1] The patient invariably feels on top of the world after this oxygen saturation treatment. Some people get a similar deep oxygenation of the blood by putting a few drops of hydrogen peroxide in water before drinking it.[2] (I strongly advise against this as hydrogen peroxide is a poison.) Neither of these deep oxygenation treatments are necessary if regular deep breathing is practised. Deep breathing is the safest and cheapest form of deep tissue oxygenation.

Scientists, using the Kirlian technique for photographing the body's electromagnetic field ('aura' to the aesthetics) have noticed that it glows brighter and extends further from the body when the lungs are full of oxygen.[3] This brightening and extending of the life field was even greater when negatively ionised air was inhaled. Negatively ionised air is found wherever water is breaking on a hard surface. Waves pounding on the beach and waterfalls cause the water molecules to split into oxygen and free hydrogen. Hydrogen with its free/surplus electron readily contributes extra energy to cellular respiration, increasing our vitality and glow of health.

CARBON DIOXIDE

This gas is one of the major waste products of cellular respiration. The burning of carbohydrate foods (bread, potato, pasta, rice, muesli, porridge, breakfast cereal, beer, Scotch) for energy, produces carbon dioxide (CO_2). Because cellular respiration never stops, carbon dioxide is continually building up and can make blood dangerously acid if not removed.

Breathing out is the major vehicle for carbon dioxide removal. Like oxygen, this gas also diffuses down a pressure gradient. The same blood that picks up oxygen from the lungs brings carbon dioxide back to the lungs. Because the concentration (pressure) of carbon dioxide in the blood is so high it readily diffuses into the lung to be blown off in the next 'out' breath. Because most of the blood vessels that serve the lung are found around its lower lobes, carbon dioxide tends to build up and sit there for extended periods when shallow (upper lobe) breathing is habitual.

Deep breathing reaches down to the lower lobes and draws the stale carbon dioxide out, leaving us feeling fresh and bright. At the end of each exhalation a holding period of three seconds is observed before inhaling again. The three second negative pressure of the empty lungs allows for maximum diffusion, or drawing off, of carbon dioxide from the blood. The lower lobes begin to fill once more. The positive pressure created by the next deep inhalation of air does not force the carbon dioxide back into the blood as so much of it is produced by cellular respiration that the blood concentrations of it are always higher than the lung concentrations.

The full effects of excessive carbon dioxide build-up in the body are described in 'The metabolism' section of this chapter. (See also Chapter 10, 'The importance of water and oxygen' and the deep breathing exercises in Chapter 11, 'Stress'.)

One interesting side effect of excessive carbon dioxide build-up in the blood is its effect on thyroid gland function. The thyroid hormone, thyroxine, is responsible for the rate at which the cells burn carbohydrate food (which has now been digested down to glucose) for energy. The more thyroxine, the faster they burn carbohydrate and the more heat and energy they produce.

One of the body's compensatory mechanisms for normalising carbon dioxide levels in the presence of shallow breathing is to slow down its production. By reducing the production of thyroxine it slows the rate at which carbohydrate is burned to produce energy and although less carbon dioxide is produced, body weight tends to increase if food intake (particularly carbohydrate) is not decreased. Food that is not burned for energy is stored as energy reserve in the form of fat.

Just as carbon dioxide slows the metabolic rate, oxygen increases it and it's not uncommon to raise a sweat while doing the deep breathing exercises described in the chapter on stress.

The advantage of the deep breathing exercises over vigorous physical exercise is that vigorous exercise stimulates the burning of carbohydrate for energy with the attendant build-up of carbon dioxide in the tissues. The deep breathing associated with vigorous exercises manages only to contain carbon dioxide build-up.

Carbohydrate metabolism is not as vigorously stimulated by deep breathing. This enables these exercises to draw out excess carbon dioxide from the blood. The slow rythmic movements of yoga and Tai Chi don't stimulate carbohydrate metabolism to the degree that football, tennis, jogging, aerobics, weight training and swimming do. As a result, they too have the net effect of normalising blood carbon dioxide levels when combined with their appropriate deep breathing exercises.

REST

An understanding of the 'brick effect' is central to an understanding of how and why our health breaks down. The brick effect holds that a given disease syndrome results from the cumulative effects of a number of less potent factors rather than one principal factor and that where a principal factor does exist it lacks potency when not augmented by the sum total of the lesser factors.

To explain: If you were to place a brick on someone's head it would more than likely cause little discomfort. A second brick would probably give a sensation of significant weight and a third would cause some pressure and discomfort. A fourth brick may well cause a headache and the removal of the fourth brick may be all that's needed to reduce it completely. To blame the fourth brick only for causing the headache is to deny the role played by the other bricks in contributing to the overall weight and pressure needed to produce a headache.

So it is with all other disease processes in the body. Seldom, if ever, is there one cause for one disease. If there was everyone would catch the 'flu during a 'flu epidemic. Even injury from motor car accidents which are clearly the result of physical impact—principal cause—can have many lesser contributing factors. A driver may lose concentration behind the wheel and hit another car because he has: (1) been working long hours lately; (2) been skipping meals; (3) not been taking vitamin supplements; (4) been suffering from the 'flu and is still working; (5) had one or two drinks after work to relax; and (6) missed lunch that day. Any one of these factors alone would not be enough to induce significant lapses in concentration. Added together they can.

Most allergies have their genesis in a genetic predisposition to allergy combined with lowered immune vitality. Lowered immune vitality can result from any of a number of factors—malnutrition being a significant one. Malnutrition itself can result from a number of things—poor diet, skipping meals, crash diets, poor digestion and absorption, to name a few. Poor digestion and absorption can result from a lack of hydrochloric acid in the stomach. Hydrochloric acid deficiency can result from vitamin and mineral deficiency; eating on the go (adrenalin); being tired due to over-work and/or over-exercising; over-eating and eating too quickly. Over-eating can be a result of malabsorption-induced hunger. Eating too quickly can result from over-commitment, which can result from dire approval seeking (inappropriate attitude). And so it goes down the line, each contributing factor being a brick which is singularly not enough to reduce immune vitality.

Because so many component factors make up a disease syndrome, the afflicted person must be viewed as a whole and treated as a whole if a cure is to be achieved. Just as any disease condition has a multiplicity of causes its treatment requires a multiplicity of therapeutic modalities. Giving a drug to suppress the symptoms of a given disease is not the answer. Diet and the drinking, breathing, working, exercising, socialising and resting habits must all be taken into account and modified where necessary.

THE THERAPY OF REST

Rest (in particular sleep) is the most potent medicine of all. No matter what the disease, be it 'flu, headache, arthritis or acne, rest and sleep are priority one if a cure is to be achieved. It is only during periods of rest, sleep and recreation that the body is able to use its energy for repair and healing. Diet, attitudes and lifestyle must also be modified if a cure of the condition is to be achieved.

Although this book holds that allergy can be, and is often, the main cause of many disease syndromes, without the contributions of malnutrition, overdoing it, and lack of rest and sleep, allergies lack the potency to do significant damage to our health. Similarly, without rest and sleep, any therapeutic modality lacks the potency needed to cure allergies. In fact any treatment modality, be it antibiotics for pneumonia, acupuncture for migraines, osteopathic/chiropractic manipulation for backache, vitamin C for a head cold, a diet for lowering cholesterol or chemo/radiotherapy for cancer, has limited effect if not accompanied by adequate rest and sleep. Rest and sleep are the imperative prerequisites of all healing modalities, at all times.

The treatment modalities used by physicians are only adjuncts to healing. They are given to aid the body's innate healing power. The body does most of the healing and to achieve this it needs energy. If its vital energies are being consumed by too much working, exercising and socialising, it cannot do the job properly. The metabolism continues to remain out of balance and the metabolic rate continues to remain low.

Twenty-two years of taking care of sick people has taught me that those who take rest seriously and get plenty of sleep get good results from treatment. Those who don't take rest seriously get mediocre results at best and often no results at all.

Detractors of the rest and sleep principle argue that because they have been able to push themselves to work and/or play at a frenetic pace all their lives, they should be able to continue doing so. Athletes and sports-oriented health buffs are the worst offenders. They seem to think that pushing the body somehow toughens it—makes it stronger. They don't recognise that the cumulative effects of a frenetic pace catches up with the body in time.

The body is not unlike a car. A new car can probably cope with a year's hard driving but two to three years could well see regular breakdowns and other signs of wear and tear. Even athletes seem to realise that pushing their car hard will cause it to wear out and depreciate its value sooner. For some reason they can't apply that same logic to their bodies. These people seldom get well.

It must be remembered that the body is capable of exhibiting only a limited number of signs and symptoms of disease. For this reason a given set of symptoms can result from a number of different causes.

For example, most of the symptoms of allergy listed in Chapter 2, 'Allergies', can also be caused by:

- stress (over-work, under-rest, over-exercise, under-sleep);
- vitamin and mineral deficiency;
- lack of oxygen (hypoxia);
- lack of fluid (dehydration); or
- negative attitudes (often caused by the above).

For this reason the above-mentioned factors must be addressed and dealt with before specific anti-candida/anti-allergy treatment is commenced.

Be patient with yourself and your physician if you're having trouble pinning down the exact cause of your particular disease. Diagnosis is not easy—so many different things can cause the same symptoms (a headache, say, can result from many different causes). By a process of elimination you will, in time, arrive at the correct answer. All it takes is patience and persistence. In my experience, those who don't give up always get well in the end.

STRESS

On top of each kidney is a gland called the adrenal. The adrenal glands have a number of roles to play in the body, one of them is to enable us to cope with the many different stresses we encounter in life. When we are under stress the adrenal glands release the stress hormones adrenalin, cortisone and testosterone.

Adrenalin is released to speed up the metabolism of all cells of the brain and body giving us the energy we need to meet the stress. It achieves this by stimulating the liver to release all its stores of glucose. It also shuts down the digestive processes by sending the blood from the digestive tract to the brain, eyes and muscles. Because of this we don't digest and absorb our food properly when we're under stress and run the risk of malnutrition if the stress is prolonged. Unfortunately, we need extra nutrients during times of stress to sustain the high revving metabolism. Imbalances in the metabolism develop when these nutrients are not forthcoming. Putting food in the stomach at this time causes the abdomen to distend giving us that same uncomfortable, bloated feeling we get from eating a food we're allergic to or feeding a gut-borne candida infection with sugar- and white-flour-containing foods.

Cortisone is released to dissolve the proteins collagen and elastin into amino acids. These amino acids are converted to glucose by the liver in an effort to prevent a glucose shortage. (More glucose is needed when we are under stress.) A glucose shortage would produce such severe metabolic imbalances as to cause serious shock, fainting and even coma. Sluggish, unhealthy livers have trouble converting amino acids quickly enough and shock and fainting spells are common in highly stressed people with unhealthy livers. (Lack of oxygen and vitamins and minerals as well as excess of alcohol, drugs and nicotine are the major cause of an unhealthy liver.)

Unfortunately for us, collagen and elastin are the major structural proteins of the skin, muscle and blood vessels. If they are dissolved faster than we can replace them the skin, muscles and blood vessels lose their tone and elasticity. In this way stress ages us prematurely (wrinkles, stretch marks, blue spider veins and purple patches in the skin). Weakened blood vessel walls are prone to leaking water and plasma proteins into the tissues, causing fluid retention. Vitamins C, A and B6 and minerals zinc, manganese and silica are the principal nutrients needed for collagen and elastin manufacture and should always be taken in supplementary form during times of stress. To be fully effective they must be taken with all the other vitamins and minerals, that is, in a complete multi-vitamin tablet.

As well as dissolving proteins to provide glucose, cortisone acts as nature's own built-in anti-inflammatory. Adrenally produced cortisone has served man well since the dawn of time, reducing the inflammations encountered from the stresses of hunting wild animals and fighting invaders. These stresses for the main part were significant but short lived. When the danger was over the adrenal glands would relax and the levels of stress hormones would return to normal. The more subtle but prolonged stresses modern man is subjected to (see Chapter 11, 'Stress') keeps high levels of cortisone in the white blood cells. This suppresses their normal function and predisposes the body to allergies and infections. Resting levels of cortisone do not have this effect.

Testosterone accelerates the processes of growth and repair of damaged tissue that results from stress. Broken bones, hair line fractures, bruises and sprains encountered as a result of over-exercise (running marathons) and heavy contact sports are examples of this. It also stimulates the sebaceous glands to produce extra sebum which pours out into the skin giving it an oily appearance. This oil acts as an insulator which retains body heat.

Increased body temperature speeds up tissue repair and protects us from the cold which, in itself, is a major stress. Unfortunately, the sebaceous glands often become so stimulated during times of stress they produce sebum faster than they can release it onto the skin. The glands swell and burst, releasing the sebum into the dermis of the skin where, being a foreign body, it causes allergic reactions that give rise to acne. (See Chapter 6, 'Asthma, skin problems, arthritis'.)

The adrenal stress hormones served ancient humans well. Adrenalin to give them the energy to cope, cortisone to reduce inflammation and provide the glucose (sugar) energy, testosterone to speed the repair of damaged tissues and beta endorphins (see Chapter 11, 'Stress') to kill the pain encountered during fighting or running barefoot over rough terrain.

So often do modern humans misuse their adrenal glands that this misuse becomes part of everyday life and hard to recognise. Hard-chargers (see Chapter 11, 'Stress') are the main culprits here. Being highly motivated people they force themselves on, even when the body has had enough and wants a rest. This pushing of themselves whips the adrenal glands, forcing them to produce more and more of the stress hormones.

Tired bodies come to rely on adrenalin for energy instead of normal cellular respiration. They rely on cortisone to suppress the inflammation of allergies that can develop in tired bodies, instead of letting normal body resistance prevent sub-clinical allergies from flaring up. They rely on beta endorphins to kill the pain that wouldn't exist if allergies hadn't flared up and to buoy the spirits that would be naturally high in a body that isn't stressed. Hard-chargers become more and more reliant on bodily produced chemical highs to maintain feelings of well-being. In time the adrenal glands become so tired they are unable to produce enough stress hormones to satisfy demand and the symptoms of stress, particularly chronic fatigue, set in. By this time beta endorphin production has also dropped significantly.

The adrenal glands are tough and can take a lot of stress before they become seriously fatigued. It takes time to wear them down. During this period of wearing down, the major symptom that the glands are tiring is tiredness on the cessation of activity. In those who have allergies, a worsening of allergy symptoms usually accompanies the onset of tiredness after activity.

Because it can take years to completely wear the glands down hard-chargers get into the habit of whipping their adrenals every time they want energy. So responsive are the tired glands that hard-chargers become lulled into a false sense of security, believing energy will always be there if they just use their willpower to push on. (See Chapter 11, 'Stress—Stress and the hard-charger'.)

Some people get so into the habit of this practice over the years they believe it's natural and can't understand it when chronic fatigue sets in and significant allergies develop. However, not all people experience the onset of their allergies at the point of adrenal exhaustion.

Some experience their onset during the wearing down period and get locked into the vicious cycle of pushing themselves to produce more cortisone to reduce the inflammatory symptoms of their allergy, not realising that the same cortisone is lowering their resistance and thus aggravating the allergy in the classic Catch 22 manner.

EXPERIMENTAL EVIDENCE

Dr Hans Selye of McGill University, Montreal, noted in his experiments with rats that removal of their adrenal glands gave rise to severe allergic reactions (anaphylaxis) when foreign substances were injected into them. Family member rats from the same cage, who had their adrenal glands intact, exhibited only minor allergic reactions when injected with the same foreign substances.

From these results Selye extrapolated that strong, healthy adrenal glands in humans were needed if humans were to cope with the stress of allergies and he was right. When the adrenal glands are tired they produce less adrenal hormones and our resistance to allergies goes down. Significant or prolonged stress tires the adrenal glands.

Doctor Herbert De Vries of UCLA in his book, *Physiology of Exercise for Physical Education and Athletics,* noted in his experiments with athletes that the human adrenal glands begin to wane after sixteen weeks of stress. He noted that in the short term the adrenal glands respond to stress by increasing in size and producing extra adrenal hormones.

This increase in size and production progressed for eight weeks levelling out at a maximum size and production for a maximum of a further eight weeks. After that adrenal gland size and hormone production fell inexorably and would not increase again unless sufficient rest was taken. Four to five weeks was needed for the adrenal glands to build themselves up to a point where they could respond positively to stress again.

Based on this adrenal rhythm Dr De Vries advised his athletes to rest for four to five weeks after every twelve to fourteen weeks of training. The stressful exercise load of Dr De Vries' athletes is no different to the stressful work load, socialising load, emotional load and commitment load that many stressed non-athletes subject themselves to. After ten to twelve weeks of stress the beta endorphins are flowing and, along with what adrenalin there is in the system, are masking the symptoms of adrenal fatigue of which physical fatigue is a significant one.

Despite the contrived feelings of well-being promoted by the beta endorphins adrenal hormone production and resistance to allergies is down. Because many people have minor allergies that under rested conditions don't manifest, they experience their allergies for the first time when under stress.

STRESS ADDICTION?

It's interesting to note the similarities that exist between the allergy addiction state and being hooked on a stressful lifestyle.

Phase 2 (adaptation phase) of the allergy addiction state is similar to the stressed state of the adrenally competent person. The allergy-addicted person feels fine so long as she/he makes regular contact with the substance she/he is allergic to. The adrenally competent, stressed person feels OK so long as she/he continues to push her/himself. Avoidance of the allergic substance and slowing down brings on the symptoms.

Phase 3 (exhaustion phase) of the allergy addiction state sees the symptoms returning so frequently and lasting so long they eventually remain permanently. No amount of contact with the allergens responsible can now alleviate the symptoms.

The adrenally incompetent, stressed person is now permanently fatigued and no amount of willpower can spur him or her on. The symptoms that used to afflict them only during periods of inactivity are now there permanently. These symptoms can be any of those listed in Chapter 2, 'Allergies'. Like the allergy-addicted person the chronically stressed person takes the view that these symptoms have appeared out of the blue for no apparent reason. Just as allergy-addicted people can't believe the habitual eating of their favourite foods is the cause of their symptoms, the adrenally exhausted people can't believe their lifestyle is the cause of their symptoms.

Those hard-chargers that see the light and slow down, frequently admit they were hooked on work, exercise, sport or socialising, or two or more of them. Being able to compare their present state of well-being with their previous chemical (beta endorphin) and hormonal (adrenalin) highs, they can see this clearly. Not that giving up hard-charging is easy; they go through much the same withdrawals that heroin addicts, smokers and the allergy-addicted (see Chapter 3, 'Allergy addiction') go through.

For some, the irritability, restlessness, depression and aggression they experience is sheer hell. They pace the floor like caged lions, curse my existence and snap at anyone who comes near.

For hard-chargers, the real challenge begins when they are well and bursting with natural energy. Hard-chargers have an innate drive to push themselves to their limits of tolerance that must be constantly monitored and vigorously controlled. Those who accept this as their new challenge remain well. Those who don't, push on to their new outer limit of tolerance and eventually experience the return of all their symptoms.

Hard-chargers must realise that the programs in this book are not a licence to push themselves ad infinitum. The programs don't make them invincible, they only extend their outer limits of tolerance, and if anyone can find their outer limits of tolerance, it's a hard-charger. (See Chapter 11, 'Stress—Stress and the hard-charger'.)

THE FLUID RETENTION DILEMMA

'Podgy muscles' is a condition many hard-chargers in time experience. Many of them complain that even despite regular workouts, runs, sport training sessions, their muscle tone is not as good as it used to be. Podgy muscles are the result of stress-based fluid retention.

The muscles become water logged and no amount of exercise will remove this water, in fact, it makes it worse. Why? Because fluid retention in the muscles is caused by calcium deficiency, which is caused by a build-up of lactic acid in the muscles.

Lactic acid builds up in muscles as a waste product of muscle metabolism. The harder a muscle is worked, the more glucose it burns for energy; lactic acid is what is left when glucose is burned for energy. Lactic acid is poisonous and must be neutralised by calcium before it can be removed from the muscles and eliminated through the kidneys.

Precious calcium reserves are soon used up and that lactic acid which is left in the muscle in its free state acts as an irritant. Nature tries to dilute the irritating effect of free lactic acid by sending extra water into the muscle. Any excess of water reduces the tone of the muscle so that its lean, muscular appearance changes to a softer, podgy appearance.

Stressed people have tight muscles. Tight muscles burn more glucose and produce more lactic acid. When heavy physical exercise (aerobics, jogging, weight training, football, swimming) is added to this, more lactic acid is produced.

Rest works wonders. Reduced lactic acid production allows calcium reserves to build up and muscle fluid levels to drop. Hard-charger health buffs are always amazed at how their muscle tone improves with rest. Amazed because their rigidly held belief is that only exercise can give rise to improved muscle tone. While it is true that the use of muscles is imperative for the gaining and maintaining of muscle tone, the 'over-use' of muscles due to over-work, over-exercise, anxiety, worry and stress causes reduced muscle tone.

Some hard-chargers also experience significant weight loss while resting. Highly stressed bodies, especially if dogged by allergies, yeast infections and vitamin and mineral deficiencies, will carry excess fluid around the abdomen, thighs, buttocks, as well as in the muscles. This fluid falls away from a resting body much to the amazement of those who rigidly believe that exercise is the only way to keep body weight down.

It takes longer for 'podgy muscles' to develop in those hard-chargers who don't have allergies, candida infections and vitamin and mineral deficiencies. These three factors are fluid retainers in their own right.

POOR POSTURE

Pain is a significant stress to the body. The adrenal glands are forced to work hard for as long as we are in pain. Back pain, neck pain and headaches are perpetuators of the stressed state. Poor posture places undue strain on the muscles of the back, shoulders and neck making them tight and eventually stiff and sore. The sensory nerves convey this state of agitation from the muscles to the brain creating, or adding to, any agitation that may already exist there. Brain agitation manifests as that stressed-out feeling of being 'uptight'. Being 'uptight' usually means tight neck muscles that are causing the shoulders to hunch up.

The muscles of the neck are attached to the vertebrae of the neck and when they tighten they pull the vertebrae together. In time the vertebrae press tightly enough against each other for the nerves that run between them to become pinched (see Fig. 16.1). Pinched nerves that emanate from the neck can cause a host of symptoms in the tissues they serve as well as pain in the neck muscles. Those that run from the neck to head can give rise to headaches and those that serve the face can give rise to involuntary twitches in the facial muscles and puffy bags under the eyes.

Those nerves that run from the neck to the nose can give rise to sinus pains, stuffy nose, runny nose and post-nasal drip (see Fig. 16.2). Pinched nerves can mimic the symptoms of allergy. Pinched nerves are one of the reasons allergy type symptoms remain in stressed people who are sticking strictly to their Anti-Candida/ Anti-Allergy Program. The other reasons are (1) long-term high levels of stress hormones in the blood which lower the body's resistance, and (2) neurokinin (see section on skin problem in Chapter 6 for an explanation of neurokinin).

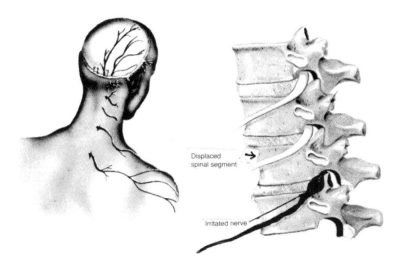

Fig. 16.1: Diagram showing neck, shoulder muscles and nerves affected by the stress of poor posture and the mechanism of the pinched nerve.

Fig. 16.2: Pinched nerves serving lung and bronchi aggravate asthma. Pinched nerves serving liver can cause nausea and headaches. Pinched nerves serving stomach can cause vomiting with headaches.

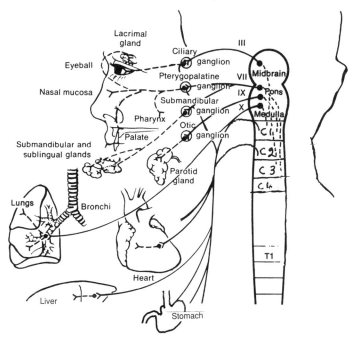

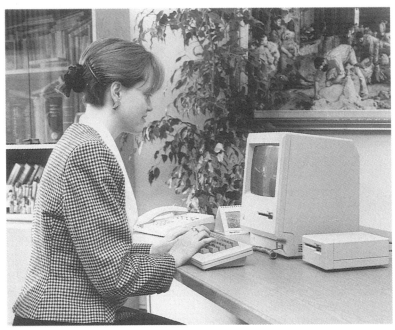

Fig. 16.3 and Fig. 16.4: Sitting up and forward (above) places great demands on neck, shoulder and back muscles, which eventually tire, giving rise to a collapsed posture (below), which further tightens them, giving rise to neck and back pain and headaches.

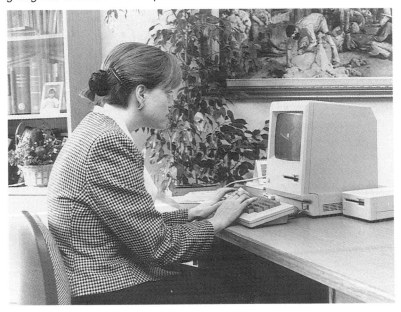

Hard-chargers are prone to bad posture. Being always on the go they tend to sit on the edge of chairs and hunch forward over desks, typewriters and computers (see Fig. 16.3 and Fig. 16.4). This in time strains the neck, shoulder and back muscles. The head weighs 7–9 kg (15–20 lb) and this perpendicular posture with a forward-bending of the head places great strain on the neck muscles, which keep the head from falling forward, back or sideways.

To get some appreciation of what this does to the neck muscles, imagine what expanding a Bullworker to 9 kg (20 lb) of pressure and holding it for eight hours would do to your arm and chest muscles. If the perpendicular, forward-bending, while perched on the end of the chair, posture is combined with a lot of rushing around and speeding in cars the muscles tighten even more. Working under pressure and taking on too much work gives rise to rushing and speeding.

Poor fluid intake and poor oxygen intake also tighten muscles. The muscles are about 70 per cent water and if these levels drop below 70 per cent the muscle tends to shrink. A shrunken muscle is a tight muscle that does not respond well to any method that is used to relax it, whether it be deep breathing exercises, massage, meditation, heat or Valium. Fully hydrated muscles expand to their normal size and are much easier to relax.

Adequate oxygen is needed to facilitate the metabolic processes of muscular expansion and contraction. Oxygen-deficient muscles (hypoxia) are more prone to fatigue, tightening and pain as any out-of-condition person knows when they suddenly take up a vigorous exercise regime. A lack of vitamins and minerals, especially the B vitamins, calcium, iron, zinc and magnesium, interfere with muscle cell metabolism and predispose muscles to spasm (tight, sustained contraction).

In addition to correct diet, deep breathing exercises, adequate fluid intake and the mental relaxation exercises, close attention must be paid to posture if tight muscles, pain and the allergy-mimicking symptoms they produce are to be overcome. Sit back in chairs. By using the support of the chair back you reduce the strain on the back and neck muscles which no longer have to work hard to keep you upright (see Fig. 16.5 and Fig. 16.6).

If having to bend forward to do paperwork take the weight of your head on your hand with the elbow supported by a pile of books (see Fig. 16.7). If your shoulder and neck muscles are already sore sit with a warm hot water bottle on them for ten minutes at night while relaxing in front of the TV (see Fig. 16.8). To thoroughly negate the stresses and strains imposed by the perpendicular forward-bending posture we need to regularly practise the opposite posture, that is, horizontal bending back.

The best way to exercise this posture is by swimming backstroke two to three times per week in warm water. Follow this with a warm shower, never a cold one (heat expands, cold contracts and tight, sore muscles are contracted muscles), with the jets of warm water being trained directly on the tightest, most painful spots. Make sure while swimming that you look at the roof, not the end of the pool. Looking at the end of the pool cranes the neck forward and strains the muscles. Don't rush, this is a time to relax. Do a length and take a rest. Breathe deeply and slowly during this time then do another length. Do not be competitive about this swimming exercise. This is a time for therapy not a time for goal setting. If you're not a swimmer then Tai Chi, yogic walking and yoga are just as effective for releasing tight neck, back and shoulder muscles. No head, neck or shoulder stands though if you do yoga.

In addition to straining neck and back muscles the posture of perpendicular forward-bending tends to round the shoulders forward so that chest expansion is restricted. This same posture forces the lower ribs down into the abdomen restricting the action of the diaphragm. Shallow breathing results, giving rise to oxygen deficiency, which tightens muscles, which in turn reduces chest expansion and perpetuates shallow breathing. A vicious circle is

Fig. 16.5: The chair back is taking the weight of the body, allowing the neck, shoulder and back muscles to relax. The arm rests are supporting the elbows, taking the weight of the arms off the shoulder muscles.

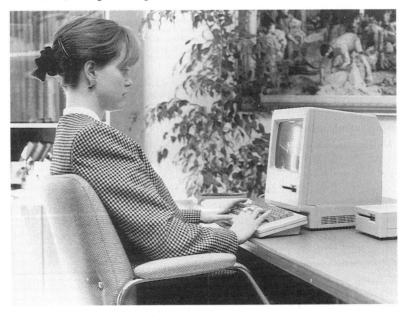

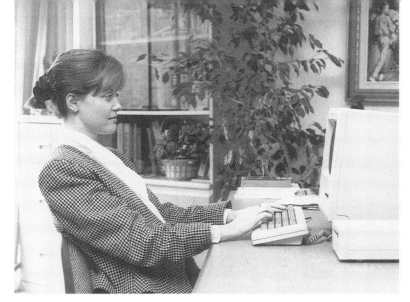

Fig. 16.6: If arm rests are not available, rest the arms on the desk.
Fig. 16.7: Taking the weight of the head on the arms reduces the workload on the back, shoulder and neck muscles by 85 per cent.

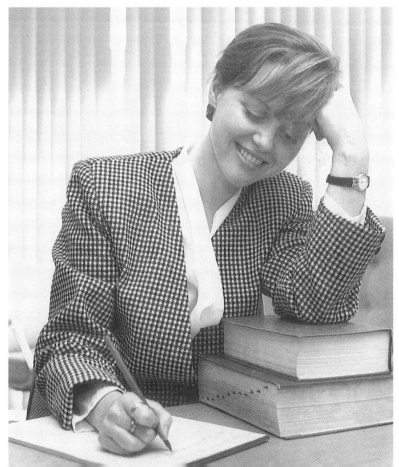

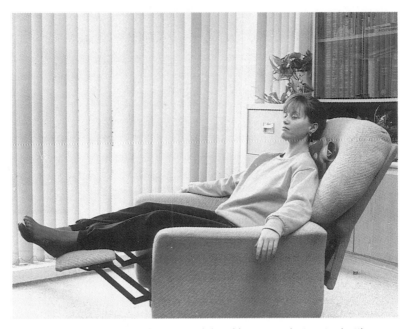

Fig. 16.8: Sitting for ten minutes at night with a warm hot water bottle applied directly to the sore spots does wonders for sore neck and back muscles.
Fig. 16.9: The correct posture for reading in an armchair.

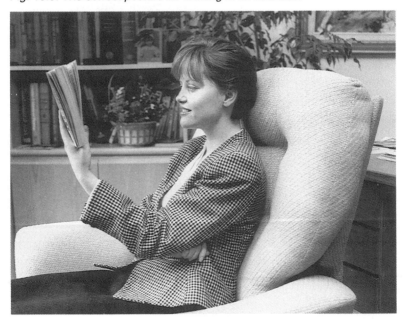

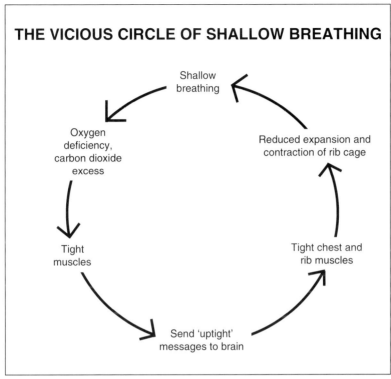

THE VICIOUS CIRCLE OF SHALLOW BREATHING

Shallow breathing

Reduced expansion and contraction of rib cage

Oxygen deficiency, carbon dioxide excess

Tight chest and rib muscles

Tight muscles

Send 'uptight' messages to brain

born which gets the sufferer more uptight and tired, which aggravates the collapsed state of the perpendicular forward-bending posture. Is it any wonder those who rush get less done, make more mistakes and have to repeat more of their work. The distraction of the pain and the lack of oxygen in their brain greatly affect concentration, comprehension and memory. In the initial stages of your muscle relaxation regimen it pays to consult your osteopath or chiropractor for heat, massage and manipulation of the muscles and vertebrae. This will accelerate your recovery.

VIRAL INFECTIONS (COLDS, 'FLU, CFS)

Viruses are tiny agents that cause infectious disease. They are the smallest known living bodies. They comprise a strip of DNA or RNA encased in a protein coat. They cannot reproduce themselves in the free state and so seek out a living cell to provide them with both the energy and the chemical building blocks needed for reproduction. Viruses are parasites whose protein coat makes contact with the cell wall and injects the strip of DNA or RNA into the cell to float through in its free state. The protein coat eventually drops away from the cell wall. Once inside the cell the DNA heads for the nucleus to try and reorganise its DNA to make the cell's metabolism conducive to the virus reproduction. In this way the virus acts as an independently existing gene. The viral RNA latches onto the cell's messenger RNA to try and change the messages it's giving to the cell's organelles and so change the cell's metabolism. Viruses are pirates whose aim is to take over a normal cell, alter its function and take from it what they can.

If the cell is strong and energetic the virus' effect is minimal—the cell is able to resist it. Control of the cell's nucleus and messenger RNA is minimal and although the cell is infected little or no harm is done to it. Healthy, energetic people can have many of these silent, unapparent viral infections and be totally unaware of the fact, as no energy is lost and no tissue damage is done. Once the virus has invaded the cell it is there for good and as long as the cell stays strong the virus will not be able to reproduce itself.

If the cell becomes weak the virus is able to gain the upper hand. It gets into the nucleus and changes the genetic instruction to the cell. The cell then yields up energy, proteins and enzymes for the manufacture of millions of more viruses whose numbers swell to the point where there is not enough room for them all. Many of this new generation of viruses emigrate to new susceptible cells where by sheer weight of numbers they have a good chance of taking it over. As this process continues the definitive symptoms of viral infection begin to manifest in the host. These symptoms differ slightly from virus to virus. The wart virus produces warts which look different to the herpes lesion of the herpes virus. The symptoms of polio are different to the symptoms of colds and 'flu, yet all these are caused by viruses.

Because all viruses rely on the host cell's energy supplies to live and reproduce they all have one thing in common: they are energy suckers and the more of them there are in your body the more energy they suck from it. Fatigue is a symptom of all viral infections.

Because there are no really effective medicines to kill viruses and because close contact between humans makes it so easy to contract them the secret is to keep the body so strong that there's enough energy to allow a few to live in your cells without detracting from the body's overall energy reserve.

The rules that apply to gaining and maintaining high energy levels are the same rules for fighting off viruses. The following should be maintained:

- adequate nutrition, which these days means a diet supplemented with a complete multi-vitamin and mineral formula;
- adequate fluid intake;
- adequate oxygen intake;
- adequate sleep;
- adequate rest and recreation;
- adequate warmth—an even warm body temperature is imperative for keeping viruses at bay (chilling slows the metabolic rate of cells allowing resident viruses to gain the upper hand; colds aren't called colds for nothing);
- containment of all allergies and yeast infections.

HOW MUCH IS ADEQUATE?

You've achieved adequate rest, sleep, oxygen and fluid intake and nutrition when you're feeling energetic. Especially when you're feeling energetic on rising in the morning. You've achieved adequate warmth if you're not catching head colds. You've contained allergy and candida infections when you're devoid of the symptoms listed in Chapter 2, 'Allergies'.

The best treatment for a viral infection is rest and warmth. Rest allows the body to direct all its energies to the task and warmth raises the metabolic rate of the cells, which gives them the heat and energy needed to contain the virus. A balanced diet, comprising three meals a day and supplementary vitamins and minerals, is needed to provide the fuel for the high metabolic rate.

VITAMIN AND MINERAL SUPPLEMENTS

Twenty-two years of taking care of sick people has convinced me of the need to supplement our diet with a complete multi-vitamin and mineral formula. Vitamin and mineral supplements form an integral part of the Metabolism-Balancing Program and the Anti-Candida/Anti-Allergy Program. Without them I find the programs get only mediocre results at best.

WHY IS THIS SO?

Quite simply the food we eat today is not as rich in vitamins and minerals as it used to be. There are a number of reasons for this:

- Vitamin content is lost from our fresh foods during transportation from the grower and during storage at the market. For instance, lettuce stored at room temperature loses 50 per cent of its vitamin C in twenty-four hours after picking and also the same amount over three days if refrigerated. The same goes for asparagus, broccoli and green beans.

- Over-cooking, especially the boiling of, fresh vegetables destroys another 25 per cent of the vitamin C, up to 70 per cent of vitamin B1 and 50 per cent of vitamin B2. And these are what we call 'fresh' vegetables.

- Poor soils. Because fruit and vegetables are usually grown on over-cultivated and exhausted soils that have been fertilised with phosphate and nitrogen fertilisers rather than trace element and mineral fertilisers (which are a lot more expensive) their vitamin and mineral content is low to start with. These days crop rotation is not practised, land is not left fallow to allow it time to regenerate. Plants grow profusely on modern day fertilisers but lack nutrient content and are usually picked before they are ripe. This limits the time they have to draw from the soil what little minerals and trace elements are in it.

  Chemical fertilisers actually create deficiencies in the plants they are supposed to be sustaining. Plants absorb nitrates from nitrogen fertilisers and the nitrates, in turn, destroy vitamin A in these plants.

- Processing of foods. For this reason canned foods are kept to a minimum on the Metabolism-Balancing, Anti-Candida or combined Anti-Candida/Anti-Allergy Programs. The foremost American authority on the nutrient content of food, Dr Henry Schroeder (in the *American Journal of Clinical Nutrition*, Vol. 24, page 562, 1971) analysed 730 common foods. He discovered that the canning of green vegetables destroys more than 50 per cent of vitamin B5 and B6. Canning of green peas and beans destroys 75 per cent of the same vitamins. Canned carrots lose 70 per cent of their calcium, canned tomatoes 80 per cent of their zinc and canned spinach 80 per cent of its iron.

  Freezing of meats and vegetables destroys the same amount of B vitamins. These are accurate measures not rough estimates. Frozen foods, although they look fresh and nutritious are very deficient in minerals as they are treated with a chelating chemical called EDTA. EDTA strips off 80 per cent of the mineral content. If this mineral content isn't stripped off frozen vegetables, they appear dull in colour after cooking. With the minerals stripped off they cook and look brightly coloured—certainly more of an inducement to buy. In the gut EDTA latches onto as many minerals as possible preventing their absorption.

The space required to describe the metabolic role of each vitamin and mineral is too great for inclusion in this text. Any good nutritional almanac will provide you with this information.

Other suggested reading includes: *Your Personal Vitamin Profile*, by Dr Michael Colgan, and *Mental and Elemental Nutrients*, by Dr Carl Pfeiffer (see 'Bibliography').

EVENING PRIMROSE OIL

This oil has been included as a supplement because it's the only food source on earth that contains almost all the essential fatty acids needed by the body. Some of these essential fatty acids can be made by the body (which is why they are not widely found in food) if it's well nourished, not under stress or assailed by drugs and alcohol. The conditions required for optimum essential fatty acid formation are rare today which is why evening primrose oil is an essential food component of the programs in this book.

The fatty acids in evening primrose oil are needed to maintain the structural integrity of the membranes of all the cells in the body. Cell membranes are subject to damage from the wear and tear of substances passing through them—bacterial, viral and fungal infections and histamine released during allergic reactions. If the cell is unable to repair its membranes, holes appear that allow the passage of foreign substances into the cell. Heavy metals, toxins from infections and the assorted flotsam and jetsam that accumulates in the body (from breathing polluted air, drinking tap water, eating processed food and the waste products of body metabolism) can float in and out of the cell. These unwanted foreign substances get themselves involved in normally occurring chemical reactions, altering their outcome, thus disrupting the cell's metabolism. Not only that, enzymes essential to the cell's function can float out further disrupting the cell's metabolism.

The body prefers to make its cell membrane from the unsaturated oils. If there is a deficiency in them it's forced to use the hard, saturated animal fats. These are not as good and the membrane becomes hard and less permeable to the admission of nutrients and the emission of waste products. The fatty acids in evening primrose oil and MaxEPA—the marine oil (lipid) concentrate—are necessary for the cell to make special chemicals called prostaglandins. These chemicals are imperative for keeping the metabolism balanced. Paticularly the metabolism of the kidneys. Fluid retention (over-weight) is a major symptom of metabolic imbalance born of prostaglandin synthesis inhibition. The fatty acids are needed to make the stress and sex hormones, the latter being particularly important for maintaining metabolic balance.

LUGOL'S IODINE

This has been included as a supplement because iodine deficiency is becoming more widespread since people have started cutting salt out of their diet. Iodised salt has been the main source of iodine for most people and as they have not been eating seafood (the only good source of iodine) two to three times per week, they have not been making up for the iodine loss. Iodine is the principal nutrient needed for the manufacture of thyroid hormone. Thyroid hormone determines the rate at which the metabolism ticks over. A deficiency in this hormone means a sluggish metabolism and low resistance to allergies, infection, cancer, high cholesterol and heart disease. A small minority of people get a mild skin rash on iodine. If this happens to you, stop taking it after fourteen days. When the skin settles down take it once a week from then on.

CHROMIUM
This mineral is one of the principals of glucose metabolism and has been described in detail in this chapter under 'Cholesterol'.

MARINE LIPID CONCENTRATE
Marine lipid concentrate (MaxEPA) contains the two essential fatty acids not found in evening primrose oil. MaxEPA, combined with evening primrose oil, provides the cells with all the essential fatty acids needed to keep the metabolism balanced. Marine lipids have a cholesterol-lowering and an anti-rheumatoid-arthritic effect.

CAN I TAKE TOO MANY VITAMINS?
To answer this question scientifically one has to say 'yes' as it is possible to have too much of anything. In reality the answer has to be 'no' as the dosages of multi-vitamin and mineral formulas are strictly monitored by the Department of Health to eliminate this possibility.

There are 5000 documented cases of vitamin overdoses in the United States. Mostly these were children gulping down sugar-coated, artificially flavoured vitamins in the belief they were lollies but in not one case was death the outcome, even though they felt nauseous and headachy for a while. This compares rather favourably with the thousands of deaths resulting from aspirin overdose (slightly more than 2000). Anyone who wants to be stupid can take massive doses of a single vitamin and this can cause metabolic disturbances of varying degrees.

VITAMIN B OVERDOSE
Although the B vitamins are water soluble it is still possible to overdose on them. Most research done on B vitamin overdose has been in relation to a single B vitamin taken by itself and has led to inaccurate results and consequent scaremongering by some re-

searchers. Massive doses of a single B vitamin (1000 mg and upwards—Formula Six contains only 50 mg) can cause toxicity in some people because the single B vitamin doesn't have its fellow B vitamins, vitamin C and the minerals to balance it and influence its action. It is for this reason that nature always includes more than one vitamin and mineral in a given food.

Therefore, taking tablets with one vitamin only in them is not recommended. For example, women who take vitamin B6 only, for premenstrual tension and fluid retention, are in danger of overloading their bodies with this vitamin and developing an adverse reaction to it if they continue this practice on a long-term basis. Whereas those who take vitamin B6 in conjunction with all the other B vitamins and all the minerals will not develop an adverse reaction unless, of course, they are allergic to the binders and fillers in the vitamin tablets.

Formula Six obeys a vital law of nature which states that all nutrients must be taken together and in correct ratios. Examples of the principle of balance abound everywhere in nature. Oxygen is a prime example. We know that oxygen is essential for the maintenance of life and that if the cells of the body are deprived of oxygen for a few seconds they begin to die. However, too much oxygen can be detrimental to life and for this reason nature has balanced the oxygen in the air we breath with another gas—nitrogen. In fact oxygen makes up only 20 per cent of the air we breath, the other 80 per cent is nitrogen and if the levels of oxygen in the air creep above 20 per cent problems of toxicity begin with symptoms of chest pain, nausea, vomiting, malaise, fatigue, numbness and tingling of the fingers and toes. If the oxygen levels increase further the alveoli cells of the lungs will become so overloaded they will collapse and die just as they would wither and die if they were receiving too little oxygen (suffocation). Should oxygen levels in a premature baby's incubator climb above 40 per cent the baby will develop retrolental fibroplasia, a condition which will cause it to go blind. Small amounts of hydrogen gas can cause severe acidity in the body but combined with oxygen in the correct ratio it provides us with life-sustaining water. Chlorine is a poisonous gas yet combined with sodium provides us with common salt.

We can therefore see that even the most essential life-sustaining elements of this earth can be toxic unless they are balanced in the correct ratio with other elements ... and so it is with vitamins and minerals. Don't be deterred from taking vitamin and mineral supplements by those who are trying to build a case against them, because the same convincing case could be built against oxygen if nitrogen was never mentioned.

Formula Six saves you the effort of trying to balance your

vitamins and minerals in their correct ratios which you would have to do if you were taking them in a single tablet form.

VITAMIN A OVERDOSE

It is true that excessive amounts of the fat soluble vitamins A and D can cause toxicity in the body but very large amounts must be ingested before any damage is done. Vitamin A toxicity could result from a daily intake of 150 000 iu every day for one or more months, but Formula Six contains only beta Carotene which the body converts to vitamin A. Nature also employs a simple method of warning that toxic levels of vitamin A are approaching with symptoms of morning sickness and loss of appetite. When the morning sickness symptoms have abated and the appetite and taste for foods containing vitamin A have returned the levels of vitamin A in the body have dropped right down and the toxic state no longer exists. It would be impossible to eat enough food to provide 150 000 iu unless you were eating whale or seal liver each day or you were making a concerted effort to gulp down fifteen 10 000 iu tablets of vitamin A. Both vehicles of vitamin A overdose would prove to be very expensive and chances are you would never persist with the exercise.

BUT DON'T VITAMINS PASS OUT IN MY URINE?

Yes, a portion of what you consume does. However, they are not being wasted for it's nature's intention that they do so. The wastes that leave the body via kidney, bladder and bowel are very toxic and capable of causing cancer in the walls of these organs and scars in the delibate kidney tubules.

If you are taking supplementary vitamins and minerals to nourish yourself there should be some left over to neutralise the waste products as they pass through the body. Vitamin C and the B vitamins neutralise the toxins in the urine (turning it yellow) thus protecting the walls of the bladder and the tubes leading to and from it. Vitamin C, E and A are very important for protecting the walls of the bowel against the toxins in faecal matter, particularly the putrefying fats. It is no coincidence that bowel cancer is second only to lung cancer as the major cancer killer. The foods we eat today don't contain enough vitamins and minerals to nourish us and protect our organs of elimination. For this reason supplementation of these nutrients is imperative.

Although it is intended by nature that we lose some vitamins and minerals through the bladder and bowel, some people do lose more than they should, because:

1. There is a lack of minerals in the food they eat or in the supplements they take. Minerals hold vitamins in the body.

2. Lack of exercise causes greater vitamin and mineral loss. (Bedridden hospital patients can lose from their bones up to 300 mg of calcium per day in the urine.) Exercise raises the metabolic rate and puts the tissues of the body to work. Working tissues (especially muscles) require greater amounts of food. Vitamins and minerals are thus retained and used in greater quantities by these working tissues.

The longer you are on a complete vitamin and mineral supplement the less you lose. As your metabolism balances, your metabolic rate increases and your health improves, you use more of the vitamins and minerals you ingest. In time only a small portion is spilling over into the urine and bowel for protection purposes.

MULTIPLE INTERACTIONS
No vitamin or mineral acts by itself, it needs to inter-react with other vitamins and minerals before it can be of any nutritional use to the body. This is why vitamins and minerals cannot be considered as therapeutic agents (in the manner of drugs) that cure specific diseases. For instance, vitamin C is not a cure for the common cold. However, it is a principal nutrient in raising the body's resistance to the cold and 'flu virus. The white blood cells (T-lymphocytes) cannot absorb vitamin C unless vitamins B12, B6, folic acid, choline and the mineral zinc are also present. Moreover, vitamin C cannot boost the virus-killing power of the white blood cell if it doesn't have these same nutrients to interact with once inside the T-lymphocyte.

If there is not enough zinc in your diet, your cells actually lose vitamin A even though you may be taking a vitamin A tablet. Vitamin A deficiency leads to improper metabolisation of iron (anaemia) which in turn affects calcium metabolism (reduced bone growth, muscle contraction and the burning of glucose for energy). When iron metabolism is disrupted vitamin B12 metabolism is disrupted, which in turn disrupts folic acid, which in turn disrupts magnesium metabolism and so it goes on and on.

By working together, vitamins and minerals get the metabolism working properly and thus correct metabolic diseases. Vitamins are only of assistance where deficiencies exist. Metabolic diseases are, in the main, the result of vitamin and mineral deficiencies.

In its 1988 report on the nutritional state of Australians the federal Department of Health found that Australian women (in particular) were deficient in zinc, calcium and iron and suggested that more seafood be eaten. My experience is that most people cannot afford the amount of seafood needed to overcome these mineral deficiencies. A complete multi-vitamin and mineral is a much cheaper way of achieving the desired result.

CAN I BECOME HOOKED ON VITAMINS?

No, you can't. Vitamins and minerals are not foreign chemicals that disrupt the body's metabolism and create addictions. They are nutrients that the body needs and wants. They have a rightful place in the body's metabolism and fulfil an important role there.

Some people assume they have developed an addiction to their multi-vitamin, mineral formula because they feel so much better while taking it and tired, run down, cranky and irritable when they are not. Feeling this way when stopping your supplements is not a symptom of withdrawal, it is a symptom of insufficient nutrients reaching your cells. The feeling of well-being experienced while on supplements is proof positive of how deficient in nutrients our modern day foods are. A vitamin and mineral supplement is simply a concentrated food and for the body to react positively to it indicates that the body needs that quantity of vitamins and minerals to function optimally. To deprive it of that food will see it fall back to its former level of function.

Taking vitamin and mineral supplements does not create dependency the way taking drugs, cigarettes, stimulants and alcohol does. In the case of vitamins/minerals/food the dependency, or need for x amount, has existed since birth and feeling better with supplements indicates that the need is finally being met. There is no comparison between the innate biological need for vitamins and minerals and the artificially contrived need for drugs, cigarettes, alcohol and chemical stimulants.

The confusion arises from the fact that some people are so used to functioning below par, they think it's normal—that the average, healthy person should and does feel that way. They misinterpret the vitality-enhancing effect of vitamin and mineral supplements as being an artificial stimulatory effect that is not normal. This belief is confirmed when they go off the supplement and slip back to feeling how they did before. As a result they struggle through the rest of their lives never knowing what good health is.

HOW LONG DO I TAKE SUPPLEMENTS?

Take them for the rest of your life. Remember, they are a concentrated food supplement and we need food from the day we are born until the day we die. Although the federal department's report indicated that only women were nutrient deficient, I have found that the significant improvement men experience on dietary supplements indicates they are just as deficient as women.

An ounce of prevention is worth a pound of cure. By keeping the body well nourished there is less chance it will fall victim to disease. The secret is to keep taking supplements while you are feeling well, so as to remain well.

HOW MUCH DO I TAKE?

Some metabolisms need less vitamins and minerals to get by than others. Some people can get by on the smell of an oily rag while others need to take their supplements religiously every day to feel as well. The supplement regime laid out in the programs in this book is sufficient for most people.

Some people need to take more. This is determined by trial and error. Go by how you feel. If the amount included in these programs is not getting the desired results gradually increase the intake quantity until you are satisfied with how you feel. It goes without saying that if you are overdoing it no amount of dietary supplements will get you feeling 100 per cent well. In these cases you need to cut down on your work, commitment, exercise and socialising load and get plenty of rest.

THE EVIDENCE

The most conclusive evidence of the need to supplement our diet with vitamins and minerals can be found in the response of the young people on my experimental program (see Chapter 8, 'Glue ear'). All of these children and young adults experienced an improvement in overall brain function and rate of physical growth, development and stamina. Mental stamina and agility also improved.

None of these children were on a diet of fast foods. They were all on regular meals of good home cooking, with occasional junk food on special occasions. If our whole grains, fresh fruit and vegetables and meats contained nutrients sufficient to meet our needs, these young people would have shown no improvement on the vitamin and mineral supplements. Clearly, those of us who are not on vitamin/mineral supplements are not functioning at full capacity.

WATER

The human body is 65 per cent water in males and 55 per cent in females (females carry more fat than males and fat is a waterless tissue). All the chemical reactions that give rise to all life on this planet take place in water. Water is the universal trigger substance of life.

Any high school student will tell you that water is a chemical compound (H_2O) made up of two simple elements, both of which are gases: hydrogen and oxygen. And yet there's still so much the scientists don't understand about water and how it works. There are so many anomalies. Water is one of the few substances that is more dense as a liquid than a solid. This is why ice floats. Water is unique in that heating it from its melting point of 0°C to 4°C makes it contract even further. Water can act as both an acid and an alkali, causing it to actually react chemically with itself under certain conditions.

The clue to some of water's strange behaviour lies in the tenuous link the 'hydrogen bond' forms between the atoms of oxygen and hydrogen. This bond makes water tremendously flexible yet very fragile. Very little external pressure is necessary to break the bonds and destroy or rearrange its pattern. Because all the chemical reactions of life must occur quickly and with little expenditure of energy, flexible water is the ideal go-between. Its fragility however can cause these normal biological reactions to go awry at times. Significant for us is the fact that water is most unstable between the temperatures of 35°C and 40°C. The daytime temperature of an active healthy body is 37°C.

Water's instability means that different people will react slightly differently under similar circumstances to a given program. For this reason some people get well sooner than others on a given program and some people will experience a steady improvement over a given period while others will experience a waxing and waning of symptoms during their progression towards improvement—the classic two steps forward, one step back pattern. Some people experience a significant improvement suddenly with a tapering off of the rate of improvement as time goes by, while others can be on the program for weeks with no improvement only to find it comes suddenly, all at once, towards the end.

There is significant scientific data to indicate that electromagnetic fields can destabilise water. The two Italian chemists S. Bordi and F. Vannel demonstrated that the electrical conductivity of water could be altered by exposing it to a very small magnet.[4] Scientists of the Atmosphere Research Center in Colorado have demonstrated that water is very sensitive to electromagnetic fields.[5] I have certainly seen evidence of this in my own practice. Sleeping on magnet-containing pillows has helped some of my patients overcome intolerable headaches and sinus problems that the anti-candida/anti-allergy and chiropractor/osteopath treatment regime was only partly able to cure. Magnet-containing knee, ankle, elbow and hand pads have helped arthritic patients while magnet-containing necklaces have helped those with asthma as have magnet-containing inner soles. I've witnessed improved responses to dietary treatment when patients have stopped wearing battery-operated and luminous wrist watches, have stopped sleeping on water beds and have moved away from high-tension electricity transmission wires.

Experiments performed by Giorgio Piccardi, Director of the Institute of Physical Chemistry in Florence, suggests that even cosmic forces can cause chemical reactions to be idiosyncratic and go off in the wrong direction or refuse to take place at all. Piccardi's interest in the possibility of outside forces affecting chemical reactions was aroused by the fact that an experimental method he devised for the removal of encrustations from industrial boilers worked well sometimes but not others.

To explore his theory he chose a simple reaction, the speed with which bismuth oxychloride (a colloid) forms a cloudy precipitate when poured into distilled water. He and his assistants carried out this simple test three times a day, until they had 200 000 separate results. These were analysed and compared with the results of a parallel series of tests made at Brussels University.[6]

Several kinds of change in the speed of precipitation showed up during the ten year experiment. There were frequent short-term, sudden changes, lasting a day or two. All of these were connected with the sun. Solar eruptions, giving rise to measurable changes in the earth's magnetic field, accelerated the speed at which the reaction took place. There were long-term changes as well and when these were plotted on a graph, they formed a curve exactly parallel to that for sunspot frequency in the eleven year cycle.[7]

Piccardi's control experiment was to do the same experiment under the protection of a copper screen. When shielded from outside influences in this way the precipitation always took place at the normal speed.

Piccardi's experiment demonstrated clearly that chemical reactions taking place in water are susceptible to electromagnetic radiation which means either the chemical or the water was affected. All available evidence points to the water.

There are other easily recognised effects the sun can have on chemical reactions and in particular those that take place in humans. Sunstroke results from a massive loss of water and salts from the body by dehydration through the skin and sometimes sunburn as well. The old Australian bush remedy of taking a large glass of water with a teaspoon of salt for a headache gains credence in the light of this. But what of the more subtle influences? Russian scientists have shown that our blood is directly affected by the sun.[8] Over 120 000 people in a Black Sea resort had the number of lymphocytes (a type of white blood cell) in their blood measured. All showed a significant drop in the number of these protector cells during times of great solar activity. The number of people suffering from lymphocyte deficiency diseases doubled during the tremendous solar explosion of February 1956.

That many of the body's functions seem to be influenced by sun-induced changes in the earth's magnetic field is given further credence by a study case of 5580 coal-mine accidents in the Ruhr that showed most occurred on the day following solar activity.[9] Traffic accident studies conducted in Russia and Germany show an increase, by as much as four times the day after a solar flare.[10] Further evidence that humans' nervous systems are sensitive to cosmic influences can be found in a survey of 28 642 admissions to psychiatric hospitals in New York. There was a marked increase in admissions on the days when the magnetic observatory reported strong activity.[11]

John Newlson demonstrated that the positions of the other planets (Mars, Jupiter, Saturn, Venus and so on) in our solar system either influence, or are at least an indication of, the sun's magnetic field. Certain planetary configurations coincide with stronger and lesser sunspot activities.[12] Does this mean that astrological equations touch life here? I have often wondered why a Virgo mother (for example) can react slightly differently to the same diet as, say, a Leo daughter, given that their body chemistries would be so similar after many years of living together and eating the same meals. I'm always explaining to family members that the nuances of difference in their reaction patterns are the result of their biochemical individuality. Could their individual horoscope (planetary alignment chart) be contributing to their chemical uniqueness? I've often wondered.

Chemical reactions within the body are certainly affected by the concentration of chemicals in the cells. Chemical concentrations increase when water levels drop, which underscores the importance of keeping the body properly hydrated at all times. Interfere with the trigger substance and you interfere with life.

Given the enormous influence the moon exerts on the contraction and expansion of the earth's oceans (that is, the ebb and flow of the tides) and given that the human brain is 80 per cent water, it's reasonable to assume that the moon has an influence on the way we respond to diets and indeed express ourselves mentally and emotionally.

From my own observation I've noticed that a patient is more likely to break a program at or about the full moon. It's interesting to note that in its report on the effect of the full moon on human behaviour the American Institute of Medical Climatology noted that crimes with a strong psychotic motivation, such as kleptomania, arson, alcoholic homicide and destructive driving, show marked increases at the time of a full moon.[13] This of course doesn't happen to everybody and not everybody breaks his or her program at the full moon. From my observations it's those who have significantly distorted metabolisms from a lifetime of wrong dietary and living habits that are prone to doing so.

Such metabolic distortions can make their mental balance precarious to start with and changes in the earth's magnetic field wrought by the forces behind the moon and sun can precipitate varying degrees of crises in these people. Happily though, as the programs are adhered to and the metabolism of the body balances, extraneous forces have less effect. A metabolically balanced person has greater control over his/her life and bodily functions.

Whatever else we, as individuals, may claim to be, we are electric machines whose vulnerable energy reserves may be mobilised and destabilised readily and by many different factors. The vulnerability of our energy reserves is inextricably bound up with the fragility and variability of our medium of electrical conduction—water.

For this reason you should not expect to react to a given program in exactly the same way twice, or as a friend or another member of your family. Don't be disappointed if they seem to be making better progress than you or you're not responding as well to a program the second time around. By accepting the uniqueness of your body chemistry and metabolism and by persisting with the program you will ultimately achieve good results. The journey might be different, the arrival will be the same.

NOTES

1. Ozone (O_3) is an allotropic form of oxygen, the molecule of which consists of three atoms. It is a common constituent of the atmosphere, is a powerful oxidising agent and is often used as a disinfectant.

2. Hydrogen peroxide (H_2O_2) is a colourless, caustic liquid, highly explosive on contact with oxidisable material. Hydrogen peroxide forms when ozone makes contact with water. It occurs naturally in rain and snow from atmospheric ozone and in mountain streams where agitated water bubbles white. Vigorously shaking a half-filled bottle of water improves its taste by producing detectable amounts of H_2O_2.

3. Ostrander, S., and Schroeder, L., *Psychic Discoveries Behind the Iron Curtain*, Prentice-Hall, Englewood Cliffs, New Jersey, 1971.

4. Bordi, S., and Vannel, F., 'Variazione Giormaliera di Grandezze Chimicofisiche,' *Geofis & Meteoral*, 14:28, 1965.

5. Fisher, W., Sturdy, G., Ryan, M., and Pugh, R., 'Some Labora-

tory Studies of Fluctuating Phenomena', in Gauquelin, *The Cosmic Clocks.*

6. Capel-Boute, C., *Observations sur les Tests Cliniques de Piccardi*, Presses Académiques Européennes, Brussels, 1960.

7. Sunspots are magnetic storms that take place on the sun. They take the form of incredible explosions of 13 million°C that start in the core of the sun and send flames shooting thousands of miles into space. From these flames streams of fast moving electrons and protons rush out into space as solar winds that buffet all the planets in our solar system causing magnetic storms in their atmospheres as well. Changes in earth weather are the most obvious signs of the effects of these magnetic storms.

8. Schulz, N., 'Les globules blancs des subjets bien portants et les taches solaires', *Toulouse Médical*, 10: 741, 1960.

9. Martini, R., 'Der Einfluss der Sonnentäligkeit auf die Haufung von Umfallen', *Zentral bl, Arbeitsmedizin*, 2: 98, 1952.

10. Podshibyakin, A. K., 'Solar Flares and Road Accidents', *New Scientist*, 25 April 1968.

11. Friedman, H., Becker, R., and Bachman, C., 'Geomagnetic Parameters and Psychiatric Hospital Administrations', *Nature*, 200: 626, 1963.

12. Nelson, J. H., 'Planetary Positions, Effect on Short Wave Signal Quality', *Electrical Engineering*, 71: 421, 1952.

13. Huff, D., *Cycles in Your Life*, Victor Gollancz, London, 1965.

Recipes

By Ludmilla Mallory, Dip. Nut.

Once again, I am honoured to have been asked to compile recipes for Phil's programs and to provide some general guidance for an easy-to-follow, but more formally structured, road to good health and well-being. As in the last book, I am also providing basic notes and explanations to better choices of the essential ingredients.

Quite a few recipes are just plain good sense and, although they may prove to be very basic for the sophisticated cook, they are included here for easy reference and to provide a foolproof method of complying with the programs for those who are not experts in the kitchen. While variety and adventure go hand in hand with good food, we feel the more daring experimentation is best left for the times when you are completely well and your immune system can cope better with the challenges this might present.

So, while your health is improving, we are asking you to try to understand how the programs work and to stay patiently and strictly within their boundaries for the prescribed time. The notes and recipes that follow are designed to make your task easier.

WEIGHT, MEASURES AND ABBREVIATIONS

All liquid and dry measures are either given in metric measurements or are based on standard metric cup.

1 cup = 250 mL
1 tablespoon = 1 T = 20 mL
1 teaspoon = 1 t = 5 mL
1 litre = 1 L = 1000 mL

All measurements are level

(A) = Contains amines
(S) = Contains salicylates
(M) = Contains monosodium glutamate

HOW TO SELECT THE RECIPES FOR THE ANTI-CANDIDA PROGRAM

1. When you first start the Anti-Candida Program, all recipes provided in this book in the Anti-Candida Program recipes are suitable.
2. As you progress with your treatment, and specific allergies become apparent, you will need to eliminate specific foods and chemicals. All recipes are marked appropriately for chemical sensitivity. Read carefully to determine if a recipe is suitable for you.

SHOPPING AND PREPARATION GUIDELINES

1. Familiarise yourself with the program thoroughly. Study the 'Food tables'. Compile a comprehensive shopping list suitable to your program and the known allergy triggers. Buy the essential foods before embarking on the programs.
2. Make it a habit to read all the labels while shopping to check the ingredients of all commercially prepared items. It will pay to be super cautious. If in doubt about some additive or ingredient, don't buy the product. Check it out with the manufacturer; make sure it is suitable for the program before buying it next time.
3. Choose your foods with care, paying attention to their freshness, types of containers and methods of manufacture.

MARGARINES

All margarines, without exception, are synthetic products, even though they are made from natural ingredients. In the process of their manufacture, using quite high temperatures, the natural molecular structures of these ingredients are altered in such a way that their digestion presents a challenge to the human organism, which has been designed to cope only with the naturally occurring molecular structures.

Long term human consumption of any denatured products will come at a cost to the body—this becomes evident at some later stage.

To avoid the many sad and unnecessary consequences of such abuse of this wondrous and wonderful machine of ours—our body—use only natural products in place of margarine. Consumed in moderation, the much maligned dairy butter and the cold pressed vegetable oils are the best alternatives. They not only taste better, they are definitely better for us.

OILS

Always choose cold pressed oils. Nowadays, even supermarkets carry good brands. However, good health food stores will have more variety. Oils not bearing the inscription, 'cold pressed', are produced by using heat during the extraction process. As a result, the oils are molecularly damaged, less nutritious, difficult to digest and generally less useful to the body. In fact, they can even be damaging. Do not buy oils sold in plastic containers. Some types of plastic chemically react with oils making them toxic to the body.

Olive oil (monounsaturated) is the most stable of all and is especially useful in the kitchen, not only for salads, but for frying as well. The 'extra virgin' cold pressed olive oil is best eaten raw in salads. The other cold pressed varieties can be used for cooking. However, sunflower, soybean, corn, sesame and walnut oils are all excellent alternatives.

Remember never to re-use the oil once it has been heated. Discard it, as it is very harmful to your health to consume it.

VINEGARS

While you are on the Anti-Candida Program, forget about the existence of these products. Use only freshly squeezed lemon juice (or lime juice) instead. In fact, even the lemon juice might have to be suspended for a while, should you be sensitive to salicylates or amines. Fresh lime juice may be substituted for lemon juice in all cases.

EGGS

Use only free range eggs. They are more easily available now and are more nutritious, coming to you from much happier hens. Do not ever throw the egg shells away, make use of them as described below.

Egg shells

Pulverised egg shells are a very good source of natural calcium, especially for pregnant, lactating and post-menopausal women. It is advisable to add $^1/_4$–$^1/_2$ t of the powder to your salad dressings, omelettes, scrambled eggs and other egg dishes.

It is not hard to prepare the egg shell powder if you have a blender. A simple routine follows below:

Collect the shells from the eggs you use. (It is easier to pulverise a number at a time.) Air dry the shells. When completely dry, crush the shells lightly and pulverise in the blender at high speed as finely as possible. Sift through a sieve to separate the egg membrane and larger pieces that did not get processed. Store in a glass jar. One large egg shell makes around 1 t of powder.

FLOURS

Select only stone-ground wholemeal flours. Plain stone-ground wholemeal wheat flour can now be purchased from supermarkets. However, do not buy the self-raising variety from supermarkets as the raising agents in them also contain additives that may be harmful to you. Use the plain variety and add your own baking powder mix (recipe provided below), unless you can obtain the flour recommended in the shopping list. It is the only one guaranteed not to have harmful additives.

The same caution applies to purchasing cornflour. In fact, for the cornflour to be of the normally accepted consistency, it must contain a number of additives to make it free-running. When in need of cornflour products, make sure you are buying a pure maize product, usually sold as maize meal, polenta or flour. For baking you will need to get the finest possible texture, so maize flour is the best. For thickening agents use arrowroot, brown rice flour or extruded rice bran.

Baking powder

Commercially available baking powder may contain harmful additives. To ensure you have none of these creeping into your baking, you will have to mix up your own baking power—all you need to do is combine 2 parts of cream of tartar with 1 part of bicarbonate of soda. Make sure the mixture is well blended before storing in an airtight glass jar. If desired, 1/2 part of arrowroot flour may be added to make the powder more free running. Just remember to use slightly larger quantities than indicated in recipes (1 level t will need to be 1 heaped t).

MILK SUBSTITUTES

Soymilk is the best substitute for dairy milk in the recipes (it can be used by both amine and salicylate sensitive people). It is available in pure form as an already prepared 'milk' (see shopping list in Chapter 14).

If it is unobtainable from your supplier as 100 per cent soya bean, make your own soymilk from the soya bean powder especially designed for such use (see shopping list in Chapter 14). Mix it according to the instructions on the packet.

Use stronger concentrations for recipes calling for cream (as a guide use 1 1/2–2 times the amount used for soymilk).

If none of the above is available:

1. The non-amine/salicylate sensitive can use coconut milk (see below) or nut milk (also see below).
2. The amine sensitive can use coconut milk, almond, cashew and hazelnut milk, or stock or water (if appropriate for the recipe).
3. The salicylate sensitive and combined amine/salicylate sensitive can use cashew milk only, stock or water (if appropriate).

Coconut milk

Not suitable for the salicylate sensitive.
Fresh coconut produces thicker, richer milk. If unobtainable, use desiccated variety.

Using fresh coconut
Remove the coconut from its hard, fibrous shell and scrape off the brown inner skin. Grate the coconut finely into a bowl, cover with 300 mL of boiling water. Leave for 45–60 minutes. Strain off the liquid, using muslin cloth and squeezing to extract as much liquid as possible. This will produce a thick, creamy liquid. It can be diluted to normal milk consistency or used as is for extra richness in recipes. The remaining strained coconut can be soaked for 12 hours and then strained again to make a thinner milk. This can be used in recipes for breads and sauces. Sauces can be then enriched by addition of thicker milk, if desired.

Using desiccated coconut
   3 cups desiccated coconut
   2¹/₂ cups boiling water

Cover the coconut shavings with boiling water, allow to stand for 24 hours. Strain through muslin cloth as above. This can be used undiluted in any recipes calling for milk.

Nut milks

The salicylate sensitive can only use cashew milk.
   1 cup raw nuts (blanched almonds [S], cashews, blanched hazelnuts [S], brazil nuts [S, A]—don't use peanuts or pistachios)
   2¹/₂ cups water

Blend dry nuts to form a meal. Gradually add water. Blend first to thick paste, then to a milky consistency.

Nut milks aren't as good for cooking as soya bean or coconut milks.

FRUITS AND VEGETABLES

When purchasing these, take all care to select only the very freshest. Anti-candida patients should pay attention to strawberries, paw paws, persimmons and all the citrus fruits. They are particularly prone to having mould growing on them if not absolutely fresh. Look for the presence of any black, brown or greeny blue spots, patches or film on the surface of the fruit. These mean mould.

STOCKS

Do not use any commercial preparations. Veal, beef, chicken, fish or vegetable stocks are easy to make. They are economical, much more nutritious and very handy to have ready for use at any time in a frozen form.

The following recipes are basic. Quantities are generous. The end product can be divided into suitable size containers (pre-measured), or poured into ice cube trays, frozen and stored in plastic bags in your freezer. Do not keep stock in your fridge without freezing for longer than two days. If you do not have any immediate use for it, take it out of the fridge, reheat, boil 2–3 minutes, cool and then freeze. Do not add salt at any stage of stock preparation. It can be added later when you are preparing your recipes. An exception is fish stock to which you should add salt.

Veal stock

Adapted (in brackets) for the amine/salicylate sensitive.
>   2 veal shanks, trimmed of excess fat and skin (have the
>   butcher open the ends of the bone on each side to expose
>   the bone marrow)
>   2 stalks of celery, cut into chunks
>   2 carrots, cut into chunks (S) (*Salicylate sensitive:* substitute
>   1 potato and 1 swede)
>   1 clove of garlic
>   1 leek, white part only, sliced
>   1 onion, cut into quarters (S) (*Salicylate sensitive:* substitute
>   1 extra leek)
>   Handful of parsley

Place the veal shanks and vegetables into a deep pot, add water to cover. Bring to boil. Reduce heat so the liquid just simmers gently. Skim the coagulated scum forming on top once or twice. Simmer for at least 1 hour, or until the meat is tender. Take the shanks out of the stock and reserve for further use (see 'Minestrone'). Strain the stock, allow to cool. Use in recipes or freeze.

Beef (or other meat/poultry) stock

Adapted (in brackets) for the amine/salicylate sensitive.

1 kg beef shin bones (have butcher cut them into suitable
    pieces), or 1 kg any suitable soup meat (not pork), or
    combination of bones and meat, or chicken (or other
    poultry) bones and carcasses, or whole (or pieces of)
    chicken or other poultry *(Amine sensitive:* skin the
    chicken)
1 carrot, cut into chunks (S) *(Salicylate sensitive:* substitute
    1 potato, diced)
1 parsnip, cut into chunks (S) *(Salicylate sensitive:* substitute
    extra celery or 1 swede)
1 leek, white part only, sliced
1 onion, cut into quarters (S) *(Salicylate sensitive:* substitute
    1 extra leek)
1 clove of garlic
2 stalks of celery, with leaves, sliced

OPTIONAL
Not for the salicylate sensitive.

1 bay leaf (S)
1 t whole peppercorns (S)

Place the bones (or other meat) into a deep pot, add water to cover.
Bring to boil. Reduce heat so the liquid just simmers gently. Skim
off coagulated scum forming on top. Add all other ingredients.
Bring to boil. Skim again, if needed. Cover loosely, maintain a very
quiet simmer for 2–2¹/₂ hours. Add more water if it evaporates
below level of ingredients. At no stage allow to boil briskly. When
cool, strain and refrigerate. The next day degrease by lifting the
solidified fat off the surface. Use or divide as needed and freeze.

OPTIONAL VARIATION (produces more flavourful, darker coloured
stock—good for use in soups, gravies and sauces): All bones and
meat may be roasted for ¹/₄–¹/₂ hour before cooking in the water.

Fish stock

Adapted (in brackets) for amine/salicylate sensitive.

1 kg fresh fish, any kind, or a combination of fish heads,
    bones, trimmings or other seafood, or seafood shells (e.g.
    green prawn heads and shells—preboil these briskly for 5
    minutes to get the bitterness out; drain well before
    including with other ingredients)
1 onion, cut into quarters (S) *(Salicylate sensitive:* substitute
    leek)
1 stalk of celery, cut into chunks
Handful of parsley

1 t lemon juice (S, A) *(Amine/salicylate sensitive:* substitute lime juice)

$^1/_2$ t sea salt

OPTIONAL

Not for the salicylate sensitive.

1 carrot, cut into chunks (S)

1 parsnip, cut into chunks (S)

Place all the ingredients into a deep pot. Add water to cover and bring to boil. Reduce heat to a gentle simmer. Skim. Simmer very, very gently, uncovered, for 30 minutes. Cool and strain through a fine sieve. Discard the strained fish and vegetables. Use or freeze as required. Use as a base for soups, sauces and as court boullion for poaching fish.

Vegetable stock

Adapted (in brackets) for the amine/salicylate sensitive.

3–4 onions, quartered (S) *(Salicylate sensitive:* substitute leek, white part only)

2–3 carrots, cut into chunks (S) *(Salicylate sensitive:* substitute swede, fennel, cabbage and/or brussels sprouts)

1 parsnip, cut into chunks (S) *(Salicylate sensitive:* omit)

3–4 potatoes, cut into chunks

4 stalks of celery, together with leaves, sliced

Handful of parsley and, if desired, any amount of shallots, leeks, any salad greens, pea pods, roughly chopped

OPTIONAL

Not for the salicylate sensitive.

1 bay leaf (S)

1 tsp whole peppercorns (S)

Place all the vegetables into a deep pot. Add water (or beef/chicken stock) to cover. Add the herbs, if using them. Bring to boil. Cover loosely and simmer gently at reduced heat for 30–45 minutes. Allow to cool for 30–45 minutes, strain. Use or freeze as required. Use as a base for soups, sauces, or add to vegetable purées.

LEGUMES

Beans, peas and lentils are very nutritious foods. They are full of proteins as well as vitamins and minerals. For these reasons they are recognised as the most important part of a vegetarian program.

Although generally rich in a variety of amino acids (essentially proteins), legumes lack the sulfur-containing amino acids to qualify them as 'complete proteins'. To derive full value out of legumes it is necessary to combine them with foods that are rich in the lacking amino acids, such as grains. Legume recipes contained in these pages are accompanied by a recommendation for supplementary side dishes for that purpose.

Certain rules have to be followed in cooking dried legumes. Nearly all beans and peas must be soaked before cooking to ensure they are digestible. This means you must remember to do it in advance of the meal. For purposes of the Anti-Candida Program it is not recommended to follow the long soaking method (12–24 hours), although it is generally a better known and common practice. Long soaking may cause slight fermentation which will not only noticeably alter the flavour of the beans but can also make them slightly toxic. Therefore, if beans are to be included in the Anti-Candida Program, they must be treated as follows:

- In a pot, cover the required amount of beans with water at least three times the volume of the beans. Cover the pot and bring to a rapid boil. Reduce the heat and allow to simmer 5–10 minutes. Take off heat, allow to stand covered for about $2^{1}/_{2}$ hours. At the end of that time, drain the beans and discard the water. Cover with an equivalent amount of fresh water and cook until tender ($1^{1}/_{2}$–2 hours) on slow heat.
- Do not add salt to the beans until near the end of the cooking time, as salt tends to harden them and to extend the cooking time. (Lentils and split peas are the exception. They can be salted at the beginning of cooking.)
- Do not add bicarbonate of soda (another common practice) to the cooking water, as it destroys vitamins.
- The 'second' cooking water (if not fully absorbed) can be drained off and used as stock or utilised in the dish being prepared.
- As beans tend to neutralise flavours, herbs and seasonings may need to be adjusted on reheating a bean dish the next day.
- Save time and energy by cooking double the amount of beans you need and store the extra in the fridge, well covered. They will keep for up to four days. Use in making salads, soups, spreads or as an accompaniment to the main meal.
- An amount of dried beans produces 2–$2^{1}/_{2}$ times the amount of cooked beans.
- Some varieties tend to foam when first cooked. Remove the scum after half an hour of cooking, and again later, if needed.

LIVER

This is a very nutritious food and forms an integral part of the Anti-Candida Program. Knowing that liver is not a favourite for many people, some ideas are offered to tempt you to change your mind about it. Apart from a choice of main meal dishes, there's a chopped liver recipe as well, to be used as a spread or sandwich filling, and an interesting way to have liver as an entry in soup.

For those who find liver difficult to tolerate, refer to a variation of the bolognese sauce for 'Spaghetti bolognese' and to 'Breakfast option 8—Savoury mince' of the Anti-Candida Program, where you can combine the liver with other meats to disguise its taste.

A note of warning: Do not use chicken livers. Depending on the feed the chickens are raised on, their livers may contain toxic substances. Lamb's liver presents no problem for amine sensitive people and is the best to use. Calf's liver may be used by all those who are not amine sensitive.

For recipes calling for minced liver, see if your butcher is willing to mince it for you. Otherwise, chop it with a sharp knife or process it in the food-processor. Do not overdo it, or it will liquify. A good method is to cook it lightly first, before processing.

Liver with avocado

Not for the amine/salicylate sensitive,
>4 thin slices of lamb's liver (or calf's [A])
>1 avocado thinly sliced (S, A)
>1/4 cup wholemeal or potato flour
>1/2 t sea salt
>Black pepper (S), freshly ground, to taste
>1/3 cup butter/olive (S, A)/other oil
>Juice of 1 small lemon (S, A) or lime
>1/3 cup beef stock (see 'Stocks', page 308)
>1/2 t dried thyme (S)
>Chopped parsley

Dredge the liver and avocado with flour seasoned with salt and pepper. Heat half the butter/oil and sauté the liver and avocado very quickly on both sides.

Transfer to a warm platter and keep hot. Heat the remaining butter/oil in the saucepan. Add lemon/lime juice, stock and thyme. When hot, pour over the liver and avocado. Garnish with parsley. Serves 2.

Liver with herbs

Not for the salicylate sensitive; adapted (in brackets) for the amine sensitive.
>250 g calf's liver, cut into 2 slices (A) *(Amine sensitive:* substitute lamb's fry)
>1 fresh sage leaf (S) or 1/2 t dried (S)
>1/2 sprig of rosemary (S) crumbled or 1/2 t dried (S)
>Handful of fresh basil (S) or 1 t dried (S)

2 handfuls of fresh parsley
1 slice of fresh wholemeal bread, without crusts
Black pepper, freshly ground, to taste (S)
1 T butter and 3 T olive (S, A)/other oil (or use all oil)
Sea salt, to taste

Trim the liver, removing any membranes or nerve tissues. Chop together the fresh herbs (or mix the dry ones and chop the parsley), put in a bowl together with freshly crumbed bread. Add a generous grinding of pepper (but not the salt). Toss the mixture well, spread it on the plate and roll the liver slices in it, coating them as evenly as possible.

Heat the butter and/or oil in a frying pan and cook the slices on both sides, sprinkling with salt on each side after it has been cooked. Take care not to prick the slices of liver. Use a spatula to turn them. Serve immediately with a sprinkling of extra parsley and basil. Serves 2.

Liver Venetian style

Adapted (in brackets) for the amine/salicylate sensitive.

250 g calf's liver (A) *(Amine sensitive:* substitute lamb's fry)
1/4 cup wholemeal or potato flour
30 g butter
1 T olive (S, A) or other oil *(Amine/salicylate sensitive:* substitute soya bean oil)
1 large onion, thinly sliced (S) *(Salicylate sensitive:* substitute 1–2 leeks, white part only)
2 T extra oil
1 T chopped parsley
Sea salt, to taste
Pepper, freshly ground (S), to taste *(Salicylate sensitive:* omit)
1 lemon, cut into wedges (S, A) *(Amine/salicylate sensitive:* substitute lime)

Trim the liver of any membranes and nerve fibres. Slice into thin strips. Coat the livers in flour, shaking off excess. Heat butter and oil in a pan, adding onions. Cook over moderate heat until soft. Remove from pan.

Add extra oil, increase the heat to high, add liver and cook, stirring continuously until it changes colour (about 2 minutes). Return onions to the pan.

Add parsley and stir. Cook for another 1–2 minutes. Season with salt and pepper and serve immediately with lemon (lime) wedges. Serves 2.

Liver dumplings in broth

Adapted (in brackets) for the amine/salicylate sensitive.

> 125 g calf's liver (A) *(Amine sensitive:* substitute lamb's fry)
> 1 small onion (S) *(Salicylate sensitive:* substitute leek, white part only)
> 1 egg yolk
> 1/4 t sea salt
> A pinch each of black pepper (S), freshly ground, thyme (S) and nutmeg (S) *(Salicylate sensitive:* these are infinitesimal amounts—so you may have them)
> 1 1/2 T chopped parsley
> 1 1/2 slices of wholemeal bread without crusts
> Milk or soymilk or water to soak bread
> 1/2 cup wholemeal flour
> 1 L stock (not fish), seasoned (see 'Stocks', pages 308–10)

Trim the liver and either mince or chop in food processor with the onion. Add the egg yolk, salt, pepper, thyme, nutmeg and parsley. Soak the bread in milk/soymilk/water to moisten and squeeze out excess liquid. Add to the liver. Add enough flour to make a soft dough (almost a batter). Bring the stock to boil. Dip a teaspoon in hot soup, then fill it with liver batter and drop the batter into the soup. Re-dip the spoon in broth before shaping each dumpling. Cover the pot and simmer gently for 10–15 minutes, depending on size of dumplings.

Chopped liver

Adapted (in brackets) for the amine/salicylate sensitive.

> 1 large onion, sliced (S) *(Salicylate sensitive:* substitute leek, white part only)
> 2 T butter
> 120 g calf's liver, sliced (A) *(Amine sensitive:* substitute lamb's)
> 2 hard-boiled eggs
> Sea salt, to taste
> Black pepper, freshly ground (S), to taste *(Salicylate sensitive:* omit)
> Parsley to garnish

Fry onions in butter until pale brown. Add the liver and fry for another 1–2 minutes. Mince, or put through the food processor, the onion, liver, 1 whole egg and the white of the second egg. Add salt and pepper and mix well. Arrange in a serving bowl, garnish with sieved egg yolk and parsley.

METABOLISM-BALANCING PROGRAM

BREAKFAST OPTION 1
Stewed fruit

Refer to the 'Anti-Candida Program—Breakfast option 7'. Any variety of fresh or dried fruit may be used (no specific restrictions apply).

BREAKFAST OPTION 4
Savoury mince

Refer to 'Anti-Candida Program—Breakfast option 8'. None of the restrictions specified in recipe apply.

BREAKFAST OPTION 5
Fish

Refer to 'Anti-Candida Program—Evening meal options 2 and 3', particularly baked fish recipes (no specified restrictions apply).

BREAKFAST OPTION 7
Wholegrain cereal

$1/3$ cup of any of the following cereals: wheat, oats, barley or rye
1 cup boiling water

The night before, stir the grain into the pan with boiling water, return to boil and simmer for 10 minutes. Take off heat, cover and allow to sit overnight. In the morning, reheat the mixture, and simmer until desired consistency (adding more water, if necessary).

Oats might only need 5 minutes, wheat and barley about 10 minutes and rye 15 minutes or more. Serve with a dollop of butter, or a little oil, and/or some fresh or stewed fruit. Serves 2.

OPTIONAL VARIATION: All the above grains may be ground before cooking, or purchased already cracked or ground. This considerably reduces cooking time. Otherwise, proceed as outlined above.

ANTI-CANDIDA PROGRAM

Easy wholemeal bread
Amine/salicylate/lactose free.
1 t sea salt
$2^{1}/_{2}$ cups water

4 cups self-raising, stone-ground wholemeal flour (see shopping list in Chapter 14)—plain, stone-ground flour can be used instead with the addition of 2 t of baking powder (see 'Shopping and food preparation guidelines' for recipe) for each cup of flour.

Dissolve salt in water. In a bowl, mix the flour and water with a wooden spoon until the dough leaves the sides of the bowl. No kneading is necessary. Place in a well-greased loaf tin and bake at 220°C (430°F) for approximately 1 hour. Test with a wooden stick. When it comes out dry, the bread is ready.

Corn bread

Amine/salicylate/lactose/gluten free.
- 1 cup pure maize flour
- 1/3 cup soya flour
- 1/4 cup rice bran (extruded)
- 1 T baking powder (see 'Shopping and preparation guidelines')
- 1/4 t sea salt
- 1/4 cup soya bean powder (milk substitute variety—see 'Shopping and preparation guidelines')
- 1 cup soymilk or water
- 1 egg, lightly beaten

Mix dry ingredients, except salt and soya bean powder. Dissolve salt and the soya bean powder in soymilk/water. Add the egg. Mix with dry ingredients until smooth. Pour into 20 cm x 10 cm (8 in x 4 in) greased loaf tin. Bake for about 30 minutes at 200°C (390°F) or test with wooden stick—if it comes out dry, the bread is ready. Very nice warm or cold. Also toasted.

OPTIONAL VARIATION: To make it lighter, use 2 eggs. Separate the eggs. Use the yolks in the soymilk/water; beat the egg whites and fold into the mixture. Proceed with baking as above.

Barley bread

Lactose free; adapted for amine/salicylate sensitive.
- 1 1/2 cups barley flour
- 1 1/2 cups brown rice flour
- 6 t baking powder (see 'Shopping and preparation guidelines')
- 1 1/2 cups water
- 1/4 t sea salt
- 2 t olive (S, A) or other oil (*Amine/salicylate sensitive:* substitute soya bean oil)

Sift flours and baking powder together. Add water with salt dissolved in it, and oil. Mix well . (You may have to use your hands to do this. Lightly oil them, then just squeeze the mixture.) Place into oiled 20 cm x 10 cm (8 in x 4 in) loaf tin. Cover with oiled foil and bake for 1 hour, possibly longer, at 180°C (350°F). Test with wooden stick—if it comes out dry, the bread is ready. Remove foil and bake for another 15 minutes for a crisper crust.

OPTIONAL VARIATION: Substitute the equivalent amount of rice flour with ¼–½ cup extruded brown rice bran—helps if you have a high cholesterol problem.

Rice bread (with carrots)

Wheat/gluten/lactose free; not for the amine/salicylate sensitive.
   125 g brown rice flour
   1 t baking powder (see 'Shopping and food preparation
      guidelines')
   1 t bicarbonate of soda
   2 eggs, lightly beaten
   150 g grated carrots (S) (or mashed banana [A], if tolerated)
   15 mg olive oil or 3 teaspoons (S, A) or butter
   ¼ t grated nutmeg (S)
   ¼ t cinnamon (S)
   ½ vanilla bean, chopped finely
   2 T soya bean powder (milk substitute variety—see 'Shopping
      and preparation guidelines')
   3 T water

Sift flour, baking powder and bicarbonate of soda together. Add all the other ingredients and mix well. Place in a greased cake tin and bake at 180°C (350°F) for about 1 hour or until a wooden stick comes out dry.

OPTIONAL VARIATION: You can add ¼–½ cup extruded brown rice bran to help lower your high cholesterol levels. You may need to add either more water or 1 extra egg to keep the right consistency.

BREAKFAST OPTION 1
Candida killer

Not suitable for the amine/salicylate sensitive. (Not in the first four weeks of the program.)
   1 large ripe avocado, sliced (S, A)
   2 T olive (S, A) or other oil
   2 T lemon juice (S, A), freshly squeezed
   ¼–½ t sea salt
   Dash black pepper (S), freshly ground
   1 large clove of garlic, crushed (more if you wish)

Optional
  1/4 t egg shells, crushed (see 'Shopping and food preparation guidelines')
  Dash cayenne (S)
  1 tomato (S, A, M), ripe, skinned and cut into cubes

Place everything into a blender or food processor. Blend until smooth. Use as often as you can as a dip, dressing, topping or sandwich filling. Candida really hates it!

BREAKFAST OPTION 4

Buckwheat kasha (Buckwheat is not related to wheat)
Adapted (in brackets) for the amine/salicylate sensitive.
  250 g raw (unroasted) buckwheat
  500 mL boiling water
  1/2 t sea salt
  60 g oil (or butter) to serve
Optional
  1 T extra olive (S, A) or sesame (S, A) or other oil

Toast the buckwheat in a heavy saucepan (either dry or with the optional oil) over medium heat until the grains turn a deep colour and emit a nutty smell. Stir constantly to prevent burning, then pour the boiling water over, add salt and bring to boil. Boil for 2 minutes uncovered. Reduce heat and simmer covered for no less than 20 minutes without opening the saucepan, allowing the steam to cook the buckwheat, by which time all the water should be absorbed and kasha tender. Take off the heat and stand covered for 10 minutes before serving. Serve with oil or butter. Serves 3–4.

  Optional variation: Serve with 1 onion (S, A) thinly sliced and fried in the oil/butter. This variation is not for amine/salicylate sensitive people.

Brown rice
Amine/salicylate free.
  700 mL water
  350 g brown rice, thoroughly washed in cold water
  1/2 t sea salt

Add the measured amount of water to drained, washed rice and bring to boil. Add salt. Cover the pot, simmer at reduced heat for 50 minutes. Take off heat and allow to stand covered for 10 minutes. Fluff the rice gently before serving. Serves 4.

OPTIONAL VARIATION: Cook as 'kasha' with addition of 3 T of olive oil (S, A) (*amine/salicylate sensitive:* substitute soya bean oil or butter), roasting the rice first, then add chicken stock instead of water. Proceed as with 'Buckwheat kasha'. You can also add sautéed onion (S) (*salicylate sensitive:* substitute leek).

Millet

Adapted (in brackets) for the amine/salicylate sensitive.

250 g millet (hulled)

1 T olive (S, A) or other oil (*Amine/salicylate sensitive:* substitute soya bean oil)

750 mL boiling water

¹/₂ t sea salt

Sauté the millet in a heavy pan with oil over medium heat until lightly browned, stirring constantly. Take off heat for 1–2 minutes. Then pour in the water. Bring back to boil, add salt. Cover and simmer for 40 minutes at reduced heat until all water is absorbed and the millet is tender. Allow to stand covered for 10 minutes before serving. Serves 4.

OPTIONAL VARIATION: You may also add sautéed onion (S) or leek as for 'Buckwheat kasha'.

BREAKFAST OPTION 7
Stewed fruit

Suitable for amine sensitive; adapted (in brackets) for salicylate sensitive.

3–4 golden delicious apples, or pears, or combination of both, peeled and quartered

Juice of golden delicious apples, diluted 50 per cent with still mineral water, to cover the apples

Rind of ¹/₂ lemon (S, A) (*Amine/salicylate sensitive:* substitute rind of 1 lime)

OPTIONAL

Not for salicylate sensitive.

Pinch of ground cinnamon or 1 cinnamon stick (S)

1–2 cloves (S)

Grated fresh ginger (S), to taste

Cover fruit with diluted apple juice. Add lemon/lime rind and, if desired (and suitable), cinnamon, cloves and ginger. Simmer gently till just tender. Cool and serve with cereal or as a dessert.

OPTIONAL VARIATION (*for amine sensitive only*): Substitute other desired fruit for apples from the 'Negligible' category in the amine chart (see 'Food tables'). Use apple juice/mineral water for stewing. Fresh peaches or apricots make a change, when in season. Occasionally, cherries from the 'Low' category may be also added.

BREAKFAST OPTION 8
Savoury mince
Adapted (in brackets) for amine/salicylate sensitive.

2–3 T olive oil (S, A) *(Amine/salicylate sensitive:* substitute soya bean oil)

1 onion (S), finely chopped *(Salicylate sensitive:* substitute leek, white part only)

1–2 cloves of garlic, finely crushed

300 g lean minced beef

1 t sea salt (or to taste)

Black pepper (S), freshly ground, to taste *(Salicylate sensitive:* omit)

1/4 cup or more of beef stock (see 'Shopping and food preparation guidelines') or water

1 T tomato paste (S, A, M) *(Amine/salicylate sensitive:* omit)

1 T chopped parsley

OPTIONAL

100 g chopped or minced calf's liver (A) *(Amine sensitive:* substitute lamb's fry)

1/2 t of any one or two well-tolerated herbs or spices such as: paprika (S), oregano (S) , thyme (S), tarragon (S), marjoram (S) *(Salicylate sensitive:* omit)

Heat the oil in a frying pan over medium heat and sauté onions until soft. Add garlic, toss for a few seconds and add beef (and liver) and all the seasonings (and herbs, if used). Mix well and cook only enough for the meat(s) to change colour. Add stock and tomato paste (if using). Barely bring to simmer. Sprinkle with parsley and serve over toasted bread with a green garden salad. Serves 2–6, depending on accompaniments.

OPTIONAL VARIATION (1): A variety of cooked, diced vegetables may be added. For example, carrots (S) or sweet corn, or green peas; also cooked legumes.

OPTIONAL VARIATION (2): 2 eggs may be added, either stirred in lightly beaten just at the end of cooking, or chopped, hard-boiled, sprinkled on top.

OPTIONAL VARIATION (3): You may serve the mince over noodles or brown rice, kasha or other cereals.

OPTIONAL VARIATION (4): Can be used as a filling in pancakes or pies.

LUNCH OPTION 1
Garden salads

When you first start the Anti-Candida Program, no restrictions are applied to the choice of your garden salads or cooking vegetables. So, unless you already know yourself to be sensitive to a particular chemical (for example, salicylates or amines), select any vegetables you wish for a salad. In your green salads, you may wish to include some vegetables that are already cooked.

However, should you be sensitive to amines or salicylates, then consult the lists of vegetables allowed for your particular sensitivity in the sections (later in this chapter) headed 'Amine free program' and 'Salicylate free program' before making or mixing a salad. There is still a wide enough choice for you to be able to make a nourishing and interesting salad.

Once you have selected the vegetables, you can choose a dressing that appeals to you (taking care to adapt it to your sensitivity, if required, as directed) from the ones that are offered below. Make sure you have a wide variety of foods and that you vary your salads from day to day.

Basic salad dressing

Adapted (in brackets) for amine/salicylate sensitive.

1 lemon (S, A), freshly squeezed *(Amine/salicylate sensitive:* substitute 1 large lime)

1 small clove of garlic, finely crushed

²/₃ cup extra virgin olive oil (S, A) *(Amine/salicylate sensitive:* substitute soya bean oil)

Sea salt, to taste

Black pepper (S), freshly ground, to taste *(Salicylate sensitive:* omit)

OPTIONAL

¼–½ t crushed egg shells (see 'Shopping and preparation guidelines')

1 T parsley (any kind), finely chopped

1 T chives, or shallots, or leeks

½ t tarragon (dry) (S) *(Salicylate sensitive:* omit)

½ t oregano (dry) (S) *(Salicylate sensitive:* omit)

1 t mustard (dry) (S) mixed with 1 T of water *(Salicylate sensitive:* omit)

Combine all the above ingredients in a jar and shake well. Serve with any garden or other types of salads.

OPTIONAL VARIATION (1): Add and shake with the above your choice of one or more, or any combination, or all of the herbs and spices listed under 'Optional' above.

321

Optional variation (2): 1–2 chopped hard-boiled eggs can be sprinkled over salad after it has been tossed with the dressing.

Basic home-made mayonnaise

Adapted (in brackets) for amine/salicylate sensitive.
  2 egg yolks (at room temperature)
  2 T lemon juice (S, A), freshly squeezed *(Amine/salicylate sensitive:* substitute lime juice)
  1/4 t sea salt
  Black pepper (S), freshly ground, to taste *(Salicylate sensitive: omit)*
  1 cup extra virgin olive oil (S, A) *(Amine/salicylate sensitive: substitute soya bean oil)*
Optional
  1 t dry mustard (S) *(Salicylate sensitive: omit)*
  1/4–1/2 t crushed egg shells (see 'Shopping and preparation guidelines')

Whip egg yolks in blender and, while blending on medium speed, add lemon/lime juice and seasonings. Continually blending, very slowly drizzle the oil into blender and beat until thick and smooth. Adjust seasonings. Add the egg shells (if using) and give it a last whirl.

Home-made mayonnaise (1)

Make up Candida Killer according to instructions and mix with 1/2 cup Basic Home-made Mayonnaise (see recipe).

Home-made mayonnaise (2)

Unsuitable for salicylate sensitive.
  1/2 cup 'Basic home-made mayonnaise' (see recipe).
  1 Lebanese cucumber (S), roughly chopped (no need to peel)
  1–2 T fresh parsley, chopped
  1–2 T fresh dill (S), finely chopped
  1/2 t tarragon (dry) (S)
  1/2 t dry mustard (S) (extra if already in the mayonnaise)
  1/2–1 t lemon juice (S, A) *(Amine sensitive: substitute lime)*

Blend for a few seconds in the blender or food processor. Pour over a garden salad of your choice. Decorate with extra dill sprigs.

Home-made mayonnaise (3)

Unsuitable for amine/salicylate sensitive.
  1/4 cup 'Basic home-made mayonnaise' (see recipe).

1 ripe tomato (S, A, M), scalded (to peel the skin off), de-
seeded and roughly chopped
1 T fresh basil leaves (S), finely chopped, or 1 t dry basil
leaves (S)
Extra lemon juice (S, A), to taste
Black pepper (S), freshly ground, to taste

Purée the ingredients in the blender/food processor. Looks and
tastes yummy over garden salad.

Home-made mayonnaise (4)

1 T 'Basic home-made mayonnaise' (see recipe)
1 t fresh chives, snipped

Mix and serve as mock sour cream over a baked or boiled potato.

'A touch of Italy' dressing

Adapted (in brackets) for the amine/salicylate sensitive,
1 cup extra virgin olive oil (S, A) *(Amine/salicylate sensitive:*
substitute soya bean oil)
1 clove of garlic, finely crushed
1 tin of anchovies in olive oil (S, A) *(Salicylate sensitive:*
substitute 4 whole dried anchovies in salt—obtainable
from Italian shops)
¼ cup freshly squeezed lemon juice (S, A) *(Amine/salicylate*
sensitive: substitute lime)
OPTIONAL
¼–½ t egg shells, crushed (see 'Shopping and preparation
guidelines')

Blend all ingredients into a purée. Goes well with steamed
cauliflower (S, A) or other cooked vegetables, as well as with
mixed greens (include some Italian lettuce—radicchio). Add
some wholemeal bread croutons tossed in a hot pan with olive
oil (S, A) *(amine/salicylate sensitive: substitute soya bean oil)*
and crushed garlic.

Oriental dressing

Unsuitable for amine/salicylate sensitive.
3 T extra virgin olive (S, A)
1 T cold pressed sesame oil (S, A)
1–2 T lemon juice (S, A), freshly squeezed
1 t fresh ginger (S), grated
1 clove of garlic, finely crushed

OPTIONAL

1 T sesame seeds, toasted (S)

2 T green onions, chopped

¼ t egg shells, crushed (see 'Shopping and preparation guidelines')

Combine in a jar and shake well. Goes well with a combination of raw Chinese cabbage (thinly sliced), snow peas (lightly steamed), bean sprouts (fresh, uncooked) or other vegetables.

Onion dressing

Not for the amine/salicylate sensitive.

1 large white onion (S), finely sliced

1 t sea salt

OPTIONAL

¼ t egg shells, crushed (see 'Shopping and preparation guidelines')

Combine and allow to stand for a minimum of 30 minutes (the longer it stands, the milder the taste). Serve over tomato wedges (S, A, M) (say 2–3 large tomatoes)

Polonaise dressing

Adapted (in brackets) for the amine/salicylate sensitive.

¼ cup extra virgin olive oil (S, A) *(Amine/salicylate sensitive: substitute soya bean oil)*

½ t sea salt

2 t white onion (S), minced *(Salicylate sensitive: substitute shallots)*

1 clove of garlic, finely crushed

¼ cup fresh lemon juice (S, A) *(Amine/salicylate sensitive: substitute lime)*

OPTIONAL

¼ t paprika (S)

¼ t egg shells, crushed (see 'Shopping and preparation guidelines')

Mix all the ingredients, allow to stand 30–60 minutes at room temperature to blend the flavours. Serve over steamed broccoli (S) or other vegetables with 2 chopped (or sieved) hard-boiled eggs as garnish.

Candida killer

See recipe in 'Anti-Candida Program—Breakfast option 1'

LUNCH OPTION 2
Bean and lentil stew
Adapted for the amine/salicylate sensitive.

   2 L water

   100 g soya or haricot beans (or any other variety), soaked as described in the 'Shopping and preparation guidelines') and drained

   100 g lentils (any variety), rinsed

   2 medium sized onions, chopped (S) *(Salicylate sensitive: substitute leeks)*

   4 T olive oil (S, A) or other oil *(Amine/salicylate sensitive: substitute soya bean oil)*

   4 cloves of garlic, crushed

   1 chilli pepper (S), finely chopped *(Salicylate sensitive: omit)*

   50 g brown rice, rinsed

   1 t cumin (S) *(Salicylate sensitive: omit)*

   1 t oregano (S) *(Salicylate sensitive: omit)*

   1 sea salt

   ½ t black pepper (S), freshly ground *(Salicylate sensitive: omit)*

   3 T coriander leaves (S), finely chopped *(Salicylate sensitive: omit)*

Bring water and beans to boil, cover and simmer for 1¼ hours at medium heat. Add lentils and cook further for 20 minutes. Meanwhile, sauté onions (leeks) in oil until light brown. Add garlic and chilli and stir fry for 1–2 minutes more. Transfer the onion (leek) mixture to lentils and beans, adding rice and all the dry spices (if using), salt and pepper (if using). Cover and simmer over a low heat for 30 minutes or until the legumes and rice are cooked, stirring occasionally to prevent sticking to the pot. Just before serving, adjust seasonings and stir in coriander (if using). Accompany the dish with a garden salad and, if wished, some steamed brown rice. Serves 4.

Beans Italian style
Adapted for amine/salicylate sensitive.

   250 g haricot, or soya, or other beans, soaked as described in 'Shopping and preparation guidelines' and drained

   2 cloves of garlic, crushed *(Amine/salicylate sensitive: use 4 cloves)*

   2 medium onions (S), finely sliced *(Salicylate sensitive: substitute leek)*

1 medium green capsicum (S), cored, seeded and thinly
   sliced *(Salicylate sensitive:* omit)
2 medium ripe tomatoes (S, A, M), roughly chopped *(Amine/
   salicylate sensitive:* omit)
1 T tomato paste (S, A, M) *(Amine/salicylate sensitive:* omit)
2 T olive oil (S, A) *(Amine/salicylate sensitive:* substitute soya
   bean oil)
2 T fresh parsley, chopped
1 t dried sage (S) *(Salicylate sensitive:* omit)
Black pepper (S), freshly ground, to taste *(Salicylate sensitive:*
   omit)
450 mL veal or vegetable stock (or water)
Sea salt, to taste

OPTIONAL
8 green olives (S), stoned and chopped *(Salicylate sensitive:*
   omit)

Combine all the ingredients, except salt, in a heavy casserole dish.
Cover and bring to boil on top of the stove. Transfer to the
preheated oven 180°C (350°F) and bake for 2 hours. Stir in salt and
bake uncovered for another 30 minutes. For proper protein
combination, serve with wholemeal noodles or bread and a green
salad. Serves 4.

Rice and potato muffins

Use in place of bread; amine/salicylate/gluten free.
½ t sea salt
¾ cup milk (or soymilk)
1 egg, lightly beaten
¾ cup potato flour
⅔ cup brown rice flour
3 t baking powder (see 'Shopping and preparation guidelines')

OPTIONAL
2 T brown rice bran

Dissolve salt in milk/soymilk. Add the egg. Sift the flours and
baking powder together, add rice bran (if using). Stir all the
ingredients together, mixing well. Pour into an oiled muffin tray
and bake for about 25 minutes at 180°C (350°F). Makes 6 muffins

OPTIONAL VARIATION: You can vary this recipe by adding some
grains. Try adding 2 T of any one (or combination) of the following
to dry ingredients: unroasted buckwheat, chopped sunflower
seeds, unhulled millet, or other favourite or permissible grains.
Proceed as above.

Millet muffins

Use in place of bread; amine/salicylate free

1¹/₂ cups millet meal

1¹/₂ cups barley flour

1 T baking powder (see 'Shopping and preparation guidelines')

¹/₄ t sea salt

1 cup milk (or soymilk)

2–3 eggs, lightly beaten

1¹/₂ T melted butter or olive oil *(Amine/salicylate sensitive:*
substitute soya bean oil)

OPTIONAL

4 T extruded brown rice bran

Mix flours, baking powder, rice bran (if using) and salt. Add all the
other ingredients. Mix well, pour into an oiled muffin tray and bake
at 180°C (350°F) for 20–25 minutes. Makes 12 muffins.

Pumpkin muffins

*May be used in lieu of bread; amine/wheat/gluten free; the amount
of salicylates per muffin is so small it won't hurt you; however, don't
eat too many at once.*

³/₄ cup pure maize flour

1 cup brown rice flour, sifted

1 T baking powder (see 'Shopping and preparation guidelines')

¹/₄ t nutmeg (S)

¹/₄ t cinnamon (S)

¹/₄ t sea salt

¹/₂ cup cooked pumpkin (S), mashed

¹/₄ cup milk (or soymilk)

¹/₂ cup melted butter, cooled (or oil)

2 eggs, lightly beaten

Mix dry ingredients together. Add all the other ingredients and mix
well. Pour into an oiled muffin tray and bake at 180°C (350°F) for
about 35 minutes. They are lovely warm. Makes 8 muffins.

OPTIONAL VARIATION: For better cholesterol control, you can
substitute ¹/₄ cup extruded brown rice bran for ¹/₄ cup of the rice
flour.

Spicy apple scones/muffins

*May be used in lieu of bread; amine/wheat/gluten free; the amount
of salicylates per muffin is so small it won't hurt you; however, don't
eat too many at once.*

½ cup arrowroot
½ cup soya bean flour
⅔ cup brown rice flour
3 t baking powder (see 'Shopping and preparation guidelines')
¼ t nutmeg, grated (S)
¼ t cinnamon (S)
½ t sea salt
¾ cup soymilk or milk or water
1 egg, lightly beaten
¾ cup apple (S), finely chopped (Salicylate sensitive: choose golden delicious apple)

Sift all flours and baking powder together, add spices, mix well. Add salt to milk, stir until dissolved. Mix all the ingredients thoroughly together, pour into an oiled muffin tray and bake at 180°C (350°F) for about 25–30 minutes. Beautiful for a Sunday breakfast. Makes 8 muffins.

OPTIONAL VARIATION: For better cholesterol control, substitute 3 T extruded brown rice bran for 3 T of the brown rice flour.

Rice pancakes
May be had with any of the lunch options; amine/salicylate/wheat/gluten free.

240 ml soymilk (or milk)
1 egg
2 T olive (S, A) or other oil (Amine/salicylate sensitive: substitute soya bean oil)
100 g brown rice flour
1 t baking powder (see 'Shopping and preparation guidelines')
½ t bicarbonate of soda
OPTIONAL
½ t sea salt

If using salt, dissolve it in soymilk/milk. Beat egg, add milk, oil. Sift dry ingredients into egg mixture and beat until smooth.

Heat oiled pancake pan. To test, sprinkle drops of water. If water bubbles skip around, the pan is ready. Cook pancakes on both sides until golden, turning just as they are puffed and bubbly, but not allowing the bubbles to break.

OPTIONAL VARIATION: For better cholesterol control, substitute ¼ cup extruded rice bran for ¼ cup of the rice flour. You may need to use a bit more soymilk/milk to maintain the consistency.

Savoury crackers

Try these in addition to bread,with soup, or with any lunch option; amine/salicylate free.

> $^2/_3$ cup wholemeal or barley flour
> $1^1/_4$ cups brown rice flour
> Sea salt, to taste
> 4 T olive (S, A) or other oil *(Amine/salicylate sensitive:* substitute soya bean oil)
> $^1/_2$ cup water

Mix flours and salt. Add oil and water and mix well. Knead for about 5 minutes or until smooth. Roll out to about 3 mm ($^1/_8$ in) thick and cut into any shapes you wish. Transfer into an oiled baking tray.

Prick all over with a fork. Sprinkle with a little extra salt (or your favourite herbs and spices—try oregano [S]). Bake for 15–20 minutes at 160–170°C (320–340°F).

OPTIONAL VARIATION: For better cholesterol level control, substitute $^1/_4$ cup extruded rice bran for $^1/_4$ cup of the brown rice flour.

Buckwheat crêpes (Buckwheat is not related to wheat)

Have with any of the lunch options, along with bread or muffins; amine/salicylate free.

> $^3/_4$ cup buckwheat flour
> $^1/_8$ t sea salt
> 3 large eggs
> 1 cup water or soymilk or milk

Sift the flour and the salt together. In another bowl, whisk together the eggs and add water/soymilk/milk. While still whisking, pour into the dry ingredients and beat thoroughly .

Allow to rest covered for a while (not less then 15 minutes, but preferably 1 hour). Stir before cooking on a hot, oiled pancake pan. Try filling these with cooked, chopped spinach (S, A) *(not for amine/salicylate sensitive)* and egg, or your other favourite fillings. Makes 18–20 thin crêpes.

OPTIONAL VARIATION (1): Substitute barley flour for the buckwheat flour.

OPTIONAL VARIATION (2): Substitute wholemeal wheat flour for the buckwheat flour.

OPTIONAL VARIATION (3): Substitute a combination of buckwheat, barley and wholemeal wheat flour for the buckwheat flour.

OPTIONAL VARIATION (4): Substitute your own favourite combination of allowed flours for the buckwheat flour.

LUNCH OPTION 3
Minestrone soup

Warning: Watch the salicylates with this recipe if you are sensitive to them, although the quantities are quite negligible, provided you substitute the vegetables as indicated in brackets.

   $^1/_2$ cup onions (S), sliced *(Salicylate sensitive:* substitute leek)
   1 clove of garlic, crushed
   2 T butter or olive (S, A) or other oil *(Amine/salicylate sensitive:* substitute soya bean oil)
   3 cups veal stock (see 'Shopping and preparation guidelines' for recipe)
   1 cup carrots (S), sliced *(Salicylate sensitive:* substitute potatoes)
   $^3/_4$ cup celery, sliced
   $^1/_2$ cup zucchini (S), diced *(Salicylate sensitive:* substitute brussels sprouts)
   $^1/_2$ cup green beans, cut 1 cm ($^1/_2$ in) long
   2 cups cabbage, slivered
   $^1/_2$ t oregano (S), dried *(Salicylate sensitive:* this amount is quite negligible for the quantity of soup. If proper care has been taken to substitute the appropriate vegetables, you may still use these amounts of herbs)
   $^1/_2$ t thyme (S), dried *(Salicylate sensitive:* negligible)
   $^3/_4$ cup cooked beans (see 'Shopping and food preparation guidelines') or uncooked fresh peas
As much as available of the veal meat off the two shanks used to make the veal stock, if using freshly made stock. Omit the meat if using the frozen veal stock.
   1 cup parsley, chopped
   1 cup tomatoes, chopped (S, A, M) *(amine/salicylate sensitive:* omit)
Sea salt, to taste

Sauté onions (leeks) and garlic in butter (oil) until soft. Add stock and bring to boil over medium heat. Add carrots (potatoes) and celery. Simmer 3 minutes over reduced heat. Then add zucchini (brussels sprouts) and green beans. Simmer till zucchini is just beginning to soften. Add cabbage and the dried herbs. Simmer till cabbage begins to soften. Add the cooked beans (or peas), diced meat off the veal shanks (if available), parsley, tomato (if using) and allow to simmer for 5 more minutes to warm the beans and meat (or until peas are cooked). Add salt. Serves 4–6 or more.

OPTIONAL VARIATION (1): If you wish to thicken this soup, use 30 g of arrowroot flour (or extruded brown rice bran) diluted in a little stock and added to the soup during the latter stage of cooking (just after the meat is added).

OPTIONAL VARIATION (2): ¹/₂ cup of small-shaped wholemeal pasta may be added 10 minutes before the soup is ready (about the time cabbage is added).

Thick potato and leek soup

Adapted (in brackets) for amine/salicylate sensitive.

   4 leeks, white part only, sliced
   1 onion (S) *(Salicylate sensitive:* substitute 1 extra leek)
   ¹/₄ cup butter or olive oil (S, A) *(Amine/salicylate sensitive:*
      substitute soya bean oil)
   5 medium potatoes, thinly sliced
   1 L stock of your choice
   1 T sea salt (or less, to taste)

OPTIONAL

   2 cups double strength soymilk (see 'Shopping and prepara-
      tion guidelines'), or dairy milk, if not during the dairy free
      period of the Anti-Candida Program

In a deep pot, brown leeks and onion (if used) very lightly in butter (or oil). Add the potatoes, stock and salt and simmer for 30 minutes, or until very tender. Purée in blender/food processor. Return to the pot and reheat. Serve with bread croutons, tossed in hot butter or oil. If using soymilk/milk, add after the soup is puréed. Can serve either hot or cold, garnished with snipped chives. Serves 8 or more.

Non-dairy cream of vegetable soup

Adapted (in brackets) for the amine/salicylate sensitive.

   4 T olive (S, A) or other oil *(Amine/salicylate sensitive:* substi-
      tute soya bean oil)
   50 g brown rice flour or extruded brown rice bran
   1.2 L water or soymilk or stock
   ¹/₄ t sea salt
   2 onions, sliced (S) *(Salicylate sensitive:* substitute leeks)
   3 stalks of celery, sliced or 100 g of permissible vegetable of
      choice, chopped
   White pepper (S), to taste *(Salicylate sensitive:* omit)

OPTIONAL

   1 clove of garlic
   Parsley to garnish

Heat 2 T of oil in a large saucepan, gently cook rice flour/bran in it. Add water/soymilk/stock and salt, bring to boil, cover and simmer 30 minutes at a reduced heat. In a separate pot, heat the remaining oil and sauté onions (and garlic if used) and celery. Add them to the soup, simmer for a further 15 minutes. Add pepper (if using). Garnish with parsley, if desired. Serves 4.

OPTIONAL VARIATION: For a different texture, purée the soup in the blender.

LUNCH OPTION 4

For recipes for muffins, see 'Anti-Candida Program—Lunch option 2'

EVENING MEAL OPTION 1

See 'Anti-Candida Program—Breakfast option 4' for instructions on how to cook 'Buckwheat kasha', 'Brown rice' and 'Millet'.

For garden salads for those who are chemically sensitive, please refer to 'Amine free program—Garden salad' and 'Salicylate free program—Garden salad' later in this chapter. For salad dressings see 'Anti-Candida Program—Lunch option 1'. For other vegetables for the chemically sensitive, please refer to 'Amine free program––Vegetables and other foods' and 'Salicylate free program—Vegetables and other foods'.

See 'Anti-Candida Program—Breakfast option 1' for the recipe for 'Candida killer'.

Basic gravy for pan-fried dishes

Adapted (in brackets) for the amine/salicylate sensitive.
   1 onion, finely sliced (S) *(Salicylate sensitive:* substitute leek)
   1 clove of garlic, finely crushed
   1 cup stock, any kind except fish (see 'Shopping and preparation guidelines')
   1 T arrowroot dissolved in 2 T stock or water
   Sea salt, to taste
   Black pepper (S), freshly ground, to taste *(Salicylate sensitive:* omit)
OPTIONAL
   1 T butter or olive oil (S, A) *(Amine/salicylate sensitive:* substitute soya bean oil)
   ¹/₂ t herb of choice (usually S) *(Salicylate sensitive:* omit)

Use preferably the same pan in which the steak, lamb, veal or chicken was pan fried. Discard excess fat from the pan. (If your meat has been grilled, heat the optional butter/oil in a shallow pan.) Fry onions and garlic in the pan until light brown. Pour the stock in, scraping the bottom of the pan gently to incorporate the pan-frying juices into the stock. Bring to simmer. Stir in dissolved arrowroot. Allow to thicken, stirring constantly. Add seasonings and herb of choice. Serve over the pan-fried/grilled meat or chicken.

Basic gravy for roasted meats

Adapted (in brackets) for the amine/salicylate sensitive.

2 cups roast juices (made by deglazing the dish from the roast with stock, either beef, veal or chicken, having previously discarded excess fat)

1½–2 T arrowroot, dissolved in ¼ cup stock (or water)

Sea salt, to taste

Black pepper (S), freshly ground, to taste *(Salicylate sensitive: omit)*

OPTIONAL

Squeeze of lemon juice (S, A) *(Amine/salicylate sensitive: substitute lime)*

Combine juices and arrowroot in a small pan. Heat, stirring until the gravy is thickened and clear. Add seasonings and lemon/lime juice (if using).

OPTIONAL VARIATION: Lightly fry 1 onion (S) *(salicylate sensitive: substitute leek)*, chopped, in the roasting pan before discarding fat. Transfer onions (leeks) into a smaller pan. Add roast juices. Proceed as above. Combine with onions (leeks) before serving.

Red sauce

Unsuitable for amine/salicylate sensitive.

1 T butter or olive oil (S, A)

1 small carrot (S), chopped or grated

1 small onion (S), chopped

1 small parsnip (S), chopped

Sea salt, to taste

Black pepper (S), freshly ground, to taste

2 cups beef stock (preferably made with roasted bones, see 'Shopping and preparation guidelines')

2 T tomato paste (S, A, M)

1½–2 T arrowroot

OPTIONAL

1 clove of garlic, crushed

Heat butter/oil. Stir fry chopped vegetables and garlic (if using), with salt and pepper until soft. Add a little of the stock and tomato paste and put through a blender. Dissolve the arrowroot in a little stock. Heat the rest of the stock and combine it with the vegetable purée. Bring to boil and while stirring, add the dissolved arrowroot. Cook until thickened. Adjust seasonings. Goes well with any kind of meat.

Sauce chasseur

Not for the amine/salicylate sensitive.
   1 T butter or olive oil (S, A)
   4 T shallots or spring onions (S), chopped
   2 medium-sized tomatoes, peeled, seeded and chopped (S, A, M)
   1 clove of garlic, finely crushed
   Sea salt, to taste
   Black pepper (S), freshly ground, to taste
   1/2 t basil (S) or tarragon (S), dried
   2 t fresh lemon juice (S, A) (or to taste)
   1 cup beef stock (see 'Shopping and preparation guidelines')
   1 T arrowroot

Heat the butter/oil. Cook shallots or onions for a minute. Stir in the tomatoes, garlic, seasonings and herbs. Cover the pan and simmer gently for 5 minutes. Add the lemon juice, stock and arrowroot, dissolved in a little of the stock. Boil rapidly for 4–5 minutes, so the sauce is slightly reduced and thickened. Adjust seasonings, to taste. Very nice served with pan-fried veal scallops.

Fresh tomato sauce

Not for the amine/salicylate sensitive.
   1 leek, white part only, sliced
   1 clove of garlic, finely crushed
   3 T olive oil (S, A)
   1 kg ripe tomatoes, peeled and roughly chopped (S, A, M)
   Handful of basil leaves (S), chopped
   Sea salt, to taste
   Black pepper (S), freshly ground, to taste

Fry leeks and garlic in olive oil until soft. Add the tomatoes and simmer 10–15 minutes. Add the basil and seasonings. This is a beautiful basic sauce for pasta, and great with any vegetables, either steamed or stir fried. Can be used for cooking cabbage rolls in, or chicken pieces.

OPTIONAL VARIATION: Instead of basil, use other herbs (most contain S) that appeal.

Spicy chilli sauce

Not for the salicylate sensitive; adapted (in brackets) for the amine sensitive.

   4–5 T olive oil (S, A) *(Amine sensitive:* substitute soya bean oil)
   3 red chillies (S), seeded and chopped
   4 shallots, chopped
   2 cloves of garlic, finely crushed
   2 T parsley, finely chopped
   Sea salt, to taste
   Black pepper (S), freshly ground, to taste

Heat the oil, add chillies, shallots and garlic. Cook for 2 minutes. Add parsley, salt and pepper. This goes beautifully over pasta and it is also excellent on steamed green beans, cauliflower or broccoli.

Italian pesto sauce

Not for the salicylate sensitive; adapted (in brackets) for the amine sensitive.

   1 T olive oil (S, A) *(Amine sensitive:* substitute soya bean oil)
   2 T pinenuts (S)
   2 cups fresh basil leaves (S) without stems
   2 cloves of garlic
   Sea salt, to taste
   Black pepper (S), freshly ground, to taste
   1/4 cup extra virgin olive oil (S, A) *(Amine sensitive:* substitute soya bean oil)

Heat 1 T of oil and toss the nuts until light brown on gentle heat. Drain and discard the oil. Process the basil leaves in blender/food processor, together with pinenuts, garlic, salt and pepper. While still processing, pour the rest of the oil in a steady drizzle until incorporated. This is lovely, not only on pasta, but on steamed vegetables like cauliflower, zucchini, or even potatoes.

Ginger sauce

Not for the salicylate sensitive; adapted (in brackets) for the amine sensitive.

   2 T butter or olive oil (S, A) *(Amine sensitive:* substitute soya bean oil)
   1 cup onion, chopped (S)
   1 clove of garlic, crushed finely
   2 t fresh lemon juice (S, A) *(Amine sensitive:* substitute lime)
   1 t freshly grated ginger (S)
   Coriander leaves (S), chopped, to taste

Heat butter/oil and lightly fry onions and garlic, until soft. Stir in lemon/lime juice and ginger. Sprinkle with coriander leaves. This is beautiful with steamed vegetables (snow peas, carrots, yellow squash) or with fish.

BBQ Sauce

Not suitable for the salicylate sensitive; adapted (in brackets) for the amine sensitive.

  4 T olive oil (S, A) *(Amine sensitive:* substitute soya bean oil)
  ¹/₂ t sea salt
  1 t paprika (S)
  ¹/₄ t cayenne (S)
  ¹/₃ cup fresh lemon juice (S, A) *(Amine sensitive:* substitute lime)

Combine all ingredients in a saucepan, bring to boiling point. Set aside to cool. This is lovely when used to baste meats and fish for your BBQ.

Dutch sauce

Not for the lactose intolerant; not for the dairy free period of the Anti-Candida Program unless a non-dairy substitute is used for the cream; adapted (in brackets) for the amine/salicylate sensitive.

  1 T arrowroot
  1 cup beef, chicken or vegetable stock (see 'Shopping and
    preparation guidelines')
  1 egg yolk
  2 T fresh cream
  Sea salt, to taste
  White pepper (S), to taste *(Salicylate sensitive:* omit)
  1–2 T fresh lemon juice (S, A) *(Amine/salicylate sensitive:*
    substitute lime)
  2 T softened butter or olive oil *(Amine sensitive:* substitute
    soya bean oil)

Dissolve arrowroot in stock. Bring to boil, cook until thickened and clear. Separately, in a mixing bowl, blend the egg yolk and cream (or non-dairy substitute) with a whisk. Gradually beat hot sauce into the mixture, until combined. Return the mixture to the pan and, continually whisking, bring to boil. Take off the heat, season to taste with salt, pepper and the lemon/lime juice. Just before serving, away from heat, beat in the butter/oil, 1 T at a time. Excellent for poached fish, steamed chicken, meat, steamed asparagus, cauliflower, broccoli and potatoes.

  Optional variation (1) *(not for the salicylate sensitive):* In the final addition of butter/oil, pre-mix the softened butter/oil with 2 t of dry mustard (S). Beat into the hot sauce, 1 T at a time. Very nice with grilled fish.

OPTIONAL VARIATION (2) *(adapted [in brackets] for the amine/salicylate sensitive):* In the final addition of butter/oil, pre-mix butter/oil with 2 T of tinned (drained of olive oil) anchovies (S, A), mashed into a purée *(amine/salicylate sensitive:* substitute dried anchovies in salt—obtainable from Italian shops). Take the pan off the heat, beat the anchovies/butter/oil mixture into the sauce, 1 T at a time. For poached fish or boiled potatoes.

Dill sauce
Not for the lactose intolerant; not for the dairy free period of the Anti-Candida Program; not for the salicylate sensitive; adapted (in brackets) for the amine sensitive.
   1 egg yolk
   4 T fresh cream (don't try and substitute non-dairy alternative—it won't work)
   ½ cup 'Basic salad dressing' (see recipe) *(Amine sensitive:* substitute soya bean oil and lime)
   Lemon juice (to taste) (S, A) *(Amine sensitive:* substitute lime)
   2 T chopped fresh dill (S) or a combination of other herbs (chives, parsley, tarragon [S])

Whip the egg yolk in blender at a low speed. Add cream and blend thoroughly. While blending, drizzle in the 'Basic salad dressing' (as for mayonnaise). Season to taste with lemon/lime juice and stir in the herbs. Fabulous with cold, hard-boiled eggs, vegetables and cold or hot fish.

EVENING MEAL OPTIONS 2 AND 3
To get the most out of fish, it must never be over-cooked. As fish, either grilled, pan fried or poached, cooks very quickly, be sure you have all your accompanying side dishes ready and waiting to be served, as once the fish is cooked, it is best eaten immediately.

Whiting (or other fish) with lemon dill butter
Adapted (in brackets) for the amine/salicylate sensitive.
   Fillets of whiting (enough for 2 servings), or 2 cutlets of Atlantic salmon, or 2 medium-sized trout (not filleted) or any other fish
   Sea salt, to taste
   Black pepper (S), freshly ground, to taste *(Salicylate sensitive:* omit)

2–3 T olive oil (S, A) *(Amine/salicylate sensitive:* substitute soya bean oil)

2 T butter

Juice of ¹/₂–1 freshly squeezed lemon (S, A) *(Amine/salicylate sensitive:* substitute lime)

2 T fresh chopped dill (S) *(Salicylate sensitive:* substitute chives or parsley)

Season the fish with salt and pepper (if using). Heat the oil in a frying pan until moderately hot. Fry the fish on both sides until just done and transfer to heated plates while finishing the sauce. Melt the butter in the same pan, add lemon juice and dill (chives or parsley). Toss in the pan for a few seconds, scraping the bottom of the pan with a wooden spatula, allowing the herbs to release flavours and blend with the pan juices. Pour over fish and serve immediately. Serves 2.

OPTIONAL VARIATION (1) *(not for dairy-free period of Anti-Candida Program, unless a non-dairy substitute is used):* Add 2–3 T fresh cream (or non-dairy substitute) to the sauce. Reduce slightly over heat, allowing the sauce to thicken.

OPTIONAL VARIATION (2): Dredge the seasoned fish in wholemeal (or brown rice) flour before frying. Add ¹/₄–¹/₂ cup of fish stock to the sauce. Simmer until lightly thickened; pour over the fish.

OPTIONAL VARIATION (3) *(not for the amine/salicylate sensitive):* Omit dill (chives) and lemon/lime juice. Add 2–3 T chopped parsley, 1 small chopped onion (S) (optional) and 1 chopped, ripe tomato (S, A, M), skinned. Cook 2–3 minutes. Adjust seasonings; serve over fish.

OPTIONAL VARIATION (4): Dredge the seasoned fish with flour (as above). Omit dill. Instead add ¹/₃ cup of almond flakes (S) *(salicylate sensitive:* substitute chopped cashews). Add the lemon/lime juice and 1 T of chopped parsley. Reduce slightly. Serve over fish.

OPTIONAL VARIATION (5): Coat the seasoned fish in a mixture of wholemeal (or brown rice) flour and wholemeal (no yeast) breadcrumbs. Fry as above. Discard the frying oil. Serve with lemon/lime juice squeezed over fish. Or prepare any of the above sauces (no cream) but cook it in a freshly melted butter (oil) in a different pan—this may be done prior to frying the fish.

Poached fish

Adapted (in brackets) for the amine/salicylate sensitive; unsuitable for the dairy-free period of the Anti-Candida Program

Sufficient quantity rich-textured, flaky fish (whole or filleted)

Sea salt, to taste

White pepper (S), to taste *(Salicylate sensitive:* omit)

Fish stock to cover (see 'Shopping and preparation guide-
   lines')
Cream, to taste
Lemon juice (S, A), freshly squeezed, to taste *(Amine/salicyl-
   ate sensitive:* substitute lime)
Parsley for garnish

Season the fish and place in a baking dish. Add warmed (not hot)
fish stock to barely cover the fish. Cover the dish with a greased
sheet of brown paper (preferable) or aluminium foil, and poach in
a preheated 180°C (350°F) oven for 10 minutes. When fish is
cooked, drain off the cooking liquid and reserve it. Bone the fish (if
necessary) and transfer to a hot serving dish. Reduce the cooking
liquid by half over a high heat. Add a little cream (to taste) and
reduce further. Adjust seasonings, if necessary. Add lemon/lime
juice to taste and cover fish with sauce. Serve immediately.
Garnish with parsley.

   OPTIONAL VARIATION: If desired, the sauce may be thickened with
arrowroot or brown rice flour.

Baked whiting with ginger

Unsuitable for the amine/salicylate sensitive.
   4 fillets of whiting (or other white fish)
   3 T butter
   1 T green ginger (S), freshly grated
   1 T lemon juice (S, A), freshly squeezed
   Sea salt, to taste
   Black pepper (S), freshly ground, to taste
   3 medium onions (S), sliced
   3 medium ripe tomatoes (S, A, M), skinned and sliced
   Parsley or chives to garnish

Place fillets in a greased baking dish. In a small pan, melt butter,
add ginger, lemon juice, salt and pepper. Mix and pour over the
fish. Cover the fish with alternate layers of onions and tomatoes. Bake for 25 minutes in a preheated 180°C (350°F) oven.
Garnish with chopped parsley or chives. This dish is nice cold.
Serves 4.

Snapper bake

Adapted (in brackets) for the amine/salicylate sensitive.
   1 medium onion (S), finely chopped *(Salicylate sensitive:*
      substitute leek)
   1 stalk of celery, finely chopped
   1/2 capsicum (S), finely chopped *(Salicylate sensitive:* omit)

2 T olive oil (S, A) *(Amine/salicylate sensitive:* substitute
   butter or soya bean oil)
1 ½ cups cooked brown rice, warm
Sea salt, to taste
Black pepper (S), freshly ground, to taste *(Salicylate sensitive:*
   omit)
1 x 1.5 kg whole snapper
1 T butter
¼ cup lemon juice (S, A) *(Amine/salicylate sensitive:* substitute lime)
½ cup shallots, chopped
1 T green ginger (S), freshly grated *(Salicylate sensitive:* omit)
1 lemon (S, A), thinly sliced (garnish) *(Amine/salicylate
   sensitive:* substitute lime)

Sauté onion, celery and capsicum in the oil, in a pan. Mix with
brown rice and season to taste. Stuff into the fish. Place the fish
into a well-greased baking dish. Melt the butter in a small
saucepan, remove from heat and add lemon/lime juice, shallots,
ginger (if using). Add salt and pepper to taste. Mix and pour over
fish. Bake in a preheated 180°C (350°F) oven for 30–45 minutes (do
not over-cook, check and baste frequently). Transfer fish onto a
serving dish. Pour the baking pan juices over and garnish with
slices of lemon/lime. This dish is also very good cold.

EVENING MEAL OPTION 5
Roast leg of lamb

Adapted (in brackets) for the amine/salicylate sensitive.
   1 leg of lamb
   1–2 cloves of garlic, slivered lengthwise
   Lemon juice, freshly squeezed (S, A) *(Amine/salicylate sensi-
      tive:* substitute lime)
   Sea salt, to taste
   Black pepper (S), freshly ground, to taste *(Salicylate sensitive:*
      omit)
   Your choice of suitable vegetables, prepared for roasting
Optional
   1–1½ t rosemary (S) *(Salicylate sensitive:* omit)
   1–2 t arrowroot or brown rice flour (for gravy)
   ½–1 cup any stock (except fish) (see 'Stocks', page 308–10) or
      water (for gravy)

Cut small slits with the tip of a knife in the lamb and insert the
garlic. Rub the meat with lemon juice and rosemary (if using) and
sprinkle with salt and pepper. Surround with vegetables (if de-

sired) or place vegetables in another pan. Roast the meat on a rack, uncovered, in a preheated 200°C (350°F) oven for 18 minutes per 0.5 kg for well done (82°C [180°F] on the meat thermometer), 14 minutes per 0.5 kg for pink (72°C [160°F] on the meat thermometer). Transfer the lamb to a warm serving platter and allow to stand for 20 minutes before carving. (Transfer the vegetables to a covered pan.) In the meantime, make the gravy.

GRAVY: Skim off all excess fat from the meat drippings, leaving any meat pieces in the pan. Stir in the stock or water. Bring to boil on top of the stove, scraping the bottom of the pan. Simmer for 1 minute. Adjust the seasonings, strain (if desired) and serve. You may wish to thicken it with 1–2 t of arrowroot or brown rice flour, dissolved in 2 T of stock/water. (For variations of gravy, see 'Anti-Candida Program—Evening meal option 1'.)

Roast lamb with herbs

Unsuitable for the salicylate sensitive; adapted (in brackets) for the amine sensitive.

1 clove of garlic, crushed
1 t sea salt
1 t black pepper (S), freshly ground
½ t powdered ginger (S)
1 bay leaf (S), crumbled
½ t dried thyme (S)
½ t dried sage (S)
½ t marjoram (S)
1 t lemon juice (S, A) *(Amine sensitive:* substitute lime)
1 T olive oil (S, A) *(Amine sensitive:* substitute soya bean oil)
1 leg of lamb

Combine all of the above seasonings, lemon juice and oil. Make slits in the lamb as for 'Roast leg of lamb'. Rub the herb mixture thoroughly into the meat. Proceed as for 'Roast leg of lamb'.

Roast beef

Suitable for amine sensitive; adapted for salicylate sensitive.

A cut of meat of your choice
Sea salt, to taste
Black pepper (S), freshly ground, to taste *(Salicylate sensitive:* omit)

For best results, the use of a meat thermometer is recommended. Preheat oven to 200°C (390°F) for all cuts, except for fillet (for fillet preheat to 230°C [450°F]). Season the meat generously. Insert the thermometer in the thickest part. Roast on a rack, standing in a roasting pan to collect the juices, until the thermometer registers 60°C (140°F) for rare, 72°C (160°F) for medium or 78°C (170°F) for well done. No basting is necessary. Transfer the meat to a warm serving platter to rest for 20 minutes before carving. Make gravy as described under 'Roast leg of lamb' or refer to 'Anti-Candida Program—Evening meal option 1—Basic gravy for roasted meats'.

Roast chicken

Adapted (in brackets) for amine/salicylate sensitive.
> 1 x 1.5 kg chicken preferably at room temperature
> Sea salt, to taste
> Black pepper (S), freshly ground, to taste *(Salicylate sensitive: omit)*
> 1 small onion (peeled) (S) *(Salicylate sensitive:* substitute 1/2 a leek, white part only)
> 1/4 cup melted butter or olive oil (S, A) *(Amine/salicylate sensitive:* substitute soya bean oil)

OPTIONAL
> 1/2 lemon (S, A) *(Amine/salicylate sensitive:* substitute lime)
> 1/2 t thyme (S), or rosemary (S), or tarragon (dried) (S) (or sprig of fresh tarragon [S]) *(Salicylate sensitive:* omit)
> And/or sprig of parsley
> And/or 1 bay leaf (S) *(Salicylate sensitive:* omit)

Preheat oven to 180°C (350°F). Rub inside of the chicken with half a lemon/lime and sprinkle with salt and pepper (if using). Add the onion/leek to the cavity (and herbs, if using) or stuff with a stuffing of your choice. Truss the chicken, brush with melted butter/oil and roast in a roasting pan (surrounded by vegetables, if desired) until the leg of the chicken moves up and down easily. Average cooking time for chicken is 18–20 minutes per 0.5 kg. Make the gravy as for 'Roast leg of lamb' or refer to 'Anti-Candida Program—Evening meal option 1—Basic gravy for roasted meats'.

AMINE SENSITIVE: As the chicken skin contains amines, the chicken has to be roasted on a rack placed into a roasting pan (to collect juices). Do not cook vegetables together with the chicken. Skin the chicken before serving and discard the drippings, as they will also contain amines. Serve vegetables and gravy cooked by other methods (see 'Anti-Candida Program—Evening meal option 1' for recipes for basic gravy and other sauces).

EVENING MEAL OPTION 6
Beef and vegetable casserole

Not suitable for salicylate sensitive; adapted (in brackets) for the amine sensitive.

500 g chuck steak, well trimmed and sliced into flat, large
  slices about 5 mm ($^1/_4$ in) thick
Sea salt, to taste
Black pepper (S), freshly ground, to taste
3–4 medium onions, sliced thickly (S)
3–4 carrots, sliced into 5 mm ($^1/_4$ in) rounds (S)
2–3 parsnips, similarly sliced (S)
5–6 large potatoes, peeled, sliced into 5 mm ($^1/_4$ in) rounds
2 T butter or olive oil (S, A) *(Amine sensitive:* substitute soya
  bean oil)
$^1/_4$–$^1/_2$ cup beef or veal stock (see 'Shopping and preparation
  guidelines') or water

In an ovenproof casserole dish, layer the bottom with meat, season
with salt and pepper, spread a layer of onion, then a layer of
carrots, then parsnips, then potatoes, seasoning lightly each
layer. Repeat the process, starting with meat and continue layer-
ing until all ingredients are used up, ending, preferably, with a
layer of potatoes. You may need to adjust quantities of vegetables,
depending on the size of your casserole dish. Top with butter (or
oil) and pour in the stock (water). Cover the dish and bring to boil
on stove top. Transfer into the oven at 200°C (390°F) for about 40
minutes, or until potatoes and carrots are tender. Serves 4.

OPTIONAL VARIATION: Chicken pieces may be substituted for beef
(amine sensitive: skin the chicken).

Lamb and vegetable stew
Not suitable for amine/salicylate sensitive.
  4 T olive oil (S, A)
  750 g breast of lamb, cut into small pieces
  Sea salt, to taste
  2$^1/_2$ cups beef, veal or other stock (not fish) (see 'Shopping
    and preparation guidelines')
  1 swede, cut into strips
  2 carrots, sliced (S)
  2 stalks of celery, sliced
  1 large potato, peeled and diced
  $^1/_2$ cup green beans, cut into 5 cm (2 in) lengths
  $^1/_2$ cup fresh peas
  3 large tomatoes (S, A, M), peeled, cut into 5 mm ($^1/_4$ in slices)
  Black pepper (S), freshly ground, to taste
  1 t lemon juice (S, A), freshly squeezed
  3 T chopped parsley

Heat 2 T of oil in a heavy pan and brown the lamb on all sides.

Season with salt and add the stock. Bring to boil, cover and simmer at a reduced heat until the lamb is tender (1½ hours). Remove the meat and reserve. Reduce the cooking juices by half on high heat. Reserve.

Combine all the sliced vegetables, except tomatoes, in a bowl and mix well. In a buttered/oiled casserole dish, arrange layers of mixed vegetables, meat and tomato slices. Season each layer of vegetables with salt and pepper. Combine the lemon juice, parsley, the remaining 2 T of oil and the reduced broth and pour over the assembled casserole. Bring to boil on top of the stove, then bake, covered, until vegetables are cooked at 180°C (350°F) (about 35 minutes). Serves 4.

For oven-baked fish recipes, please refer to 'Anti-Candida Program—Evening meal options 2 and 3'.

EVENING MEAL OPTION 7

For a recipe for Bean and Lentil Stew, please refer to 'Anti-Candida Program—Lunch options 2 and 3'.

EVENING MEAL OPTION 8
Bolognese sauce

Unsuitable for the amine/salicylate sensitive.
  1 medium-sized onion (S)
  1 large stalk of celery
  1 medium-sized carrot (S)
  3 T olive oil (S, A)
  250 g minced veal/beef
  3 large ripe tomatoes (S, A, M), chopped
  1 cup stock (see 'Shopping and preparation guidelines'), any
     kind (except fish)
  1 T, or to taste, tomato paste (S, A, M)
  1 T chopped parsley
  1 bay leaf (S)
  Pinch nutmeg, freshly grated (S)
  Sea salt, to taste
  Black pepper (S), freshly ground, to taste
OPTIONAL
  1 t dried oregano (S)

Finely chop the onion, celery and carrot. Heat the oil in a heavy pan. Sauté the chopped vegetables (not the tomato) for 10 minutes. Add the minced meat and sauté for 10 minutes, stirring with a wooden spoon. Add tomatoes, stock, tomato paste, herbs and seasonings. Bring to simmer, cover and cook on gentle heat for 1 hour. Add more stock, if necessary. Taste and correct seasonings. Serve over wholemeal spaghetti, or other shapes of pasta. Serves 2–4.

OPTIONAL VARIATION: This is a good dish for adaptation if you wish to include liver. A good proportion is 175 g veal/beef mince and 75 g calf's or lamb's liver, minced. Also, if desired, you can include 1–2 cloves of garlic, finely crushed.

EVENING MEAL OPTION 9
Spinach lasagna
Not suitable for amine/salicylate sensitive.

6 sheets of lasagne pasta
4 t olive oil (S, A)
1 bunch of spinach (S, A), torn off stalks
Double quantity of the 'Bolognese sauce' (see recipe), but using only half the quantity of stock (i.e. 1 cup of stock for double quantity of everything else)
60 g butter or olive oil (S, A)
80 g wholemeal or brown rice flour
500 mL milk or soymilk
Sea salt, to taste
Black pepper (S), freshly ground, to taste
Pinch nutmeg (S), freshly ground
2 egg yolks

Cook pasta, two sheets at a time, in plenty of salted water with 2 t oil. When tender, transfer into a bowl of cold water with the remaining 2 t oil. Steam spinach with a small amount of boiling salted water just long enough to wilt it. Drain well, squeezing water out of it and chop roughly. Have the meat sauce ready.

MAKE A WHITE SAUCE: Melt the butter (heat the oil) in a saucepan, add flour and cook for 1 minute. Gradually add the milk/soymilk and bring to boil. Cook until the sauce thickens. Season with salt, pepper and the nutmeg. Take off heat. Stir in the egg yolks.

ASSEMBLE LASAGNA AS FOLLOWS: Place 2 drained pieces of pasta over the base of a shallow ovenproof dish; trim, if necessary, to fit. Spread half the meat sauce over the pasta, then cover with a third of the white sauce. (Both sauces will be easier to handle if made the day before and refrigerated.) Spread the chopped spinach over the white sauce. Top with two more pieces of drained, trimmed pasta. Spread with the second third of white sauce, then the remaining bolognese sauce, then with the remaining drained and trimmed pasta and the last third of the white sauce. Bake in a moderate

(180–200°C [350–390°F]) oven for approximately 40 minutes. Allow to stand for 10 minutes before serving.

Vegetable lasagna

Not suitable for the amine/salicylate sensitive.
Cook as above but omit the spinach layer, if desired. Instead of the bolognese sauce use the following:

 1 small eggplant (S, A), diced
 Sea salt, to sprinkle the eggplant liberally
 2 T olive oil (S, A)
 1 onion, sliced (S)
 200 g green beans, cut into 2 cm (³/₄ in) lengths
 200 g zucchini (S), sliced
 1 cup chopped, ripe tomatoes (S, A, M), skinned
 2 T tomato paste (S, A, M)
 1 t dried basil (S)
 1 t dried oregano (S)
 Sea salt, to taste
 Black pepper (S), freshly ground, to taste
 60 g chopped walnuts

Place the diced eggplant in a colander, sprinkle with salt. Leave to stand for ¹/₂–1 hour. Rinse well and pat dry with paper towels. Heat oil in a saucepan, add onion and cook until soft on a moderate heat. Add eggplants, green beans and zucchini and cook for 5–7 minutes. Add tomatoes, tomato paste and herbs and seasonings. Stir, cover and simmer over lower heat for 30 minutes. Cool before assembling the lasagna in a similar manner to 'Spinach lasagna'. Sprinkle the top with chopped walnuts and bake as for 'Spinach lasagna'.

For proper food combining and inclusion of sufficient protein, accompany 'Vegetable lasagna' with a green salad and a legume (beans, lentils) dish of your choice.

EVENING MEAL OPTION 10
Marinara sauce

Unsuitable for the amine/salicylate sensitive.
 500 g green, unshelled prawns
 250 g scallops
 1 cup fish stock, hot (see 'Shopping and preparation guidelines')
 1 T fresh lemon juice (S, A)
 8 oysters

1 tin of flat anchovy fillets in olive oil (S, A)
2 T olive oil (S, A)
5 large, ripe tomatoes, peeled and chopped (S, A, M)
2 cloves of garlic
1 T tomato paste (S, A, M)
1 T chopped parsley
Sea salt, to taste
Black pepper (S), freshly ground, to taste

Shell and de-vein prawns. Cut scallops in half and cook in fish stock and lemon juice for 1 minute. Drain and combine with the rest of the seafood in a bowl. Drain anchovies on paper towel and chop finely. Heat oil in a heavy pan, add tomatoes, garlic, tomato paste and anchovies. Stir well and cook for 5 minutes. Add seafood and cook 5 more minutes. Add parsley, salt and pepper. Stir well and serve over wholemeal spaghetti or other shapes of pasta.

OPTIONAL VARIATION: Substitute the suggested seafood with 500 g of shelled seafood of your choice or buy premixed marinara seafood mix. Cook as above.

DESSERTS
Fruit salad
For a selection of permissible fruits and preparation guidelines please refer to the 'Amine free program' and 'Salicylate free program' later in this chapter.

You may dress your fruit salads by any one or combination of the following: 1–2 t lemon juice (S, A) (amine/salicylate sensitive: substitute lime); 1–2 t cold-pressed apricot kernel oil (A) (amine sensitive: substitute soya bean oil); purées of either peeled pears or paw paw, to taste.

Stewed fruit
See 'Anti-Candida Program—Breakfast option 7'.

SNACK
Popcorn
For those who are not allergic to corn, a delicious, healthy gluten free snack is popped corn. It is easy to prepare (as most would know).

Just heat 1 T of oil in a pan (big enough for expansion!). Add enough corn to cover the bottom of the pan in one or two layers. Cover and shake gently until popped. Herbs and spices can be added. Also melted butter.

AMINE FREE PROGRAM

GARDEN SALAD

The following vegetables and nuts can be used: asparagus, capsicum, carrot, celery, corn (M), cucumber, French beans, green peas, lettuce, lima beans (cooked), onions, leeks, chives, shallots, spring onions, radish, soya beans (cooked), zucchinis, American chestnuts, buckeye nuts, horse chestnuts, pinenuts, pistachios (not for Anti-Candida Program), almonds, beech nuts, cashews, coconut (raw not dried or desiccated), macadamia nuts, sunflower seeds.

After four weeks on the amine-free garden salad the following vegetables and nuts may be added once per day, two days per week only: cauliflower, broccoli (M), olives, brazil nuts, filbert nuts, peanuts (though not the ones in the red skin). Peanuts, pistachios, melons and dried fruit all contain mould and are not to be included in any salad if you are on the Anti-Candida Program.

A salad dressing of sunflower, soya bean, almond, cashew or macadamia oil with freshly squeezed lime juice and the powder of pulverised egg shells (to sweeten) may be used. (Egg shells are rich in calcium—good for kids, people with osteoporosis, pregnant and breastfeeding mothers.)

Olive oil may be used as the base of the salad dressing after four weeks, but only once per day, two days per week and not on successive days.

VEGETABLES AND OTHER FOODS

Use in soups, stews, casseroles or stir fried, baked, roasted or steamed: cabbage, celery, corn (M), French beans, green peas, kohlrabi, lima beans, onions, potatoes (steamed), soya beans, turnips, zucchinis.

Use only sunflower, soya bean, almond, cashew or macadamia oil for stir frying.

After four weeks off all amines the following vegetables may be added once per day, two days per week, but not on successive days: broccoli (M), cauliflower, olives.

The full range of herbs and spices may be used. The only condiments that are not to be used are Bonox, meat extract, soya sauce, Vegemite, Marmite, Promite, Bovril and Oxo. As well as being high in amines these condiments are high in MSG.

Beef, veal, chicken and lamb (fresh from the butcher only) may be eaten, as may all seafood and fish except: canned or smoked salmon (fresh is OK), mackerel, herring, sardines (canned or dried) and tuna (fresh or canned).

After four weeks off all moderate, high and very high amines, processed meats such as chicken liver, ham, salami, canned salmon and fresh tuna may be had once a day, two days per week, but not on successive days. Pickled and smoked meat and fish, like corned beef or smoked salmon, salami and ham are not permitted on the Anti-Candida Program.

Goat, rabbit, hare, venison, buffalo (bison), turkey, goose, quail, duck, pheasant, guinea fowl are all amine free and may be had with the amine free vegetables. No sausages or hotdogs—there are too many chemicals in them. Pork and bacon are high in amines and therefore are off the program.

FRUIT SALAD

Use apple, apricot, blueberry, gooseberry, lime, peach, pear, rhubarb, strawberry, blackcurrant, cherry, grapefruit, honeydew melon, mandarin, redcurrant, rockmelon. You may also use sunflower seeds, pinenuts, pistachio, American chestnuts, buck-eye nuts, almonds, beech nuts, cashews, macadamia nuts, coconut (raw, not dried or desiccated).

No melons to be had if you're on the Anti-Candida/Anti-Allergy Program. Melons grow on the ground and tend to be infected with soil mould (cephlasporium). After four weeks off all amines the following fruits and nuts may be added to the fruit salad once per day, and not on successive days: kiwi fruit, orange, passionfruit, paw paw (papaya), tangerine, dates, brazil nuts, filbert nuts, peanuts (though not the ones in the red skin).

No dates or any other dried fruit, peanuts or pistachios if you're on the Anti-Candida/Anti-Allergy Program.

A dressing of apricot kernel oil and lime juice may be had if desired. Any of the above fruits may be stewed (no sweetener or flavourings added).

SALICYLATE FREE PROGRAM

GARDEN SALAD

The following vegetables and nuts may be used: bamboo shoots, brown lentils (cooked), cabbage, celery, choko, dried beans (cooked), dried lentils (cooked), chives, dried peas (cooked), garlic, green beans, green peas, lettuce, mungbean sprouts, shallots, potato (peeled and cooked), cashew, poppyseed.

A salad dressing of soybean or cashew oil, with garlic, poppy seed or chives and/or shallots, can be had over the salad.

After four weeks off all moderate, high and very high salicylates the following vegetables and nuts may be introduced, but only once per day, two days per week, and not on successive days:

asparagus, beetroot, black olives, carrots, kohlrabi (cooked), mushrooms (M) (not for Anti-Candida Program), onions, raw tomato (M), sweet corn (M), sweet potato (cooked), walnuts, yellow and green chillis (fresh, not dried and small quantities only), brazil nuts, coconut (not dried or desiccated), hazelnuts, macadamia nuts, peanuts (not for Anti-Candida Program), pecans, pinenuts, pistachios (not for Anti-Candida Program), sesame seeds, sunflower seeds.

After four weeks off moderate, high and very high salicylates, lemon juice may be added to the salad dressing. Sunflower, soya bean, olive oil from black olives and sesame seed oil may also be used. If you're unsure of the source of your olive oil, don't use it. This salad dressing is to be had once per day, two days a week only, and not on successive days.

VEGETABLES AND OTHER FOODS

Use in soups, stews, casseroles, or stir fried, baked, roasted or steamed: bamboo shoot, brown lentils, brussels sprouts, cabbage, celery, choko, dried beans, dried peas, garlic, green beans, green peas, kohlrabi, leek, potato (peeled), red cabbage, red lentils, soya beans, swedes.

Use only soya bean oil for cooking. After four weeks off moderate, high and very high salicylates you may add the following vegetables once per day, two days a week only, not on successive days: asparagus, baby squash, beetroot, broccoli (M), carrot, cauliflower, marrow, yellow and green chilli, pumpkin, spinach, sweet corn (M), sweet potatoes, turnips, mushrooms (M) (not for Anti-Candida Program), onion and parsnips.

The same meats and seafood permissible with the amine free vegetables may be had with the salicylate free vegetables. Fresh pork may be had on the salicylate free program, though not pork derivatives such as bacon, sausages and ham. The only permitted condiments are as follows: soya bean, olive (from black olives only––don't use if not sure), sunflower and sesame oil may be used for cooking after four weeks total avoidance of salicylates. Use these oils only once per day, two days per week, and not on successive days. Don't cook with them if you've had them as a salad dressing that day.

FRUIT SALAD

Use banana, cashew, golden delicious apple (peeled), paw paw (papaya), pear (peeled), pomegranate, poppyseed.

After four weeks off the salicylates the following fruits and nuts may be added to the fruit salad once a day, two days a week only, and not on successive days: custard apple, kiwi fruit, lemon, loquat, mango, pear (with peel), persimmon, raw fig, red delicious apple (not jonathon, which is also red), rhubarb, tamarillo, brazil nuts, coconut (raw, not dried or desiccated), hazelnuts, macadamias, peanuts (though not the ones in the red skin), pecans, pinenuts, pistachios, sesame seeds, sunflower seeds, walnuts.

No dried fruits, peanuts or pistachios are to be had if you're on the Anti-Candida/Anti-Allergy Program. No melons for at least three months.

A dressing of soya bean oil and lemon juice may be had twice per week after four weeks on the salicylate free program, or purée one or two suitable fruits (for example, banana, pears and paw paw). Make sure that fruit like paw paw, lemons or persimmons are very fresh and that their skins are mould free if you are on the Anti-Candida Program. Wash fruit very carefully.

Any of the above fruits may be stewed (no sweeteners added). The only permissible flavouring is vanilla bean.

The nuts may be put through the blender and poured over the fruit salad or fruit stew as a purée. They also may be had whole. Nut butters that are guaranteed free of all additives may be had on the salad or stew. They may be added to the salicylate free fruit salad/stew after four weeks off salicylates, but only twice per week.

The peanuts in red skins are not to be used. No peanuts or pistachios if you're on the combined Anti-Candida/Anti-Allergy Program.

COMBINED AMINE AND SALICYLATE FREE PROGRAM

GARDEN SALAD

This garden salad is the same as the salicylate free salad, with the total exclusion of tomatoes and mushrooms, which are high in amines and contain MSG as well.

Pecan nuts are also totally excluded from the combined amine and salicylate free garden salad. Use only those salad dressings from the salicylate free garden salad, but excluding lemon as lemon is high in amines and must be deleted from the combined amine salicylate free salad dressing.

VEGETABLES AND OTHER FOODS

Use the same cooking vegetables and oils as for the salicylate free list, except no spinach, mushrooms or cooked tomato.

The same meats, poultry and seafood as for the amine free list. This means no pork, bacon, ham, pork, sausages or any other pork derivative. The only permitted condiments are as follows: garlic, parsley, saffron, tandori, salt.

FRUIT SALAD

Use: golden delicious apple (must be peeled), pear (peeled), pomegranate, cashews, poppyseed.

Any of the above fruits may be stewed (no sweetener or flavourings added).

A salad dressing of soya bean oil (cashew nut or poppyseed oil if you can get your hands on them) can be used or purée one of the suitable fruits.

After four weeks on the combined amine and salicylate free fruit salad/stew the following fruits and nuts (whole, puréed or as nut butter) may be added, but only once a day, two days per week, and not on successive days: custard apple, kiwi fruit, loquat, mango, passionfruit, paw paw (papaya), persimmon, red delicious apple (not jonathon which is also red), rhubarb, tamarillo, cashews, hazelnuts, macadamias, peanuts (though not the ones in the red skins), pinenuts, sesame seeds, sunflower seeds.

Be careful with persimmons—make sure the skin is mould free if on the Anti-Candida Program. Wash very carefully.

Peanuts are not permitted on the Anti-Candida/Anti-Allergy Program because they grow in the soil and can have soil mould (cephlasporium) growing on them. Peanuts are technically legumes.

Nuts are OK because they are fruits that grow from a flower on a tree. An exception is pistachio nuts—they are prone to mould and it is practically impossible to wash them successfully.

Food tables

BEEF

If you are allergic to beef, stay off veal, as well as all steaks, calves' liver, brains and ox heart. Also, empty the contents of any capsule onto a spoon and take it straight with a little water. All capsules are made from beef gelatin. Beef emulsifier is used in many commercially prepared breads, cakes, biscuits, pastries and lollies. Don't eat ox or buffalo. Read all labels carefully.

COCONUT

If you are allergic to coconut don't eat anything containing palm oil or palmoline. Most fast foods are deep fried in palm oil. Read all labels carefully, especially on such foods as cakes, biscuits, breads. Do not use coconut-based body oils, especially suntan oils; the smell of it is enough to cause a reaction.

CORN

Corn is used in a great variety of foods. We have included in our listing foods in which corn *may* be used. Not every brand of all these kinds of foods necessarily contain corn but many of them do. Any food listed here must be considered as containing corn unless you can prove otherwise by phoning the manufacturer. Explain that you have allergies and get a categoric guarantee that the product in question is free of corn or any other substance you may be allergic to.

Foods containing corn: Cornflour, corn meal, corn oil like Mazola, cornstarch, corn sugars, corn syrups, popped corn, fresh corn, canned corn, frozen roasting ears, fritters, glucose syrup, baking mixes (cakes, puddings), commercial batters for frying, bourbon and other whiskies, commercial pastries and cakes, some breads, some sweets, chop suey, commercial biscuits, icing sugar mixture, corn flakes, cream puffs, deep fat frying mixtures, some toothpastes, gelatine desserts, gravies, chewing gums, gin, ice-cream, some liqueurs, monosodium glutamate, some margarines, spreads, sauces for sweets and meats, sherbets, soups (creamed, thickened, vegetable), canned mixed vegetables, wines (some American wines are corn free), ales, aspirin and other tablets, bacon, baking powders, beers, carbonated beverages, bleached wheat flour, catsups, cheeses, chilli, instant coffee, cream pies, milk in paper cartons, peanut butters, canned peas, powdered sugar, preserves, puddings, custards, rice (coated), salad dressings, dried fruit confectionery, French dressing, Fritos, frostings, fruit (canned and frozen), fruit juices, frying fats, glucose products, graham crackers, grape juice, hams (cured/tenderised), bath and body powders (inhalants), popcorn, starch, jams, jellies, meats (bologna, sausages), Similac, string beans (canned and frozen), soybean milks, powdered sugar, syrups (commercial preparations: cartose, glucose, Karo, Puretose, Sweetose), talcums, instant teas, vanilla, vinegar (distilled), vitamins (tablets, lozenges, suppositories, capsules), Zest.

NOTE: It is necessary to check ingredients on all commercially prepared products.

CONTACTS: Adhesives, envelopes, stamps, stickers, sticky tapes.

EGGS

EGGS ARE FOUND IN: baking powders, batters for French frying, Bavarian cream, boiled dressings, bouillons, breaded foods, breads, cake mixes, cakes, custards, doughnuts, dried eggs, dumplings, egg albumin, French toast, fritter glazed rolls, fritters, frostings, glazed rolls, griddle cakes, hamburger mix, hollandaise sauce, ice-cream, ices, icings, macaroni, macaroons, malted cocoa drinks (Ovaltine, Ovomalt, and many others), marshmallows, meat jellies, meatloaf, meat moulds, meringues (French torte), noodles, omelettes, pancake flours, pancakes, pasta, pastes, patties, pretzels, puddings, quiche, salad dressings, sauces, sausages, sherbets, some dessert mixes, souffles, soups (noodle, mock turtle, consommés), spaghetti, Spanish creams, tartare sauce, timbales, waffle mixes, waffles, wines (are 'cleared' with egg white).

NOTE: It is advisable to determine whether egg is used in your own brands of pastries, puddings and ice-creams. Dried and powdered eggs are often overlooked when enquiry is made. Some fancy breads contain egg. When in doubt enquire at bakeries. It is necessary to check ingredients on all commercially prepared products.

How to substitute egg in cakes: (1) Replace eggs with 1 tablespoon of gelatine. Dissolve in cold water, then add boiling water to make 1 cup. Equal to three eggs. (2) Use 1 tablespoon of golden syrup to ½ pint of warm milk. Equal to three eggs (not for Anti-Candida Program).

FISH

If you are allergic to one fish in a family, you'll probably be allergic to the others as well. The following is a guide to fish families:

Decapod family: Crab, crayfish, lobster, prawn, shrimp.
Pelecypod family: Clam, cockle, mussel, oyster, scallop.
Cod family: Cod (scrod), haddock, hake.
Croaker family: Croaker, drum, sea trout, silver perch, weakfish.
Flounder family: Flounder, halibut, plaice, sole, turbot.
Herring family: Menhaden, sardine, sea herring, shad.
Mackerel family: Albacore, bonito, mackerel, skipjack, tuna.
Sea bass family: Groper, sea bass, red schnapper.

FRESHWATER SPECIES
Catfish family: Bullhead, catfish.
Perch family: Sauger, walleye, yellow perch.
Pike family: Pickerel, northern pike, muskellunge.
Salmon family: Salmon, trout.
Sunfish family: Black bass, bluegill, crappy, sunfish.

SINGLE FOOD FAMILIES
Each of these foods is in a separate family: Anchovy, bluefish, carp, eel, lake whitefish, mullet, ocean catfish, ocean perch, shark, smelt, sturgeon, swordfish, tilefish, whitefish.

INHALANTS THAT HAVE FOOD CORRELATIONS

Oats: Common oats is a grass, the spores of which are frequently in the air in spring and autumn. Many people are allergic to these spores (sinusitis, hayfever, conjunctivitis). Sensitivity to common oats is lowered by removing all oats from the diet, and avoiding all contact with: muesli, porridge, Guinness stout, oatmeal soap, oatmeal skin preparation.
Rye grass: Avoid Ryvita, rye bread.

OTHER GRASSES: Those with a sensitivity to a number of grasses and pollens do better if they stay off herbal teas, most of which are of grass and pollen origin. Although herbal teas are better for you than ordinary tea and coffee, if you are allergic to grasses and pollens they can do more harm than tea and coffee.

AIRBORNE MOULDS: Sensitivities to airborne moulds, including those that live in air-conditioning systems of large offices (namely alternaria) and those found in the soil (cephlasporium) can be lowered by staying off the foods listed under yeasts and moulds in the food table.

GLUTEN

FOODS CONTAINING GLUTEN: Wheat, rye, oats, barley, triticale, MSG, most commonly used drug medications in tablet form.

SOME GLUTEN FREE FOODS: Rice, soya bean, maize, millet, buckwheat, arrowroot, tapioca. NOTE: Unfortunately cornflour is adulterated with wheat and other gluten-containing flours. Use only pure maize flour.

JUNK FOOD

This includes all the packaged, bottled, canned, plastic- or celophane-wrapped and cardboard-boxed foods on the supermarket shelves that contain added sugar (sucrose, dextrose, glucose, maltose, fructose) and white flour; also additives such as metabisulphite (223, 224), monosodium glutamate (621), benzoic acid (210), and tartrazine (102). Read all labels carefully. You'll find you are eliminating about 90 per cent of all the foods on the supermarket shelves.

Exceptions are: canned fish (sardines, tuna and salmon in brine), dried herbs and spices, preservative-free and sugar-free tomato paste, butter, natural cheddar cheese, fresh full-cream milk and unsweetened full-cream yoghurt.

Canned fruit, vegetables, beans, lentils, vegetarian nut meats and fruit juice, with no added sugar, white flour, syrups, sauces and preservatives, are borderline. Also borderline are preservative-, sugar- and syrup-free home-bottled fruit and vegetables, as are frozen fruit and vegetables which have not been treated with EDTA. Dehydrated vegetables are devoid of vitamins and are definitely out.

When fresh fruit and vegetables are out of season the sugar-, white flour-, preservative-free tinned, frozen or home-bottled fruit, vegetables, beans and lentils may be used.

Categoric junk foods

Takeaways such as: hamburgers, deep-fried chicken, fish and chips, hot dogs, frankfurters, sausages and sausage rolls, pies and pasties, and pizza.

Packaged foods

Salami, devon, luncheon, sausages, ham, bacon, pre-cooked and frozen foods (TV dinners), canned or packaged soup, all packaged and canned convenience foods, such as baked beans, spaghetti, casseroles in sauces or gravy; all biscuits, cookies, cakes and refined butters (peanut, cashew) with sugars and preservatives in them (have unrefined nut butters from the health store instead); processed cheeses and mayonnaise (make your own, see 'Recipes') Wholemeal bread, muesli, rolled oats and brown rice, even though packaged, are nutritious and may be eaten freely.

Confectionery

Lollies, sweets, candy, snack bars; glazed and sulphited dried fruit (pure, preservative-free, sun-dried fruit are OK); milkshakes, flavoured milks, soft drinks, cordials; cakes, custards, desserts, puddings, chocolates of all sorts; jellies, jams, marmalades (un-sweetened, preservative-free conserves from the health store are OK); Milo, Ovaltine, cocoa, Drinking Chocolate, coffee and chicory essence, condensed milk, coffee whitener, coffee and milk prepa-rations, skim milk powders, long-life milk; sweet or savoury waffles, treacle, maple sauces; ice blocks, ice cream; all sweet sandwich spreads and toppings; cheese cake, cheese deserts, cheese dips (make your own, see 'Recipes'); pretzels, flavoured potato crisps (plain Kettle Chips are OK now and then)

Five per cent junk food means a maximum of five items and preferably less of junk per week. Junk food is vitamin and mineral deficient and full of chemicals. Worst of all it lacks the 'life force' of fresh food and so robs you of 'zing' and 'glow'. It predisposes you to over-weight, tiredness, premature ageing and diseases such as diabetes, cancer, heart and circulatory problems.

Fresh is best; have fresh food whenever possible.

MALT

Malt is a product derived from barley and other grains. It is primarily used as a flavouring and colouring agent. It is a major ingredient in beer, ale, malt liquors and non-alcoholic products such as horehound beer.

Foods containing malt: Most baked goods such as brown bread, pancake and waffle mixes; some biscuit and cake mixes; cracker biscuits like Saos; some confections like caramels, fancy ice-cream; butterscotch; some lollies; some commercial cakes; baby cereal; malted milk; infant formulas; potato crisps (Smith's plain variety is malt free); malt extract; malted syrups; malt vinegar; flavoured milk; some coffee substitutes; other malted drinks like Milo, Aktavite, Ovaltine.

Malt free foods: *Drinks:* Nestles chocolate and strawberry Quik; *cereals, biscuits, sweets:* Only brands stating that they contain no malt should be consumed, so it will be necessary to check the labels on these foods. If a label contains maltodextrone or maltodextrin then it contains malt.

METABISULPHITE

Metabisulphite (sulfur dioxide) is an additive mainly in acidic foods and beverages to prevent undesirable growth of bacteria, food discolouration and to help maintain vitamin C in fruit juice. This preservative does not occur naturally.

Metabisulphite is contained in the following foods:

Beverages: Orange- or yellow-coloured soft drinks in glass bottles; cordials; bottled drinks containing fruit juice. Check on all commercial fruit juice packs; some are preservative free.

Fruit: Dried tree fruit such as apples, apricots, pears; fruit bars. Sultanas, currants, raisins do not contain metabisulphite and prunes are not preserved with it either. 'Fresh' fruit salad from commercial outlets may have metabisulphite added to maintain appearance. Some fresh fruit are dusted with metabisulphite, so be careful.

Vegetables: Dried vegetables; instant mashed potato; some types of potato crisps; pickled onions; pickles; commercially prepared chipped potatoes for cooking.

Meat, fish, poultry: Sausages, sausage mince; frankfurters, chicken loaf; devon, brawn; uncooked fresh prawns; prepared meals in clubs and restaurants, especially roasts.

Dairy products: Fruit yoghurt, cheese pastes and many cheese mixtures.

Miscellaneous: Vinegar, salad dressings, dessert toppings, flavourings, essences, syrups, jams, cider, wine, beer, pickled onions. Most fast food products have some metabisulphite.

MILK

Milk is found in baker's bread (most contain milk), baking powder biscuits, Bavarian cream, bisques, boiled salad dressings, butter, butter sauces, buttermilk, cakes, candies, cheese, chocolate, chowders, cocoa drinks and mixtures, condensed milk, cooked sausages (devon, luncheon), cookies, cream, cream sauces, creamed foods, curds, custards and puddings, doughnuts, dried or evaporated milk, food fried in butter, foods prepared au gratin, fritters, gravies, hamburgers, hard sauces, hash, hot cakes, ice-creams, junket, malted milk, mashed potatoes, meatloaf, milk chocolate, milk desserts, oleomargarines (cooking margarines), omelettes, Ovaltine, Ovomalt, packet cakes, pie crust made with milk products, prepared flour mixtures (biscuits, cakes, doughnuts, muffins, pancakes, pie crusts, waffles), salad dressings, scrambled and scalloped dishes, sherbets, soda crackers, soufflés, soups (particularly creamed), spumoni, sweets made with milk, whey, yoghurt, zweiback

MONOSODIUM GLUTAMATE

Monosodium glutamate (MSG) is usually used in foods as a flavour enhancer. In nature it is a building block of all protein.

NATURALLY OCCURRING MSG: Tomatoes, wine, mushrooms, cheeses (for example, parmesan, camembert, blue vein, brie, gouda, gruyere, and rocquefort), grapes, broccoli, prunes, sweet corn, soy sauce, Marmite, Vegemite, worcestershire sauce, brandy, sherry, liqueur, port, rum and Bonox. To avoid MSG in foods it is very important to read labels on food products very carefully.

FOODS CONTAINING ADDED MSG: Chinese, Japanese, Asian foods; fried rice from these places with spicy sauces; take-away pizza, especially spiced and seasoned; take away seasoned chicken; commercial savoury foods; packet or canned soup; canned and luncheon meats; meat and fish pastes; canned vegetables in sauce; flavoured potato crisps; savoury biscuits; cocktail onions; gherkins; soy sauce; mixed seasonings and spiced seasonings; stock cubes; stuffing mixes; gravy makers; frozen prepared dishes; pies, sausage rolls, frankfurts; prepared Italian food; most prepared foods in restaurants and clubs, especially roasts, garden salads, fruit salads, fruit punch. Garden and fruit salads bought at fast food outlets often have MSG on them to prevent browning. Most soups, sauces and snack foods. Most Pizza Hut products.

SOYA BEANS

BAKERY GOODS: Breads, cakes, many pastries, K-biscuits, several brands of crisp crackers.

SAUCES: Oriental Show You Sauce, La Choy Sauce, Lea & Perrins Sauce, Heinz Worchestshire Sauce.

CEREALS: Sunlets, Cellu Soy Flakes.

SALAD DRESSINGS: E-P-K French dressing, many other salad dressings, many brands of oil.

MEATS: Pork link sausages, lunch meats.

CANDIES AND SWEETS: Hard candies, nut candies, caramel, lecithin (invariably derived from soya bean and is used in candies to prevent drying and to emulsify the fats), custards.

MILK SUBSTITUTES: All soymilks, Sobee, Mull-Soy.

BUTTER SUBSTITUTES: Oleomargarines.

ICE-CREAM: Some brands.

SOUPS: Check the labels!

VEGETABLES: Fresh soya sprouts served as vegetable in some Chinese dishes, soya bean noodles, macaroni and spaghetti, Reezon season, Crisco, Spry and other shortenings, oleomargarine and butter substitutes, some cheese, tofu, natto and miso, dry lemonade mix, dry ready-to-eat cereals (such as Honey Comb, Buck Wheats, Super Sugar Crisps). Many other foods contain soya beans or soya flour—check all labels.

BEVERAGES: Coffee substitutes.

CONTACTS: Varnish, paints, enamels, printing ink, candles, celluloid, cloth, massage creams, linoleum, paper sizing, adhesives, fertiliser, nitroglycerine, paper finishes, blankets, grease, Gropup dog food, French's fish food soap, automobile parts, fodder, glycerine, textile dressings, lubricating oil and illuminating oil. Many new contacts are to be expected each year with the introduction of new products.

WHEAT

BEVERAGES: Cocomalt, Ovaltine, postum, beer, bourbon, gin, malted milk, whisky.

BREADS: Biscuits, crackers, muffins, rolls, and the following breads: corn, gluten, graham, pumpernickel, rye, soya, white, all commercial breads; rye products are not entirely free of wheat.

CEREALS: Bran Flakes, Corn Flakes, Crackers, Muffets, Puffed Wheat, Rice Krispies, Shredded Wheat, Wheatmeal Porridge, Semolina, Farina, Pep, Ralstons Wheat Cereal, Triscuits, Wheatena and many others.

FLOURS: Some brands of buckwheat flour, cornflour, graham flour, lima bean flour, rice flour, potato flour contain wheat and others don't; phone the manufacturer and check before using.

PASTRIES AND DESSERTS: Cakes, cookies, doughnuts, pies (including frozen), chocolate candy, candy bars, puddings.

MISCELLANEOUS: Bouillon cubes, cooked mixed meat dishes, gravies, hot cakes, ice-cream cones, malt products or foods containing malt, most cooked sausages (wieners, bologna, liverwurst, lunch ham, hamburger), matzos, mayonnaise, pancake mixtures, sauces, synthetic pepper, some yeast, thickening in ice-creams, waffles, wheat cakes and wheatgerm. Foods prepackaged or thickened with flour, batter or breadcrumbs, vegetables canned in sauce, commercial meat rolled in flour, hot cakes, glucose syrup, noodles, rusks, dumplings, zweiback, vegetable salad, commercial thickened pie fillings, macaroni, spaghetti, vermicelli, soups, sauces and stews thickened with these flours. Packet puddings and pie fillings, pastry mixes, artificial cream, packet or canned soups.

HOW TO SUBSTITUTE WHEAT FLOUR IN YOUR BAKED PRODUCTS: For 1 cup of flour (120 g), try substituting one of the following combinations: 1/2 cup (60 g) pure maize meal/flour and 1/2 cup (60 g) soya bean flour; 1/2 cup arrowroot and 1/2 cup soya bean flour; 1/2 cup brown rice flour and 1/4 cup (30 g) potato flour; 3/4 cup (90 g) potato flour (by itself); 3/4 cup rice flour (by itself). Commercially available breadcrumbs, even if specifically made with wholemeal flour (for those who can tolerate wheat), are not suitable for the Anti-Candida Program because they will contain yeast.

Therefore, for recipes calling for breadcrumbs, use your own home-baked bread made with any of the wheat flour substitutes. Slice the bread thinly, dry slowly in a warm oven. Then put the dry bread through a food processor. Store in an airtight glass jar. Millet meal, brown rice bran or ground nuts and seeds can also be used in place of breadcrumbs.

SENSITISING CHEMICALS IN FOODS

BENZOIC ACID: Naturally occuring in many foods that contain salicylate. Also added as a preservative to fruit juices, cordials and soft drinks.

SORBIC ACID: Preservative added to fruit juices, cordials, dried fruit, dried vegetables, cheese slices, pickled food.

NITRATE/NITRITE: Preservative added to processed meat; for example, ham, bacon, corned beef, sausages and salami.

PROPRIONIC ACID: Preservative added to bakery items; for example, bread, crumpets.

ANTIOXIDANTS (BUTYLHYDROXYANISOL, BUTYLHYDROXYTOLUENE): Preservative added to commercial fatty foods; for example, vegetable oils, margarine, snack foods (Twisties, Cheezels, chips), chewing gum, ice-cream, instant potatoes.

AZO DYES/COLOURING (TARTRAZINE, ANNATTO, ERYTHROSINE): Colourings added to processed foods; for example, pastries, cakes, biscuits, candies, soft drinks, cordials.

YEASTS, MOULDS, FERMENTS

YEAST: Most breads, hamburger and hotdog buns, rolls, doughnuts, coffee cakes, crackers, pastries, pretzels, commercial cakes, cookies and cake mixes, meat fried in cracker crumbs, gerbers oatmeal, barley cereal; B complex and multiple vitamins containing B complex; products containing B5, B12, vitamin D (some multi-vitamin and mineral tablets are guaranteed free of yeast—these are OK); all products containing brewer's yeast or derivatives—these include Vegemite, Promite, Bonox, Marmite, some wines and beers.

FERMENTS: Vinegar or any food containing vinegar—that is, salad dressings, mayonnaise, pickles, catsup, sauerkraut, olives, most condiments, sauces like barbecue, tomato, chilli, horseradish, green pepper sauces, mince pie preparations and many others; beer, wine, champagne, gin, whiskies, vodka, rum, brandies, tequila, root beer, ginger ales, as well as all substances which contain alcohol: that is, extracts, tinctures, cough syrups, other medications; fermented dairy products, cottage cheese, natural, blended, pasteurised cheeses, yoghurt, buttermilk, sour cream; milk drinks which have been malted, cereals and candies that have been malted; soya sauce; tofu, miso; soured breads, including pumpernickel and similar others; pickled or smoked meats and fish, including sausages, bacon, ham, salami, devon, hotdogs, corned beef, pickled tongue.

MOULDS: Truffles, mushrooms; dried fruit—some may be mould free, but others will have commercially acceptable amounts of mould on the fruit while drying; most melons, especially rockmelon; canned fruit, juices and vegetables; peanuts.

NOTE: Be careful in restaurants with the sauces and gravies.

AMINES AND SALICYLATES

These are naturally occurring chemicals in fruit, vegetables and other foods which can build up in the system causing a poisoning effect that mimics allergy. This effect differs from true food allergy, which results from the production of antibodies against a given food with the subsequent release of histamine and consequent inflammation. Amines and salicylates build up over time and irritate nerve endings, causing many allergy symptoms via nerve inflammation rather than via histamine.

Amines and salicylates don't show up on standard allergy tests. Sensitivities to them are diagnosed by their trial and error removal from the diet.

Amines and salicylates are cumulative and derive from many sources. Most often they build up over time from a collection of foods until the body's threshold of tolerance is reached. At this point a given food may trigger a reaction and be blamed as the sole cause of that reaction.

Total load

True food allergy is driven by the all or nothing law whereby a little will always cause definitive reaction. Amine and salicylate poisoning acts by the build-up principal. The more of them your body harbours the worse you feel. By reducing the total load in your system, you not only feel better but you will help reduce your sensitivity to all true food and inhalant allergens.

Suggested treatment plan if you are amine and/or salicylate sensitive

Stay off all those foods on the very high, high and moderate amine and salicylate lists—eat only from the low and negligible lists minus those foods you showed up allergic to on allergy tests. Do this for at least four weeks. For most people this is enough time to lower the levels and heal the inflamed nerve ends. Now reintroduce the foods (though not too many at a time) from the moderate list, once per day, on no more than two days (not successive) per week. Hold it at this level for four weeks then slowly build up to the high list—again only two days per week. If after four weeks you're still OK, start having amine/salicylate foods three to four times per week and from the very high lists on special occasions only.

If you're going out to a dinner party or restaurant where only well-cooked, spicy foods are the order, go back onto the low and negligible list foods for three to four days before and after the event. Make this your life's routine from now on.

363

Check your cosmetics, and skin- and hair-care range to make sure they do not contain high salicylate fruit and vegetable products. Salicylates can be absorbed through the skin.

Be flexible

Listen to what your body is trying to tell you. The more you practise this the better you'll become at it and in time you'll be impressed with the accuracy of your decisions.

If you get the feeling that, say, amines only are your problem, then stay on salicylates. If vice versa then go with that. If after four weeks you feel confident about going back on one but not the other, then go with that. Everyone is different. You need to experiment so don't make rigid rules. Your body knows what's best so let it define the action. Just listen to its subtle cues.

At first glance, the prospect of removing amines and salicylates from your diet may seem complex and daunting. Don't be put off by this. As you continue to read this section and familiarise yourself with the amine and salicylate lists and recipes you will find the issue will become less complex and easier to understand. Soon you will have an easy-to-stick-to routine worked out whereby you will know what foods are allowed and what derivation of the appropriate recipes are for you. All it takes is patience and persistence.

Don't be deterred by the fact that your diet will be bland for a while. Time passes surprisingly quickly and by going without your favourite spices and seasonings you'll soon be feeling great. Only 5 per cent of people have a total sensitivity to amines and salicylates, so we'll assume you're in that 95 per cent who can tolerate varying degrees of them.

Remember, your degree of tolerance will vary from day to day according to your stress level. Overwork, overexercise, late nights, lack of sleep, being hungover, and infections (viral, bacterial or fungal) can lower your tolerance to amines and salicylates and are frequently the triggers of your sensitivities to them in the first place. Overeating or bingeing while tired or suffering from a cold, hangover, or an attack of thrush is a frequent cause of amine/salicylate sensitivity. Don't attempt to reintroduce these foods if you are in any of these states.

Pregnancy and lactation also make the body more sensitive to amines and salicylates, most likely as a protection mechanism for the developing baby. Women remain more prone to these sensitivities throughout the childbearing years and can't afford to stress their immune systems with strict weight-loss diets, especially high-salicylate, cigarette and coffee/tea crash diets. Don't assume a wheat allergy if, in a hungover state, you react badly to your morning toast and jam, especially if it's burnt toast. It could quite easily be the amines or salicylates you are reacting to.

AMINES

These chemicals form as a result of protein breakdown and/or fermentation. This is why they're so prevalent in processed foods. Aged food produces amines which is why all food must be bought and eaten fresh, especially high-protein food such as meat, fish and chicken. The ripening process of some fruit, like banana and avocado, produces significant amines. The browning of foods (grilling, baking, roasting, toasting, pan frying) produces amines and, along with food ageing, can give rise to the incorrect diagnosis of food allergy. Many a food-sensitive person has erroneously diagnosed wheat allergy because they reacted to Weet-Bix, or toast or bread that was a few days old. Many of these people find they can tolerate fresh bread when the brown upper crust is removed. Some of the very amine-sensitive can tolerate only fresh white bread and, whereas white bread is not good it's better than no bread at all.

Very few people are allergic to red meat, although many react to barbecued meat and leftovers. Microwaving, boiling, stewing and steaming produces far less amines. Undercooking (for example, rare steaks) produce less again. Don't write meat off until you've tried these cooking methods.

Amine sensitivity is aggravated by constipation. Take psyllium husks and if necessary *Cascara segrada* capsules so that the bowels move every day. Semi-digested protein food lying around and fermenting in a sluggish gut greatly raises the blood amine levels, limiting the number of foods you can enjoy.

Amines are powerful vasodilators in those who are sensitive to them—they dilate blood vessels. For this reason they can cause migraines and should be suspected when all headache treatments fail.

The following abbreviations are used in the amine list

(S) = Also contains salicylates.
(M) = Also contains MSG.
(S, M) = Also contains salicylates *and* MSG.

Any foods not listed are free of amines and may be had if you have not shown up allergic to them.

Fruit

NEGLIGIBLE: Apple (S), apricot (S), blueberry (S), gooseberry (S), lime, peach (S), pear, rhubarb (S), strawberry (S).
Low: Blackcurrant (S), cherry (S), grapefruit (S), honeydew melon (S), mandarin (S), redcurrant (S), rockmelon (S).
MODERATE: Dates (S), kiwi fruit (S), orange (S), passionfruit (S), paw paw, tangerine (S).

High: Avocado (S), banana, fig (S), grapes (S, M), lemon (S), pineapple (S), plum (S), raspberry (S).

Vegetables

Negligible: Asparagus (S), cabbage, capsicum (S), carrot (S), celery, corn (S, M), cucumber (S), French bean, green pea, lettuce, lima bean, onion (S), potato, radish (S), soybean, turnip (S), zucchini (S).

Moderate: Broccoli (S, M), cauliflower (S), dill pickle (S), olives (S).

High: Eggplant (S), mushroom (S, M), tomato (S, M).

Very high: Sauerkraut, spinach (S).

Nuts

Negligible: Acorn (S), American chestnut (S), buckeye nut (S), horse chestnut (S), sunflower (S), sesame seed (S), pinenut (S), pistachio (S).

Low: Almond (S), beech (S), cashew, coconut (S), macadamia (S).

Moderate: Brazil (S), filbert (S).

High: English walnut (S), mackernut (S), pecan, sweet pignut (S).

Very high: Black walnut (S), butternut (S).

Meats, chicken and fish

Low: Beef, chicken, lamb.

Moderate: Chicken liver, ham, salami, salmon (canned), tuna (fresh).

High: Bacon, mackerel (canned), pork, sardines (canned), frankfurters, hotdogs, meatloaf.

Very high: Beef liver, caplin (salted), chicken skin, fish marinades, processed fish meat (fish fingers, fish sticks, fish paste), herring (dried, pickled, salted, smoked), herring roe, mackerel (dried), sausages, tuna (canned).

Cheese

Negligible: Cottage cheese.

Very high: Brie (M), camembert (M), cheshire, cheddar cheese, cracker barrel, Danish blue, Dutch gloucester, edam, emmental, English cheshire, gouda (M), gruyere (M), jarlsberg, leicester, liederkratz, limberger, mozarella, munster, parmesan, processed cheese, provolone, roquefort, romano, stilton, Swiss, wensleydale,

Sweets

High: Milk chocolate, white chocolate.

Very high: Dark chocolate.

Condiments

HIGH: Bonox (S, M), meat extracts (S, M), soya sauce (M), Vegemite (S, M).

VERY HIGH: Marmite (S, M), Promite, Bovril, Oxo.

Drinks

MODERATE: Ale (S), champagne (S), sake (S), stout (S).

HIGH: Beer (S), chianti (S), claret (S, M), drinking chocolate, fruit wines (S), port (S, M), red wine (S, M), sherry (S, M), white wine (S, M).

SALICYLATES

These are nature's insecticides. They are there to protect the plant from micro-organisms and insects which they readily poison. Humans, being a lot bigger than insects, can ingest a lot more of the plant food before the irritating effects of salicylate manifest themselves. Degrees of tolerance differ significantly, with allergic people being the least tolerant. Children, being smaller, can tolerate even less. When their nerve ends are salicylate-irritated they can become quite hyped up, easily frustrated, aggressive and lacking in concentration. A summer spent on stone fruit can see them ratty and restless by the time school starts again in February. Mango madness is no myth, as many parents know. Various skin rashes and a worsened asthma condition usually accompany this end of summer intractability. Nature concentrates her pesticide on the outside of plants for greater protection, so peeling fruit and discarding the outer leaves of such things as lettuce helps to reduce salicilate intoxication.

Salicylate content is high in perfumes, scented toiletries, eucalyptus oils, some medications and flavourings. The latter are why so many kids become revved up on sweets, ice-creams, soft drinks and cough mixtures.

Hyperactive anti-social children and those with learning difficulties respond well to a low salicylate diet though should be wormed before the diet commences. Worms can mimic the effect of amine and salicylate poisoning, especially if the children also have eczema, hives, psoriasis and asthma. The sudden withdrawal of salicylate foods will not affect their growth and development. These chemicals are not found in the staple foods of meat, fish, poultry, potato, wheat (bread) and rice.

The following abbreviations are used in the salicylate lists:

(A) = Also contains amines.
(M) = Also contains MSG.
(A, M) = Also contains amines *and* MSG.

Any foods not listed can be considered free of salicylates and may be had if you have not shown up allergic to them.

Fruit

NEGLIGIBLE: Banana (A), pear (peeled).

LOW: Golden delicious apple (peeled), paw paw (A), pomegranate.

MODERATE: Custard apple, lemon (A), loquat, mango, pear (with peel), persimmon, red delicious apple, rhubarb, tamarillo, kiwi fruit (A), raw fig (A).

HIGH: Avocado (A), grapefruit, granny smith apple, jonathan apple, lychee, mandarin, mulberry, nectarine, peach, tangelo, watermelon, dried fig (A), passionfruit.

VERY HIGH: Apricot, blackberry, blackcurrant, blueberry, boysenberry, cherry, cranberry, currant (dried), date (A), grape, grapevine leaves (as used in Lebanese food) (A, M), guava, loganberry, orange (A), pineapple (A), plum (A), prune (A, M), raisin dried, raspberry (A), redcurrant, rockmelon, strawberry, sultana, youngberry.

All dried fruit is too high in salicylate for consumption by sensitive persons.

Vegetables

NEGLIGIBLE: Bamboo shoot, cabbage, celery, lettuce, potato (peeled), swede, dried beans, dried peas, brown lentils, red lentils, rice.

LOW: Brussels sprouts, chive, choko, green beans, green peas, leek, mungbean sprouts, red cabbage, shallots, potato with skin.

MODERATE: Baby squash, asparagus, beetroot, broccoli (A, M), carrot, cauliflower (A), marrow, mushroom (A, M), onion, parsnip, pumpkin, spinach (A), sweet corn (M), sweet potato, turnip, raw tomato (A, M), kohlrabi, black olive (A), yellow and green chilli.

HIGH: Alfalfa sprouts, broad beans (A), cucumber, eggplant (A), watercress, stewed tomato (A, M).

VERY HIGH: Capsicum, champignon, chicory, endive, gherkin (A), radish, tomato products (A, M), zucchini, green olive (A), red chilli.

Nuts

NEGLIGIBLE: Poppyseed.

LOW: Cashews (A).

MODERATE: Peanut butter, brazil nuts (A), coconut (A), hazelnuts, macadamia (A), peanuts (A), pecans (A), pinenuts (A), pistachio

(A), sesame seeds (A), sunflower seeds (A), walnuts (A).
HIGH: Peanuts with red skins (A).
VERY HIGH: Almond, water chestnuts.

Sweets

NEGLIGIBLE: Carob, cocoa (A), maple syrup, white sugar.
LOW: Caramels, golden syrup.
MODERATE: Molasses.
HIGH: Jellies.
VERY HIGH: Honey, liquorice, peppermints, Minties, Koolmints, Steam Rollers, Allens Strong Mints, chewing gum.
NOTE: Artificial colourings, flavourings and preservatives are salicylate based. Read all labels carefully to see if the product contains any artificial flavourings, colourings or preservatives.

Herbs, spices and condiments

NEGLIGIBLE: Poppyseed, beef stock cubes, fennel.
LOW: Garlic, malt vinegar, parsley, saffron, soy sauce (A, M), tandori (A), vanilla.
HIGH: Allspice, bay leaf, cardamon, carraway, cinnamon, cloves, ginger, nutmeg, pepper (black), pepper (white), pimento, white vinegar (A), coriander, Bonox, basil (dried), yellow and green chilli, celery herb, chicory, fenugreek, red chilli, fresh endive, commercial soups, sauces and salad dressings.
VERY HIGH: Aniseed, canella, cayenne, cumin, curry, dill, five spice, garam masala, mace, Marmite (A, M), mint, mixed herbs, mustard, oregano, paprika, sweet paprika, rosemary, sage, tarragon, tumeric, Vegemite (A, M), worcestershire sauce (A, M), thyme, fish paste, pickles, tomato sauce, flavouring syrups.

Drinks

NEGLIGIBLE: *Coffee:* Decaffeinated; *Other:* Aktavite (A), Milo (A), Ovaltine (A), milk; *Alcohol:* Gin, whisky, vodka.
LOW: *Coffee:* Harris instant, Bushells instant, Andronicus, Bushells Turkish, Robert Timms instant, Pablo instant; *Tea:* Camomile; *Cereal coffee:* Ecco, Bambu, dandelion.
MODERATE: *Coffee:* Harris Mocha, International Roast instant, Moccona instant, Nescafe instant, Reform (cereal); *Tea:* Decaffeinated, fruit, rosehip; *Other:* Coca-Cola (A), fruit juice, tomato juice, rosehip syrup; *Alcohol:* Beer, brandy (A, M), cider (A), sherry (A, M).
VERY HIGH: *Tea:* All brands, peppermint; *Cereal coffee:* Nature's Cuppa; *Alcohol:* Liqueurs (A, M), port (A, M), rum (A, M), wine (A, M).

Medications

Oil of wintergreen, artificially coloured vitamins, aspirin, any medication containing aspirin or salicylic acid (see aspirin list).

Medications containing aspirin

This is a list of medications containing aspirin, plus any other cross-reacting drugs which will provoke your symptoms. You should totally avoid these:

ASPIRIN AND ALOXIPRIN: Alka-Seltzer, Aspalgin, ASA Arthritis Strength Aspirin, Aspro and Aspro Clear, Asprodeine and Asprodeine Soluble, Bayer Aspirin, Bex Powders and Tablets, Bi-Prin, Bufferin and Bufferin 500, Codiphen, Codis, Codox, Codral Blue Label and Red Label, Codral Cold Tablets, Codral Forte, Decrin Powders, Disprin, Doloxene Co, Ecotrin, Ensalate, Morphalgin, Orthoxicol Cold and Flu Capsules, Ostoprin 100, Palprin Forte, Percodan, Perpain, Rheumat-eze, Rhusal, Salicylamide, Solcode, Solprin, Solvin, SRA, Veganin, Winsprin.

NON-STEROIDAL ANTI-INFLAMMATORY DRUGS (NSAIDs): Arlef (Flufenamic acid), Arthrexin (Indomethacin), Brufen, Butazolidin, butazone, Clinoril (Sulindac), Dolobid (Diflunisal), Feldene (Piroxicam), Fenopron, Indocid, Inflam, Naprogesic (Naproxen Sodium), Naprosyn, Naxen, Orudis and Orudis–SR (Ketoprofen), Ponstan (Mefenamic acid), Rafen, Rheumacin, Voltaren (Diclofenac Sodium).

NON-SALICYLATE MEDICATIONS: Codeine, Panadeine, Panadol.

NOTE: Always check labels as there may be other medications containing aspirin and related compounds. Please show this chart to any physician who may be prescribing medication for you.

FOOD FAMILIES

If, after having removed amine- and salicylate-containing foods, definitive allergy symptoms still remain, it's time to consider the possibility that you are allergic to family members of those foods you showed up allergic to on the cytotoxic food test. Few people are allergic to the family members of their particular food allergens.

For this reason, you would consider the removal of family members as your very last option in your quest for optimum health.

Look at rest quota, fluid intake, oxygen intake, vitamin and mineral intake, attitude, stress levels and the possibility of hard-charging as reasons for your lack of response before deleting family members from your diet. Even human error in the cytotoxic food and skin sensitivity tests should be considered a possibility before sensitivity to food members.

If too many foods are removed from the diet, the problem of malnutrition can arise and this can cause all the same symptoms of candidiasis, allergy, stress and fluid retention.

The only exceptions to this rule are the nightshade family and the plantain family. An allergy to one member of the nightshades invariably includes the rest of the family—go off the whole family if you are allergic to one. And if you show up allergic to plantain grass on the skin sensitivity test, go off bananas as well.

ARROWROOT FAMILY: Dashean, poi, taro root.

BANANA FAMILY: Arrowroot (musa), banana, plantain.

BIRCH FAMILY: Hazelnuts.

BOVINE FAMILY: Beef, beef emulsifiers (cakes, biscuits—read all labels carefully), buffalo (bison), butter, cheese, gelatine, gelatin capsules, ice-cream, lactose, lamb, milk (spray dried), milk products, mutton, oleomargarine, renin (rennet), Rocky Mountain sheep, sausage casings, sheep (domestic), suet, yoghurt.

BRAZIL NUT FAMILY: Brazil nuts.

BUCKWHEAT FAMILY: Buckwheat, garden sorel, rhubarb, sea grape.

CACTUS FAMILY: Prickly pear, tequila.

CAPER FAMILY: Capers.

CAROB FAMILY: Carob.

CARROT FAMILY: Angelica, anise, caraway, carrot, carrot syrup, celeriac (celery root), celery (seed and leaf), chervil, coriander, cumin, dill, dill seed, fennel, finocchio, Florence fennel, gotu kola, lovage, parsley, parsnip, sweet cicely, water celery.

CASHEW FAMILY: Cashew, mango, pistachio, poison ivy, poison oak, poison sumac.

COMPOSITE FAMILY: Absinthe, boneset, burdock root, cardoon, celtuce, chamomile, chicory, coltsfoot, costmary, dandelion, endive, escarole, globe artichoke, goldenrod, Jeruselem artichoke, artichoke flour, lettuce (head and leaf), pyrethrum, romaine, safflower oil, salsify (oyster plant), santolina (herb), scolymus (spanish oyster plant), scorzonera, sunflower seeds and oil, southernwood, sesame seeds (homous oil), tahini, tarragon, vermouth (cragweed).

CRUSTACEAN FAMILY: Crab, crayfish, lobster, prawn.

EBONY FAMILY: Permission.

FUNGI FAMILY: Baker's yeast, brewer's yeast, mould (in cheeses), citric acid, morel, mushroom, puffball, truffle, antibiotics.

GINGER FAMILY: Cardamon, East Indian arrowroot, ginger, tumeric.

GOOSEBERRY FAMILY: Currant, gooseberry.

GOOSEFOOT FAMILY: Beetroot, ceae, chard, kochia, lamb's quarters, silver beet, spinach, sugar beet, tampala, thistle.

GOURD FAMILY: Marrows, butternut, buttercup, cantaloupe, casaba melon, caserta, chayote, Chinese preserving melon, cocozelle, crenshaw, crookneck, cucumber, cushaw, gherkin, golden nugget, honeydew melon, hubbard varieties, loofah, muckmelons, pattypan, Persian melon, pumpkin, squashes, turban, vegetable spaghetti, watermelon, zucchini.

GRAPE FAMILY: Grape, brandy, champagne, cream of tartar, raisin, wine, wine vinegar, muscadine, dried currant, sultana.

GRASS FAMILY: Bamboo shoots, barley, bran, bulgur, cane sugar, citronella, corn meal, corn oil, corn sugar, corn syrup, corn (mature), cornstarch, cornflour, gluten, graham flour, hominy grits, lemon grass, malt, maltose, millet, molasses, oats, oatmeal, patent, popcorn, raw sugar, rice, rice flour, rye, sorghum, sweet corn, triticale, wheat, wheatgerm, whole wheat, wild rice.

HEATH FAMILY: Blueberry, cranberry, huckleberry, wintergreen.

HOLLY FAMILY: Bearberry, mate, pokeberry.

HONESUCKLE FAMILY: Elderberry.

IRIS FAMILY: Saffron.

LAUREL FAMILY: Avocado, bay leaves, cassia bark, cinnamon, sassafras.

LEGUME FAMILY: Alfalfa (sprouts), beans, black eyed peas (cowpea), carob, carob syrup, chickpea (garbanzo), coumarin, fava, fenugreek, gum acacia, gum tragacanth, jicama, kudzu, lecithin, lentil, licorice, limabeans, mungbean (sprouts), navy beans, pea (green and field), peanuts, peanut oil, peanut paste, peanut butter, pinto bean, red clover, senna, snow peas, soyflour, soy grits, soymilk, soy oil, soya bean, string bean, kidney bean, tamarind, tonka bean.

LILY FAMILY: Aloe vera, asparagus, chives, garlic, leek, onion, ramp, sarsaparilla, shallot, yucca (soap plant).

MACKEREL FAMILY: Albacore, bonito, mackerel, skipjack, tuna.

MADDER FAMILY: Woodruff, coffee.

MALLOW FAMILY: Cottonseed, maple syrup, maple sugar, okra.

MAY APPLE FAMILY: May apples.

MINT FAMILY: Basil, oregano, horehound, marjoram, mint, peppermint, sage, savory, thyme.

MOLLUSC FAMILY: Gastropods, abalone, snail, cephalopods, squid, pelecypods, clam, cockle, mussel, oyster, scallop.

MORNING GLORY FAMILY: Sweet potato.

MULBERRY FAMILY: Breadfruit, fig, mulberry, hops.

MUSTARD FAMILY: Broccoli, brussels sprouts, cabbage, cauliflower, Chinese cabbage, collards, colza shoots, couve tronchuda, curly cress, horseradish, kale, kohlrabi, mustard greens, mustard seed, radish, rape, rutabaga (swede), turnip, upland cress, watercress.

MYRTLE FAMILY: Allspice, cloves, guava, cherry guava.

NIGHTSHADE FAMILY: Belladonna, cayenne, chilli, eggplant, ground cherry, hyoscyamus, paprika, pepino (melon pear), pepper (capsicum), pimento, potato, tobacco, tamarillo, tomato, tree tomato.

NUTMEG FAMILY: Mace, nutmeg.

OAK FAMILY: Chestnut.

OLIVE FAMILY: Green olives, black olives, olive oil.

ORCHID FAMILY: Vanilla.

PALM FAMILY: Coconut, coconut oil, date, date sugar, palm cabbage, sago starch, any product containing palm oil or palmoline.

PAW PAW FAMILY: Papain, papaya, paw paw.

PEPPER FAMILY: Peppercorn, black pepper, white pepper.

PHEASANT FAMILY: Chicken, eggs, peafowl, pheasant, quail.

PINE FAMILY: Juniper berry (gin), pinion nut, pignolia.

PINEAPPLE FAMILY: Pineapple.

PLUM FAMILY: Almond, apricot, cherry, nectarine, peach, persimmon, plum (prune), wild cherry.

PURSLANE FAMILY: New Zealand spinach, purslane.

ROSE FAMILY: Apple, black raspberry, blackberry, boysenberry, cider, crabapple, dewberry, loganberry, longberry, loquat, pear, pectin, pommes, purple raspberry, quince, raspberry (leaf), red raspberry, rosehips, strawberry (leaf), vinegar, wineberry, youngberry.

RUE FAMILY: Angostura bitters, citrange, citron, grapefruit, kumquat, lemon, lime, murcot, orange, pummelo, tangelo, tangerine, mandarin.

SAPODILLA FAMILY: Chicle.

SOAPBERRY FAMILY: Lychee nuts.

SPURGE FAMILY: Kassava meal, tapioca.

STERCULIA FAMILY: Chocolate, cocoa, cocoa butter, cola bean.

SWINE FAMILY: Bacon, ham, lard, pork (hog), pork gelatin, pork sausage, scrapple.

TEA FAMILY: Tea.

WALNUT FAMILY: Black walnut, butternut, English walnut, hickory, pecan.

Bibliography

Alexander, P. J., *Overweight, Dieting and Disease Explained*, Davont Pty Ltd, Sydney, 1984.

Anderson, J. R., *Muir's Textbook of Pathology*, Edward Arnold Ltd.

Bernard, M. E., *Staying Rational in an Irrational World*, McCulloch, Melbourne, 1986.

Buist, R., *Food Chemical Sensitivity*, Harper & Row.

Cheraskin, E., *New Hope for Incurable Disease*, Arco Publishing, New York, 1971.

Cheraskin, E., *Psychodietetics*, Bantam, New York, 1976.

Colgan, M., *Your Personal Vitamin Profile*, Blond & Briggs, London, 1983.

Crook, W., *The Yeast Connection*, Professional Books, Jackson, Tennessee, 1983.

Davis, A., *Let's Get Well*, Unwin Paperbacks, London, 1976.

De Vries, H. A., *Physiology of Exercise for Physical Education and Athletes*, Wm C. Brown, Iowa, 1986.

Dyer, W., *Pulling Your Own Strings*, Avon, New York, 1978.

Dyer, W., *Your Erroneous Zones*, Avon, New York, 1976.

Ellis, A., & Harper, R., *A New Guide to Rational Living*, Wiltshire Book Company, North Hollywood, 1977.

Forman, R., *How to Control Your Allergies*, Larchment Books.

Gibran, K., *The Prophet*, Heinemann, London.

Griffiths, S., *Allergy Overload*, William Collins.

Herriott, James, *The Herriott Omnibus Series* (four titles: *All Creatures Great and Small*, *All Things Bright and Beautiful*, *All Things Wise and Wonderful* and *The Lord God Made Them All*), Pan Books, London, 1970s (various).

Hoag, Cole & Bradford, *Osteopathic Medicine*, McGraw-Hill, New York, 1969.

Hoffer, A., *Orthomolecular Nutrition*, Keats Publishing, New Canaan, Connecticut, 1978.

Osol, A., *Gould Medical Dictionary*, McGraw-Hill, New York, 1972.

Pearson, D., & Shaw, S., *Life Extension—A Practical Scientific Approach*, Warner Bros.

Pfeiffer, C. C., *Mental and Elemental Nutrients*, Keats Publishing, New Canaan, Connecticut, 1975.

Schauss, A., *Diet, Crime and Delinquency*, Parker House, Berkeley, California, 1980.

Schroeder, H. A., *The Trace Elements and Man*, Devin-Adair.

Selye, H., *The Stress of Life*, McGraw-Hill, New York, 1978.

Smith, A. L., *Microbiology and Pathology*, Tenth Edition, C. V. Mosby Pty Ltd, Saint Louis, 1972.

Tepperman, J., *Metabolic and Endocrine Physiology*, Year Book Medical Publishers, Chicago, 1980.

Truss, C., *The Missing Diagnosis*, C. Truss, PO Box 26508, Birmingham, Alabama 35226, 1982.

Williams, R., *Nutrition Against Disease*, Bantam, New York, 1971.

Index

Page numbers in *italics* refer to illustrations. Page numbers in **bold** refer to main entries.

Mail order service

Should you experience difficulty in procuring any of the products recommended in this book, then you may phone Phillip Alexander's clinic in Sydney on:

(02) 9981 2225 or
(02) 9982 7135

and we will post them to you as part of our mail order service.

Mail order service

Should you experience difficulty in procuring any of the products recommended in this book, then you may phone Phillip Alexander's clinic in Sydney on:

(02) 9981 2225 or
(02) 9982 7135

and we will post them to you as part of our mail order service.